BIRTH DAY

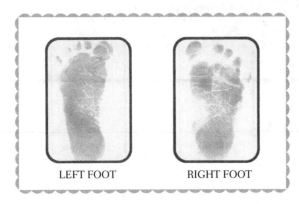

LEFT FOOT   RIGHT FOOT

Claire's footprints, June 14, 1990

BIRTH DAY

A PEDIATRICIAN EXPLORES THE SCIENCE,
THE HISTORY, AND THE WONDER OF CHILDBIRTH

MARK SLOAN, M.D.

Ballantine Books
New York

Published in the United States by Ballantine Books, an
imprint of The Random House Publishing Group, a division
of Random House, Inc., New York.

BALLANTINE and colophon are registered trademarks of
Random House, Inc.

Library of Congress Cataloging-in-Publication Data
Sloan, Mark, M.D.
Birth day : a pediatrician explores the science, the history, and
the wonder of childbirth / Mark Sloan.—1st ed.
p. cm.
Includes bibliographical references and index.
ISBN 978-0-345-50286-5 (hardcover : alk. paper)
1. Childbirth—Popular works. I. Title.
RG525.S618 2009
618.4—dc22   2009000662

Printed in the United States of America on acid-free paper

www.ballantinebooks.com

2 4 6 8 9 7 5 3

Book design by Simon M. Sullivan

For Elisabeth, Claire, and John, without whose love
I would have no story to tell;

for my mother, Peg, who birthed seven big-headed Sloan babies,
and my father, Barney,
who got Mom to the hospital on time, every time;

and

for James Bernard Sloan,
the brother I never knew

My mother groaned, my father wept,
Into the dangerous world I leapt;
Helpless, naked, piping loud,
Like a fiend hid in a cloud.

—WILLIAM BLAKE (1757–1827)

When I was born, I was so surprised
I couldn't talk for a year and a half.

—GRACIE ALLEN (1895–1964)

It has been my privilege to care for thousands of new-born babies and their parents in my pediatric career. In order to respect confidentiality in the relative handful of cases described in *Birth Day*, I have changed names and some identifying details. My family members, on the other hand, are exactly as portrayed. They have promised not to sue me.

CONTENTS

Part IV · Looking at Babies

PART I
On Being Born

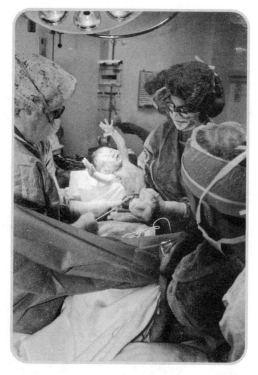

John's birth, December 31, 1991

Chapter 1
Twenty Babies: An Unexpectedly Quick Introduction to Vaginal Birth

I delivered twenty babies in the summer of 1977. I was hardly more than a baby myself, just turned twenty-four and starting my third year of medical school. At that point I was toying with the idea of becoming a family practitioner or a general surgeon. Babies didn't much figure into my future.

This is how my obstetrics rotation was supposed to work: a medical student was typically paired with an intern, who in turn was under the direct supervision of a senior resident. The senior resident did the complicated cases—forceps deliveries, cesarean sections, and such—while the intern handled the routine vaginal births. My role as a medical student was more or less like Cinderella's in her pre-princess days: do the dirty work, like IV starts and blood draws, and stay in the shadows to avoid the wrath of the overworked intern and resident. A "good" student—one with the sense to do his work quietly while openly admiring the skills of his elders—could expect the chance to deliver an uncomplicated baby or two as his reward.

Two things conspired to make this particular rotation different. The first was that it was early July, a traditionally scary time to have a baby in a large teaching hospital, since the interns are only a week out of medical school and generally have less experience delivering babies than the women whose babies they're delivering. The second thing was that, for reasons I can't recall, the OB resident staff was a few bodies short of a full complement. This meant that the interns and residents had to cover many more patients than usual, which didn't leave them much time for supervising green medical students embarking on their first hospital rotation.

And so one sweltering Chicago morning I stood in my crinkly white coat before Mitch, a stocky, gruff senior resident with a startled head of jet-black hair and a permanent dusting of cigarette ash down the front of his scrubs. We were in the hallway outside the maternity ward. Gurneys with moaning women aboard rattled by like Model Ts on an assembly line, pushed by a corps of tough-looking nurses. Mitch had paused between a C-section and a vaginal birth to give me my orders: I was to join Ben, a brand-new intern from a tony private medical school, on what Mitch called the "firing line"—a row of wheeled labor beds separated by unadorned canvas curtains.

Mitch clamped his hand on my upper arm like a bailiff leading a felon into court and marched me through the labor room's swinging doors to Bed 4, where a tiny nurse with Popeyesque forearms was helping a hugely pregnant woman out of a wheelchair.

"Okay, you had some OB training in your physical assessment class, right?" Mitch asked. No, I told him, I hadn't. My physical assessment class had been at the veterans' hospital down the street. There, I had watched men with terminal lung cancer chain-smoke cigarettes through their tracheostomy tubes, had seen others who had lost limbs to diabetes or D-Day land mines, and had personally examined what a senior resident described as the case of the year—a cabdriver who got scurvy (scurvy!) from a decades-long diet of plain White Castle hamburgers and Coke, period. Not only had I not seen a baby born at the VA, I told Mitch, I hadn't seen a single female patient. The woman climbing onto the bed in front of us would be the first woman I had ever touched with medical intent.

Mitch scratched the stubble on his cheek. "Well, you've *read* about childbirth, haven't you?" I said that I had. Just the night before, in fact: half a chapter, with diagrams. Took me twenty minutes.

"No problem, then." He slapped me on the back. "Just sit

there"—he motioned me to a rolling stool between the woman's now propped-up legs—"and call me when you see a head." Then he left.

I sat there for two hours. I killed time by rearranging the contents of my pockets, cleaning my stethoscope, and, once I had overcome my shyness, talking to the woman who was to produce the head I had been ordered to be on the lookout for.

Her name was Tonya. She was two months younger than I was, and in between contractions I learned that for the last five years she'd been a secretary at an insurance company downtown. This was her third child—her oldest, a girl, was just two and a half—and she absolutely hated childbirth. She compared the pain of having a baby to the pain of being stabbed, which she had been, twice—both times being cases of mistaken identity, she assured me. But childbirth was worse, she said, because "it's like they won't take the knife out." Childbirth and knifing: two experiences I had never had. I took Tonya's word for it.

Our conversation gave way to long stretches of silence as Tonya's labor intensified. She panted as her contractions came, her hands gripping the metal siderails of the bed with such force that I thought she'd bend them. Between contractions she stroked her belly with her hands, her eyes closed.

Ben, the intern, came and went in a sweaty blur, muttering to himself as he lurched up and down the row of beds. He shook my hand on one pass. "Everything okay here?" he asked in a strangled voice. "Good," he said absently, not waiting for an answer. He patted my shoulder and scuttled out the labor room door. I went back to my pockets, moving my reflex hammer, tuning fork, pens, and alcohol wipes from one side to the other and back again while I waited for something to happen.

A sudden eruption of curses drew my attention. Startled, I looked down between Tonya's legs and saw the top of a tiny head peeking out from her vagina. I shouted for Mitch and then Ben, but neither responded. The nurse who'd been working the firing line was gone, too—off helping them, I supposed.

A pale student nurse appeared behind her clipboard at the foot of Tonya's bed. "I think they're doing an operation," she said. Her eyes widened at the sight of Tonya's baby's head. "Maybe I should go look for them?" She dropped her clipboard in my lap and took off at a half-trot. The double doors swung shut behind her. Now it was just me, the swearing Tonya, and the top third of a birthing baby's head.

I remembered a picture in my night-before's reading where the obstetrician has his hand placed confidently on the emerging newborn's head. So I did that. I put my gloved right hand on Tonya's baby's head. It was warm and wet, and squishier than I had imagined it would be. Contact made, I exhaled for the first time in what seemed like an eternity.

My relief was short-lived. I had mastered the art of placing my hand on a birthing baby's head, but what came next? Would the baby just kind of fall out of Tonya on its own, I wondered, or was I supposed to grab on to that puckered patch of scalp and pull? I silently cursed myself for not finishing the chapter. Caught between pulling and not pulling, I chose a middle, temporizing route. Like the Dutch boy at the dike, I put my hand on the baby's head and pushed back, hoping to persuade it to pause just long enough for Mitch or Ben to come and save me.

Tonya's curses were getting personal now. She had finished damning her absent husband for putting her through this agony not once, not twice, but *three* times, and now she turned her attention to me. "Get that damn baby out of me!" she shrieked, glaring at me over the top of her belly. "Get it out now or I'll cut you!"

Dutch boy be damned. I was losing the battle. There was now an entire head under my hand, face and all. Amniotic fluid bubbled from its nose. Its mouth opened and closed in some horrible parody of breathing. Caught between threats of mayhem and my feeble attempt to hold back eons of childbirthing evolution, I closed my eyes and surrendered myself to whatever came next.

Suddenly a pair of hands pushed me aside. Mitch reached in, grabbed the baby's head and yanked with so much force that I was afraid he was going to tear it off. He pulled the head sharply downward—the right shoulder appeared at the top of the birth canal—then up, and the left shoulder popped out from below. The rest of the body followed, like a rabbit pulled from a magician's hat. Mitch plopped the baby in my lap—a big, squalling, slippery boy—and then clamped the cord with a pair of long hemostats and cut it in two. A minute later he tugged on the remnant of the umbilical cord and out came the placenta.

A nurse wrapped the baby in a white receiving blanket and handed him to Tonya, who cried and smiled and cootchie-cooed her thirdborn, seeming to have forgotten for the moment about killing me. His name was Robert, she said, because he had his grandfather's cleft chin.

"That wasn't so hard now, was it?" said Mitch, as he jotted a note on Tonya's chart. I didn't answer him—couldn't, really. I just sat on the stool with my mouth hanging open, dumbstruck. My scrub shirt was soaked in sweat. There was blood on my socks and shoes. Mitch stripped off his gloves and tossed them in a trash can at the foot of Tonya's bed. He yanked me into the hall, where two more mothers-to-be in wheelchairs waited. "Okay, then," he announced. "Time for the next one."

Had I been a little more observant—and less panicked—I would have noticed that Robert's head had rotated one way as I held it, and then back again as his body emerged. I would have pondered the pushing, pulling, and pain of having a baby, and the torpedoish shape of the baby's head as he lay in my lap. I would have marveled at Tonya's rapid transition from swearing attempted murderess to doting new mother, and at her ability to ignore the gaping wound in her vagina, the one that Mitch came back to sew up after he'd moved me on down the line to watch for another head. What I had witnessed, had I had the time to process what I had seen, was a highly compressed history of the last several million years of human evolution.

· · ·

One would think, given eons of evolutionary tinkering, that *Homo sapiens* could have come up with an easier way to birth its babies. What's the point of putting mother and child through such a painful, risky ordeal? Why aren't we more like other species, most of whom get the business of reproduction over with quickly and easily? Why can't we just spawn like salmon, lay eggs like chickens, or bud like yeast? More to the point, why can't we give birth the way gorillas do?

The female gorilla is a study in childbirthing efficiency. When labor begins, she simply ambles off to the edge of her group and has her baby in a half hour or so, with few visible signs of discomfort. She does this without help; the other members of her group usually ignore her. Compared to a human birth, which lasts an average of eighteen painful hours the first time around and almost always requires assistance from those nearby, gorillas have it easy. If Tonya had been born a gorilla, I think she would have preferred childbirth to getting stabbed.

Gorilla birth is made relatively easy by a fact of obstetrical anatomy: mom is big, fetus is small. Because the female pelvis is so roomy compared to the fetus that must pass through it, birth is a straightforward process. The gorilla fetus starts and finishes labor in the same position—head down and facing forward, toward its mother's abdominal wall. No twists or turns, no shifting orientation as it negotiates its exit. Just down, down and out.

Human childbirth, though, is more like an Olympic bobsled run. There are two participants with well-defined roles: a mother who does the pushing and a fetus who steers the course. There's a well-marked start and finish, and in between there are banked turns and the real possibility of disaster. Down at the finish line there's a throng of cheering supporters, some of them ready to assist when things get tricky, others simply milling around with cameras and champagne.

Childbirth isn't exactly like a bobsled run, of course. There are no helmets or spandex racing suits, for one thing, and it's usually not snowing on the participants. Childbirth is also a bit slower. A bobsled in midrace can reach 70 miles per hour. A fetus at its zippiest hits a top speed of roughly .00000025 mph. Of course, that's only in a woman's first labor; things can go twice as fast in subsequent deliveries.

Obstetricians divide childbirth into three stages. In the first stage, the cervix, which, along with the vagina, makes up the soft tissues of the birth canal, thins and dilates. The second stage, officially known as the expulsion of the fetus, is the birth itself. The delivery of the placenta constitutes the third and final stage. The second stage is the most prolonged and painful, and the course the fetus travels is, compared to the straightforward path taken by its gorilla cousin, an oddly curvy one.

The human female pelvis is an anatomical puzzle. The birth canal of the gorilla is more or less a compressed cylinder, like a cardboard toilet paper roll with its sides gently squeezed. From top to bottom, the roll is uniformly widest in the front-to-back dimension. The modern human birth canal, though, puts a twist on this ancient design. The upper third of the birth canal in humans is widest in the side-to-side dimension, while the lower two-thirds is widest from front to back, like the gorilla's. It's as if our ancestors took the gorilla's gently squeezed toilet paper roll and, over much time, pinched the upper third sideways, so that the top and bottom of the birth canal are now perpendicular to one another. This is the winding road the human fetus must navigate to get out—a tricky route that leads to a world of childbirthing woes.

Like the gorilla, a typical human fetus spends its third trimester in a head-down position, chin tucked on chest, arms and legs crossed, waiting for the signal to start its run to daylight. But here the differences begin: unlike the gorilla fetus, which faces forward, toward its mother's abdomen, the human fetus faces backward, toward its mother's spine. When labor begins, instead of simply dropping into the soft tissues of the birth canal as the gorilla does, the human fetus turns its head sharply to the side, as though making an over-the-shoulder check of the competition. The sideways-facing head then enters the pelvic inlet—the opening of the bony pelvis, the framework of bones that surrounds the cervix and vagina—and, spurred on by uterine contractions, begins its descent. On its way to being born, the fetus flexes, extends, and rotates its body, executing a complex series of maneuvers not seen in any other primate.

Why is human birth so filled with twists and turns? Every other large primate, from baboons to chimpanzees and bonobos, has its babies like the gorilla: a straight shot from womb to world. If human birth is a torturously slow bobsled run, the rest of our large-primate cousins are on a rope-straight downhill ski race. Why are we so different?

Until the mid-twentieth century, the only attempts to explain human birth's difficulty were framed in theological terms: the commonly held (and, as we'll see in a later chapter, scripturally questionable) view that childbirth pain was visited upon millennia of women in divine retribution for Eve's temptation of Adam. But as archaeologists discovered more and more fossilized human ancestors, they learned that the path to painful childbirth was not so much a divine curse as it was a complex compromise between what we once were and what we've since become.

Millions of years ago, all large primates gave birth pretty much the way gorillas do today. The maternal pelvis was big enough to allow a small-brained fetus to pass through with relatively little difficulty. But as the ancestors of modern humans split away from the rest of the primate kingdom, childbirth started to get complicated.

The split came about when our distant ancestors came down from the trees and moved out onto the grassy central African savannah. It was a smart move—the savannah offered vast new opportunities for food and water, far from the competing bands of treebound primates who would become today's monkeys and apes. But it also brought new dangers. The grasses were tall; the tree-swinging, knuckle-walking style of locomotion that worked so well in the jungle now limited visibility, leaving our forerunners vulnerable to the big-toothed predators that patrolled the savannah.

So they stood up. Bipedal (two-legged) locomotion offered the distinct advantage of allowing prehumans to see over the grass, making it easier to spot distant food sources and approaching dangers. Over much time, natural selection for upright walking changed the shape of the skeleton, particularly the pelvis. "Lucy," the famous *Australopithecus* skeleton found in Kenya's Olduvai Gorge in 1974, shows that by three million years ago those changes were well under way. Her pelvis was wider than an ape's, and her pelvic inlet had already taken on the oval, sideways-oriented shape characteristic of a modern human female.

But Lucy wasn't completely modern. Much of her pelvis was still apelike, and with *Australopithecus* being a small-brained species it's likely that the fetus passed through the birth canal much the way today's gorilla fetus does: head down and body facing its mother's abdomen from start to finish. There was one major difference, though. Because of the wider, oval-shaped inlet, the fetus would have had to turn its head to the side when it entered the birth canal—just as modern human fetuses do.

So, the first major change in human childbirth came about as a response to upright walking. As Lucy and her descendants mastered that task, they began to use their freed-up hands to make tools for cutting and scraping, and, eventually, weapons. Evolution soon favored those with the nimblest tool-making minds. Brains became bigger, and once again the female pelvis had to adapt.

Given the fact that the *Australopithecus* pelvis was still relatively roomy, it took thousands of generations before the fetal head got large enough to become an obstetrical problem. That crisis point was reached about 1.5 million years ago. As the fetal head enlarged, the maternal pelvis could grow only so wide in its attempt to accommodate; beyond a certain point, an awkward, wide-based gait would make it difficult for females to flee predators. Faced with a problem that could kill either or both of them and end the human race before it started, mother and fetus displayed that most human of traits: they compromised.

Here's the problem in a nutshell: newborn babies, then and now, have heads that are just a bit too big to fit down the birth canal in the round fetal state. Take a look at a newborn's head—his ears reach out nearly to his shoulders. If that head-to-shoulder ratio never changed, an average adult would have about a size 20 head, and there isn't enough polyester in all of China to make a world full of baseball caps that big.

Getting that big fancy tool-maker's noggin out of the womb with minimal damage to mother and fetus became one of the great engineering challenges of human evolution. It was more or less the same challenge faced by a man who gets carried away building a boat in his garage.

Imagine that the man starts out with a simple boat in mind, maybe a kayak or a canoe, something he can paddle around the park lagoon on a Sunday morning. As the project unfolds, though, his imagination catches fire. Why just a simple little tub, he thinks? Why not a sailboat, or a ketch, or a schooner? So he adds bulwarks and gunwales and a crow's nest. Soon he's upgraded his little canoe to an oceangoing yacht capable of winning the America's Cup.

One problem, though. His boat is now way too big to fit out the garage door. The man is left with two options: make the boat smaller, or the opening bigger. In the end he does a little of both— he lowers the crow's nest and widens the doorway—and one morning, to much fanfare, the SS *Show Off* squeezes ever so carefully out the door and into the big lagoon of life.

That, minus the crow's nest, is the story of the coevolution of the human head and the female pelvis.

First, the garage. By the time our direct ancestor, *Homo erectus,* had begun to displace *Australopithecus* a million and a half years ago, the bones of the pelvis had done about all the compromising they could with the fetus. Any bigger or wider and the resulting awkward running gait would have turned *H. erectus* females into saber-toothed tiger lunch. Yet the uterus continued to be a work-shop for evolutionary dreamers—a place where astonishing new features were continually being added to brain and body, all with-out much thought to an exit plan.

It's not surprising, since the uterus pays no direct price for its ex-travagances. With only the soft abdominal wall to restrict its growth, the uterus can expand outward almost infinitely. As any woman who has given birth to full term twins knows, there seems to be no limit to how big a woman's belly can get.

And yet it never explodes. The abdominal skin grows so taut over the course of a pregnancy that an earth-visiting alien (or a cu-rious human child) might assume that the fetus simply pops out through its mother's navel. But as the abdominal skin strains to contain the growing fetus, the first of many maternal adaptations—and the only one visible from the outside—kicks in. The *dermis,* the stretchy, collagenous middle layer of the skin, breaks down slightly, allowing room for a bit more fetal expansion. Most postpar-tum women carry the evidence of this adaptation etched in their skin: those long, thin, purple-to-silvery scars known as stretch marks.

Unfortunately, no matter how exuberant the growth and expan-sion in the uterus gets, nature puts strict constraints on how big the exit can be. At first glance, the bones of the pelvis present an insur-mountable obstacle to birthing an increasingly large-headed fetus. After all, bones don't give, they break—and broken maternal bones aren't conducive to the survival of a species. But, like the captain of the SS *Show Off* and his altered garage, humans developed a few tricks along the way to give the fetus a bit more room.

A truism about childbirth: there's a hormone for everything. In the case of the big-head, small-pelvis dilemma, that hormone is *re-laxin,* a protein produced in small amounts by the ovaries through-out a woman's life. Researchers are still working out its many functions, but this much is clear: as soon as a woman becomes pregnant, relaxin production skyrockets. Rather than try to coax flexibility from the rigid bones themselves, relaxin targets the ligaments that fasten them together—in particular, those that bind the pubic bones and keep the sacroiliac joints tight. As its name suggests, relaxin causes the ligaments to relax and soften over the course of pregnancy, so that when labor begins, the fetus pushes its head against a once-rigid pelvis that now gives a bit. The garage door gets a little bigger.

But another major obstacle remains. There's still the matter of persuading the cervix, the cork that has kept the fetus safely bottled up for nine months, to open up—*way* up—and launch that big-headed boat.

Mitch, my OB resident, was not a man with a passion for teaching. He was a few months away from joining a private practice in the suburbs, and he resented student intrusions on his daydreams about the cushy life that awaited him. "You've got books, don't you?" was his stock answer to just about any question I might have on the subject of childbirth.

Still, teaching medical students was in his contract, and so, from time to time, Mitch would begrudgingly impart some fine point of obstetric care upon whichever student happened to be nearby.

My turn came one groggy postcall morning as we finished rounding on the women admitted during the night. Mitch sat in the hallway with his feet propped on a linen cart, silently munching a bagel as I finished up a chart note. Suddenly he reached across the table that separated us and snatched the pen from my fingers. "Time for some education," he said. "Let me see your hand." He grabbed my index and middle fingers and spread them widely, painfully apart. "Okay, that's about right," he said. "Follow me."

Puzzled and in pain, I closed my fingers and followed Mitch to the cramped office space the OB residents shared. He pulled a sheet of paper from a dented file cabinet and then, with a sweep of his hand that sent a cluster of abandoned coffee cups rolling, cleared a spot on a folding table in a corner of the room.

"Take a look at this," he said, tapping the paper. There wasn't much to see—just a series of mimeographed circles, one larger than the next, ten of them in all. Mitch pointed to the smallest circle. "This one's a centimeter wide," he said. "Not much can fit through that." I nodded agreeably. Was I supposed to take notes? I pulled another pen from my scrub shirt pocket, just in case.

"This one," Mitch continued, "is two centimeters." I nodded again, pen at the ready. He stifled a yawn. "You could maybe fit a Barbie doll head through that."

Mitch slowly worked his way through the other circles, estimating the action figure, body part, or newborn animal that might fit through an opening that big. Three centimeters: a G.I. Joe helmet. Five centimeters: a human spleen, if you squeezed it a bit. I was starting to see a pattern.

Mitch took a break to hunt down his styrofoam coffee cup, the one with his name scratched in the side. He poured some cold, thick coffee into it and downed it in one noisy gulp. Then he turned it upside down and smacked it on the eight-centimeter circle. It fit perfectly, minus the spreading coffee stain. "Doesn't work with a ceramic mug," he said. I nodded in sage agreement.

"Now this one," he said, pointing to the second-biggest circle, "this one's nine centimeters." He paused, bobbing his head twice in a solemn nod. "*Almost* big enough for a human baby to fit through, but not quite." He grabbed my fingers again and stretched, this time almost tearing the web between them. "Your fingertips are now exactly ten centimeters apart." He plopped them onto the largest circle. It was a painful, perfect fit. "And that is usually, and I emphasize *usually*, big enough for a baby's head to fit through."

With that, Mitch dropped my hand, grabbed his clipboard, and headed for the office door. "Any questions?" he asked. I shook my head, rubbing my sore fingers under the table. "Okay, then," he said as he left. "Class dismissed."

Alone in the office now, I studied the paper with the circles. Gingerly, I placed my fingertips on it again. This time, without the aid of Mitch's wishbonelike stretch, they were exactly nine centimeters apart.

•   •   •

With his paper circles and finger stretching, Mitch taught me the basics of cervical dilation, the process by which the cervix—the lower end of the uterus—opens to allow the fetus to squeeze through. Mitch's choice of lessons was more practical than educational, though. By the end of my first week on the ward, I had developed a reputation in his mind as an alarmist, a student who called too early and too often for assistance. But now, armed with my nine-centimeter finger span, I could accurately "size" the cervixes of laboring women on the ward, the better to know when to yell for help. My performance improved. Soon after our lesson, Mitch stopped referring to me as "Chicken Little."

It would be years before I learned to appreciate the cervix as something more than a ring of tissue that had to stretch wider than my finger span to let a baby out. Far from being a passive organ forced open by the birthing fetus, the cervix plays an active role in pregnancy, labor, and delivery. Mitch's doll-and-coffee-cup comparisons hardly did it justice.

Shaped more or less like a thick, elongated doughnut, the cervix in a nonpregnant woman acts as a valve, controlling what goes into, and comes out of, the uterus. The cervical *os*—the hole in the doughnut, if you will—stays closed most of the time. The os keeps most foreign material out of the uterus (sperm and a number of sexually transmitted organisms being notable exceptions), while opening ever so slightly each month to let out old blood and uterine tissue during menstruation. It's a thankless task. If a healthy nonpregnant woman gives any thought to her cervix at all, it's probably when it comes time to have that awkwardly located organ screened for cancer.

Once a woman becomes pregnant, though, the cervix's somewhat humdrum existence as keeper of the uterine gate becomes critical. Its job shifts from a simple valve to a cork in a bottle, holding the fetus in the uterus until it's time to be born. Unlike a cork, though, the cervix executes a precisely timed series of changes from conception to the moment of birth that allow it to lock the fetus in place while simultaneously preparing its escape.

The cervix is composed mainly of collagen, smooth muscle cells, and a stretchy protein called *elastin*. Early on, the cervix manufactures more collagen, densely cross-linking and packing it together; the added strength helps keep the fetus inside the uterus—its "cork" function. But as pregnancy progresses, the cervix begins to weaken itself. It produces special enzymes that slowly kill off the collagen and smooth muscle cells that gave the cervix its early pregnancy strength. The dead cells are replaced by water, which makes the cervix softer—or "riper," as obstetricians describe it.

When labor begins, and often well before, pressure from the fetal head causes the elastin layers to stretch. The cervix begins to dilate. Uterine contractions then push the fetus's head against the cervix, accomplishing full ten-centimeter dilation in an agonizingly short matter of minutes to hours. After birth, the cervix reverses field and slowly builds itself back up again, retreating to its everyday life as a gatekeeper—at least until the next pregnancy rolls around.

The thing that shocked me most about Tonya's delivery, apart from the cursing, the threats, and the sudden appearance of that head, was how she thrashed around at the very end. Tonya was a big-muscled woman. Her biceps were as large as mine, and her legs were thick and solid. "Arnie"—not her husband's name—was tattooed on the inside of one muscular thigh, and later, after Mitch saved the day and I resumed breathing, I wondered what had become of poor Arnie after he fell from Tonya's affections.

Tonya had started labor in the same position as the woman in the half-read chapter of my OB textbook—flat on her back, with a pillow or two to support her head. Somewhere between arrival and delivery, a nurse had hoisted Tonya's feet into a pair of metal stirrups, knees bent, so that her legs splayed outward at 45-degree angles. The better for me to watch for the head, I knew.

But Tonya became increasingly uncomfortable in that position as her labor approached its climax. She tried more than once to sit up or roll onto her side, but the no-nonsense nurse who patrolled the labor beds quickly wrestled her onto her back.

The two of them went a few rounds as Tonya's contractions waxed and waned, exchanging harsh words and hard stares until the nurse finally pulled out her trump card. "That's the safest position for your baby," the nurse snapped. "You wouldn't want to hurt your baby, now, would you?" They glared at each other for a moment, then Tonya sighed and laid her head back on the pillows. "Son of a bitch," she muttered to the ceiling.

Tonya did finally deliver flat on her back, with her feet in the stirrups, just as the nurse and my textbook said she should. But to the very end she rolled and writhed and shifted her bottom. Holding on to her baby's head while Tonya bucked and weaved was a challenge, like landing a jet on an aircraft carrier in an ocean storm—or so it seemed to my neophyte baby-catching self.

Looking back on it later, I couldn't understand why Tonya wouldn't hold still. Sure, having a baby was a painful thing, but couldn't she see that all that moving around was just making things worse? Shouldn't her concern for her baby have outweighed everything else? Too busy to give it much more thought, I subscribed to Mitch's hurried explanation: pain makes people do weird things.

It took me years to understand how right Tonya had been, and how wrong the rest of us were. All her rocking and shifting wasn't so much a reaction to the pain as an instinctive, important part of labor itself. It turns out that the position that's most comfortable to the mother, which can vary from moment to moment as labor progresses, is usually the one that allows a fetus to pass most easily through the birth canal as well. On an intuitive level, Tonya knew what she was doing.

Tonya gave birth in the lithotomy position, so named for its use in surgery where stones (*lithos* in Greek) are removed from the bladder, kidneys, or gallbladder. Flat on the back, knees flexed, feet up in stirrups—it's the birth position of choice among many modern obstetricians, and only a few modifications removed from the completely flat *dorsal decubitus* position that first became popular in the late seventeenth century.

The lithotomy position is an awkward, uncomfortable-looking way to lie down, and I'm sure many a laboring woman has wondered whose idea it was in the first place. Blame it on the Sun King. Louis XIV, the king of France from 1643 to 1715, was something of a voyeur. He found childbirth fascinating, and in order to observe it firsthand, he commanded that a viewing table be built so that he could watch his mistress give birth to their child.

This was an astonishingly bold decree. Men were routinely banned from the birthing room in those days, with the exception of obstetricians and male midwives, and even they weren't allowed to see a whole lot. In the name of decency, the mother's perineum—the part of the pelvis that includes the vagina and rectum—was usually kept hidden under her dress or a layer of blankets; doctors worked mainly by feel, often crouching in front of a standing patient. Even an absolute monarch had his birthing room limits—rather than gawk over the obstetrician's shoulder as his mistress gave birth, Louis allegedly watched the proceedings from behind a curtain.

Once it became known that the flat-on-the-back dorsal decubitus position was the king's favorite, the practice quickly spread to the nation's physicians. Traditional birthing positions—variations on squatting, crouching, and the use of a birthing chair—were abandoned, at least in those areas of the country where doctors were likely to attend a birth. Soon, since the French were the cream of Europe's obstetrician crop, the rest of the Continent followed suit.

As if royal endorsement weren't enough, the dorsal decubitus position got an additional boost from technological advances in obstetric care. Forceps were invented around 1600, and the up-on-the-table, flat-on-the-back position was perfect for an instrument-packing obstetrician to see, or feel, what he was doing. As childbirth became increasingly medicalized and obstetricians displaced traditional midwives in the birthing suite, the dorsal decubitus position became enshrined as the ideal birthing position—one that was best, and safest, for mother and baby. Its real origin, as a convenient viewing station for king and doctor, was soon forgotten.

And so things stayed until well into the twentieth century, at least in the more "advanced" parts of the world. The lithotomy position and its variants became so firmly entrenched that by the time I entered medical school, there was no discussion of any alternatives, and no hint in my textbook that women, all the way back to Eve, had ever given birth in any other way.

But even in the mid-1800s, a few obstetricians questioned the practice of flat-on-the-back childbirth. In 1857, a London-based physician named Rigby set out to determine the "natural" labor position by analyzing reports of British women who had accidentally labored alone, without medical intervention. He ultimately gave up, bewildered by the variety of positions his subjects assumed in the absence of obstetric input. "There is no natural position in labor," he wrote, "any more than for [the writhings of] a man . . . with a West India dry belly," the severe abdominal pain that resulted from drinking lead-laced Caribbean rum.

George Engelmann (1847–1903), a St. Louis obstetrician, was a keen observer of women in labor, and a lot more patient than Rigby. He realized early in his career that no matter what he had been taught in his obstetrics training, lying flat was an inefficient way to have a baby. "It was not until I had . . . begun to study the positions assumed," he wrote, "that I began to understand that there was a method in the instinctive movements of women in the last stage of labor. I have seen them toss about, and sought to quiet them; I bade them have patience, and lie still on their backs; but, since entering upon this study, I have learned to look upon their movements in a very different light."

Engelmann noted that "although *dorsal decubitus* is the position which is taught by the laws of modern obstetrics, nature does not seem to have designed that woman should in this way free herself from her burden." The angle of the birth canal alone made him doubtful: a woman laboring on her back actually has to push her fetus uphill. In genteel nineteenth-century language he went on to point out that humans do not voluntarily lie down when having a bowel movement—which, like childbirth, involves the use of the abdominal muscles and gravity—so why should a woman do so to have a baby?

Engelmann was also an avid ethnologist; he soon turned his interest in the study of human cultures to the labor practices of "the savage races." In 1882, he published *Labor Among Primitive Peoples,* a compilation of his findings gleaned from foreign obstetricians, missionaries, and far-flung army medical officers. Engelmann found that in each of the forty-seven cultures he studied, from rural Ireland to Abyssinia to "the Hottentots of the Cape of Good Hope," laboring women preferred to sit, stand, squat, or kneel during labor, and to change positions frequently. They also used various tools—posts, ropes, knotted cloths, slung hammocks, bricks, stones, piles of sand, birthing chairs or stools, and willing companions— as aids in finding a comfortable position. His most striking finding: not one of the cultures used the dorsal decubitus position. In fact, they all actively *avoided* it. The "savages," he concluded, knew what they were doing.

Engelmann was no backwoods doctor. He was one of America's foremost obstetricians, a founding member of the American Gynecological Society and president of the International Congress in Gynecology and Obstetrics. But his conclusions about birth position—that a woman in early labor should be "guided . . . in the position assumed . . . by the dictates of her instinct," and that ultimately she should deliver in a kneeling, squatting, or semirecumbent position (i.e., with the head of the bed well propped up)—went largely ignored.

A century later, Engelmann was vindicated. Studies done in the last two decades have shown that women allowed to assume the position they find most comfortable during the first stage of labor— from the onset of contractions to the full dilation of the cervix—

can enlarge their pelvic outlets by as much as 30 percent. Not surprisingly, these women tend to have easier births. On average, they have fewer episiotomies, a slightly shorter second stage—from complete cervical dilation to the birth of the baby—and less severe pain than do women lying on their backs. The conclusion reached by several recent studies: let mothers give birth in the position they find most comfortable.

Tonya, then, was just trying to follow George Engelmann's recommendations. And we, a modern hospital staff still working in the shadow of Louis XIV, stopped her. But things are improving. If Tonya were delivering in the hospital I work in today, she'd be encouraged to stand, squat, walk the halls, shower, hang on to a labor bar, whatever made her most comfortable. She'd also be offered a large inflated "labor ball" to sit on—the Western equivalent of squatting, since very few modern American women have the leg power to adopt the traditional labor squat that Engelmann's correspondents observed.

Finally, as her contractions inched Robert into the world, Tonya would deliver in a semirecumbent position, surrounded by friends and relatives, with a nurse midwife in attendance. Not exactly a "primitive" birth, but close enough to make George Engelmann proud.

This, then, is how a mother compromises: her skin stretches, her ligaments soften, her cervix builds itself up and then tears itself down again. During labor she shifts positions in ways that maximize the available space for her fetus to pass through the birth canal. So what does the fetus, the too-big boat in the garage, do to help?

Let's start with that oversized head. The fetal skull could well carry a label: "Some assembly required." Unlike the rigid adult cranium, the skull of a fetus is really a set of loosely joined springy plates. Before labor begins, the fetal skull looks like a map of ancient earth—continents of bone running up against one another, but not yet fused into a solid adult-style head. A large anterior fontanel (the "soft spot") sits on top of the skull, where the plates come together, while a smaller posterior fontanel lies toward the back.

When labor begins, the fetus's head turns into a slow-motion battering ram. With each contraction it pushes against the cervix, causing it to dilate. As the birth canal's opening grows larger, though, the head actually grows smaller—or at least longer and skinnier. The bony plates crowd together, then slide over each other slightly, creating the longer, thinner "conehead" that often alarms new parents. The brain, a damage-resistant organ with the consistency of thick pudding, goes along for the ride, changing shape right along with the skull.

Run a finger over a newborn's head. If the baby was born by a scheduled cesarean section—and thus never entered the birth canal—the top of the head is usually smooth. No coning, no unusual lumps or bumps. Now do the same with a vaginally born baby, and you'll often feel a hard ridge running along the top from front to back, connecting the fontanels. That ridge is called an "overriding suture," and it's a sign of continental collision: the edge of one bony plate lying over the top of its neighbor. The ridge is sometimes disconcertingly prominent, but it's only temporary. Within a few days of birth, the plates slide back into place and the head returns to its original round, parent-pleasing shape.

The springy skull's knack for changing shape as it moves through the birth canal, and the ability of its bony plates to slide over one another, decrease the width of the head by as much as half an inch. When you're dealing with a not quite four-inch-wide exit, that can be a huge difference.

Once the head has successfully passed through the birth canal, an even bigger problem follows: the shoulders, which are an inch or so wider still than the head. Once again, nature figures out a way to squeeze them through. The bones of the shoulder girdle—primarily the collarbones—are springy, like the skull. They bend, twist, and compress as labor progresses. If that doesn't do the trick, they break.

One in every thirty or so babies fractures a collarbone (or two) during birth. What looks like a design flaw, though, is really a clever, last-ditch size-reducer. Once broken, the edges can slide over each other, as the skull plates do. The shoulder breadth becomes a few millimeters narrower. Remarkably, a fractured collarbone doesn't seem to hurt a newborn nearly as much as it does an adult. The fracture is treated by slinging the arm to the baby's side with some fishnet gauze. Simple pain medications like acetaminophen alleviate what little pain a baby seems to experience from the break. The fracture heals quickly, and only rarely causes any lasting harm.

After all the bending and twisting and occasional fracturing that nature dishes out, the obstetrician or nurse midwife executes one final maneuver to extract those broad shoulders: she delivers them one at a time. When Mitch shoved me aside at Tonya's bed and grabbed on to Robert's head, he first pulled it downward until the upper shoulder popped out of the birth canal, then pulled up to deliver the lower one. That angled, one-at-a-time shoulder shrug saves both fetus and mother the extra trauma that would result if the shoulders were forced to emerge simultaneously.

A more profound, though less obvious, compromise between the human fetus and maternal pelvis was made a long time ago. Run a finger along a baby gorilla's skull and you'll find it's very different from a human baby's—there's no soft spot, no overriding suture, and little, if any, "coning." The gorilla's skull plates can't slide over one another, because they finish fusing together well before birth. Not that a gorilla needs a flexible skull, anyway—remember, the gorilla birth canal is so spacious that a fused-skulled fetus easily passes through.

Another striking difference between humans and other mammals is our level of physical development—or lack of it—at birth. A newborn horse can run; a dolphin can swim. A gorilla baby can cling to its mother's fur and crawl to her waiting breast. In some monkey species, the newborn actually assists at its own birth. Once its arms are free of the birth canal, the half-born baby uses its hands to push the rest of its body out of its mother—a feat that would earn a human baby a year's worth of tabloid front pages. Human babies are born helpless. They can't sit, stand, or walk. They can't see clearly, find food, or even hold their own heads up. Our newborns require the most parental care, and for the longest period of time, of any mammalian species.

These two key differences between human and ape newborns—the "primitive" human skull with its soft spots and disconnected bony plates, and the complete dependency on adults for every aspect of newborn care—are actually part of the same childbirth compromise. In the million or so years after Lucy and her *Australopithecus* relatives went extinct, our ancestors' brains nearly tripled in size. In evolutionary terms, this was frighteningly fast. The female pelvis, despite radically redesigning itself to accommodate the demands of upright walking and the ever larger human brain and head, simply could not keep up.

So, once the maternal pelvis and fetal head had done all the compromising they could, our ever resourceful ancestors did the next best thing. As the fetal head approached the size of no return, they birthed their babies prematurely, in earlier and earlier stages of development. This kept the head size more or less constant, and allowed for relatively safe passage down the birth canal, but it also resulted in a newborn who was neurologically half-baked—floppy, bewildered, and totally vulnerable. More and more of the head growth and neurological development that once happened in utero (and still does in gorillas), now takes place after birth. Primate anatomist R. D. Martin has estimated that humans really have a twenty-one-month "gestation"—nine months in the womb and another twelve months outside it, just catching up to the physical skills most apes possess shortly after birth.

Another way to look at it: if Martin is correct, a human mother would have to give birth to a twenty-three-pound baby—the size of an average one-year-old human—with a head 30 percent bigger around than a newborn's, all just to have a child with the physical skills of a newborn gorilla. Given the alternative, that first year of diapers and strollers and walking the floor at night isn't such a bad deal.

The trend toward difficult labor and helpless babies had other, far-reaching implications for human evolution. As we'll see in later chapters, giving birth to such big-headed, wrong-way-facing newborns requires the help of birth assistants, of which, in Tonya's case, I was a particularly pathetic modern example. And, as raising those helpless babies became more of a community project, fathers were gradually drawn into what had long been the sole turf of women—the care of newborns.

None of this—gorillas, hormones, the king of France—mattered much to me back in '77. I was too busy trying to keep my head above water on a hospital ward that, thanks to the shortage of doctors and nurses, teetered between way too busy and pure chaos. The early days of my rotation passed in a blur of moaning women, crying babies, IVs, and blood tests, all of it fueled by my first experience with coffee, the drug of choice for the *What, me sleep?* medical set.

Things had not started well. In addition to Tonya's delivery and the Chicken Little thing, I was something of a klutz in that first week or two. One night I tripped on a bedrail and ripped a phone out of the wall as I went down, waking the dozen women sleeping on one wing of the postpartum ward. Later that same night, I destroyed the blood samples I had painstakingly collected from them when I failed to secure the tiny sample tubes properly in the lab centrifuge. Five minutes later I opened the lid to find a paste of blood and pulverized glass splattered all over the inside of the machine. A centrifuge, I learned, is not an easy thing to clean.

By the final morning of my Summer of Babies, though, I was a transformed man. My klutzy phase had ended; Chicken Little was long gone. Buoyed by an unbroken string of complication-free vaginal deliveries, I had become, at least in my own head, a certified junior obstetrician. Not that I wanted to *be* an obstetrician, mind you—the tight squeeze of childbirth was a bit claustrophobic for my taste, and I already found myself drawn more to newborns than to their laboring mothers.

But I had reached that rarefied level of confidence occupied mainly by true believers and medical students, those whose self-assurance is exceeded only by their inexperience with real-world complications. In my mind, I could do anything when it came to birthing babies, and I pitied those who could not. It never occurred to me that Mitch was assigning me only the easiest, least risky cases.

Mitch leaned against a door frame that morning, clipboard in hand, adding the names of the latest batch of laboring women to the scratched-out list of those who had gone before them. A group of new students in clean white coats, those who would relieve me and my beleaguered colleagues the next day, passed by on a self-guided tour of the ward. They looked at Mitch expectantly, waiting, I suppose, for some words of wisdom to prepare them for tomorrow.

"This is where they're born," he said without looking up from his list. He jerked his head in the direction of the postpartum unit. "That's where they go when they're done." A silent moment passed. Mitch finally looked up from his scribbling. "See you *tomorrow*," he said with a dismissive wave. The students flocked away, disappearing down the hall in the direction of Mitch's head jerk like a covey of white-jacketed quail.

I watched them go with a knowing smile, like a grizzled, battle-weary Marine on Iwo Jima watching his green replacements come ashore. Pathetic wretches—how could they know what they were in for?

"Sloan!" Mitch barked. "Take beds three and four. Nice, uncomplicated ladies. Already had a couple kids apiece, so they know what they're doing." I slipped into my rumpled white coat and got to work.

I turned my attention to Bed 3, where a short, dark-haired woman lay panting between contractions. This was her fourth pregnancy, according to her chart, and as is true of many "multips"—OB slang for a multiparous woman, meaning one who has given birth in the past—she wasted no time in having this one. When I examined her I found that her cervix was already dilated to my nine-centimeter finger span. Twenty minutes later, she gave birth.

It was a textbook delivery, I must say. I guided the head with my hand as it emerged from the birth canal in a gush of fluid. I calmly did the pull-down-and-then-up maneuver to free the shoulders. The rest of the body followed an instant later, and there I sat with a slippery baby girl in my lap. I cut the cord, and a short time later the placenta passed easily.

A student nurse—the same one who had abandoned me the morning of Tonya's delivery—took the baby to a nearby table and swaddled her in a cotton receiving blanket. I spoke with the baby's mother for a few minutes. She had weathered the delivery well and was happy to have a girl to go with her three rambunctious boys. She thanked me for my help, even described my delivery technique as "gentle." Damn, I was good. I nearly floated over to Bed 4.

The woman in Bed 4, Danuta, was an anomaly in our inner-city maternity ward. She was tall, thin, and very pale, with a long blond braid tucked inside the back of her hospital gown. Alone except for her rosary and prayer book, she spoke no English. Javier, our over-worked interpreter from Mexico City, simply shrugged when he was called in to help. He spoke two languages, he said, and neither of them was whatever it was she was speaking.

What Danuta was speaking was Polish, and then only a little of that. She was quiet, almost eerily so, for a woman in labor. What little I learned of her I gleaned from the thin chart that lay open on the table next to her bed. She was a recent immigrant from Krakow, newly arrived in Chicago's large Polish community. She had two older children, aged eight and ten, and she'd arrived at the emergency room doors an hour before, accompanied by a man who claimed to be a relative. He knew nothing about her health, he told the admitting nurse, and then he disappeared into the street. Now Danuta was lying in Bed 4, laboring quietly, half a world away from home. Where were her husband and children now, I wondered. Chicago? Poland? I couldn't tell from her papers, and she was in no mood for untranslated chit-chat.

I did my best to explain what I was going to do. What must she have thought, I wonder now, of the overconfident young medical student hovering at the foot of her bed, pantomiming his intentions with a pair of widely spread fingers?

Fortunately for me, Danuta had been through this twice before. She understood the need to have her cervix checked, and allowed me to examine her. With my gloved hand in Danuta's vagina, I felt the rim of her cervix—not yet fully dilated—and her baby's smooth, bald scalp. "Eight centimeters," I told her, holding up eight fingers as a kind of Esperanto visual prop. She looked at me uncertainly, wondering, I think, whether I was estimating the hours till her delivery or perhaps the number of babies that I thought were in there. "Milek," she said in return, pointing to her belly, which I took to be either the baby's name or the Polish word for "eight." "Milek," I repeated, waggling my eight fingers. She nodded, then grimaced as a contraction took hold.

Her quietness was unsettling—with Tonya I'd known exactly where I stood in terms of her discomfort. From time to time I'd ask Danuta with an up-or-down thumb gesture how she was doing. Her stock response was a simultaneous sideways nod and shrug, the universal sign for "can't complain, though I probably should." Between our infrequent signing exchanges she prayed, her rosary beads wound tightly through her clenched fingers.

A half hour later Danuta's praying grew louder and faster. I examined her again—this time she was fully dilated, and a tiny patch of pink scalp was peeking from the birth canal. "Push!" I shouted, miming a man pushing a car up a hill. "Push!"

Mitch's head appeared from a bed around the corner. "Everything okay here?" he asked. "Yes!" I called out with the self-assured voice of a man at the peak of his powers. "No help needed here! Everything's fine!"

I covered the baby's head with my hand as it emerged, ready to guide it into a new life in Chicago. The head had a funny feel to it—softer than I was used to, and the skull's suture seemed unusually deep, more a fleshy valley than a hard ridge. I barely had time to marvel at the diversity of the human head when I felt a warm eruption under my glove. I pulled my hand away to find a ribbon of blackish-green paste shooting from the middle of Danuta's baby's head. I stared, dumbfounded, as the ribbon of goo continued to grow. There was only one conclusion I could draw, given that my experience was limited to straightforward, uncomplicated births: Milek's head was exploding.

"Oh my god!" the student nurse shrieked from over my shoulder. "It's a butt!"

The news of the appearance of Milek's buttocks where his head should have been passed around the corner at the speed of light. Two bellows, like a duet of wounded buffalo, sounded in response. Mitch, and then Ben, converged on Bed 4 in a matter of seconds. Mitch pushed me aside as he had at Tonya's delivery, but this time with a little more force. "Jesus, Sloan!" he shouted. "Don't you know a breech when you see one?" The question was rhetorical. He didn't wait for my answer.

I don't remember how Mitch got little Milek out of his mother, but somehow he did. Looking at an obstetrics text now, I figure he must have gently guided Milek's bottom out of the birth canal, just far enough so he could free the legs. Then, when the shoulder blades were just visible, he would have pulled the arms down and out one at a time, leaving only Milek's head inside the birth canal. Finally, with Mitch's fingertip maneuvering the upper jaw, the head would have followed. Feet first, head last: a perfectly upside-down birth.

I didn't see any of it, though. From my stool in the rear of the room I could only see backs: Ben's, Mitch's, and those of several nurses and students who had gathered around to watch. I sat there motionless, wondering if I had managed to kill poor Danuta's baby. Finally, after a minute that seemed to drag on forever, I heard a baby's strong cry. Mitch stood up and placed the squalling baby in his mother's arms. He turned and took a little bow for the staff, then winked and nodded at me in a way that left me wondering if maybe—just *maybe*—he'd known about the breech all along.

I had a harder time recovering from that birth than either Milek or Danuta did. They were both fine and home in a couple of days. But my house-of-cards confidence had come tumbling down. I had been lulled by the normalcy of most births into thinking that that's all there was to it: the lady gets in the bed, you do a few examinations, and then poof—a baby falls in your lap. When the butt came first, I wasn't ready. I failed the test.

That evening, after I had signed off for the last time to the on-call team, I stopped by the office to say good-bye to Mitch. He was wearing a suit and tie, the first time I had seen him in anything but scrubs. His hair was neatly combed, too—another first. He was taking his girlfriend to the symphony, he said in response to my stunned expression, and bloody shoes just wouldn't do. He was in a hurry. "Walk out with me," he said, and I followed him down the hallway to the exit.

Out on the street in the thick air of a Chicago summer evening, Mitch put an arm around my shoulder and squeezed, like an uncle about to give important career advice. I sighed and dropped my head, waiting for some final words of wisdom before getting on with the rest of my medical life. "You know," he said, in what passed for him as a kindly voice, "if you can't tell a baby's head from its ass, maybe you're in the wrong business." He squeezed my shoulder again, then slipped into the crowd passing in front of the hospital. He didn't look back.

Mitch was right, if crudely so. I didn't know it at the time, but I had performed my last delivery. My next rotation was pediatrics, and I loved it from the start. I would throw in my lot with the babies.

Chapter 2
The First Five Minutes

Amy Lincoln is halfway born. After eighteen hours of labor her head is on the out-in-the-world side, the side where her father, Jack, a pipefitter by trade and a man witnessing the birth of a child for the first time, watches with ever widening eyes. The rest of Amy—chest and shoulders squeezed tightly in the birth canal, feet in the womb—is still inside her mother, Beth.

In this brief moment Amy is neither fish nor fowl. She's not really a fetus anymore—her mouth is open, searching for air, even though she's still a few seconds away from taking her first breath. Yet with her pulsing umbilical cord still attached to her placenta, she's not a full-fledged baby, either.

If we could look inside Amy's body as she hovers between worlds we would be witness to one of life's great miracles. There is no time in life, not even the moment of death, that can compare to the human body's transformation in the first five minutes outside the womb. Birth is about radical, creative, life-affirming change. It is about adaptation on a nearly unbelievable scale. Abrupt, rapid-fire transitions are the order of the day: dark to light, warm to cold, wet to dry. Amy's fetus-body was marvelously well designed for the task of life in the womb; within five minutes of birth she'll leave all that behind.

But Jack can't see any of that. He just sees a head with red hair like Beth's, and he wonders what's taking so long for the rest of his baby to show up.

The pause in Amy's birth is intentional. She's gotten tangled up in her umbilical cord during labor, and now, as her head emerges, I can see that a loop of cord is tightly noosed around her neck. That accounts for the worrisome drop in Amy's heart rate over the last few minutes—the reason I've been called to attend her birth.

The midwife tells Beth not to push for a moment—easier said than done, judging from the incredulous *I'm-about-to-explode-here!* look on her face. Moving quickly, the midwife clamps the cord in two places and cuts it, releasing Amy's neck from its grip. The danger passes. Amy's heart rate stabilizes.

Freed to resume pushing, Beth bears down with all her might. Amy's right shoulder emerges from the birth canal, then the left follows. A gush of fluid and a burst of baby and suddenly Amy's all here, gulping her first breaths of air in the midwife's lap, an official out-in-the-world human being.

But she's not quite the baby her parents were expecting. The Amy that Beth and Jack have carried in their mind's eye these past nine months is pink and cuddly, smiling and content, with Cupid's-bow lips and a little Gerber baby curl sticking up from the top of her head. This Amy, the one newly placed on Beth's abdomen by the midwife, is, well, none of that. She's pale blue and slippery, covered in blood, amniotic fluid, and a little meconium—newborn poop. The place on her head where the curl should be is matted and lopsided, the scalp pushed to one side like a bad toupee. She's bandy-legged and pigeon-toed, squinty-eyed and squalling. Beth and Jack look over to me, not sure whether they should be alarmed. I smile and nod encouragement. *Just wait.* In the decades since Tonya's wild delivery and Mitch's parting advice, I've learned to do just that.

And sure enough, in a few short minutes, everything changes. Amy calms down, her initial frantic cries soothed by Beth's touch and familiar voice. Her color shifts from blue to purple to pink. She opens her eyes and looks at the world, fixing first on Beth's face and then on Jack's. She squirms her way to Beth's waiting nipple, opens her mouth, and takes it in as though she'd been doing this all her life. And just like that, aided by the kind of new-parent vision that's blind to blood, goo, and odd-looking heads, Amy Lincoln becomes the cherubic pink fluff-bundle of her parents' dreams.

Amy's transformation from battered-looking ex-fetus to the baby her parents were expecting is dramatic, but those of us present at a birth see only the external, cosmetic part of the story. The real action takes place inside Amy herself, hidden from view. It is nothing short of miraculous that the vast majority of babies make their way through this incredible transition without a hitch. Nearly three thousand births into my career, those first few minutes of life are still the most amazing of them all.

It's a whole different world in the womb. Apt analogies are hard to come by. I once read an account of childbirth that compared the emerging fetus to a surfacing scuba diver. Both of them move from a watery environment to an air-filled world, the author wrote. Each carries an oxygen supply—an air tank for the diver, a placenta for the fetus. At the moment of transition they simply toss aside their now obsolete underwater gear and take a big gulp of fresh air.

That analogy only goes so far. If a diver really were like a fetus, his lungs would be filled with seawater, his air tank would be connected to his belly button, and half his blood supply would be floating in a sac outside his body. On his way up from the depths he'd squeeze the extra blood back into his body, force the water out of his lungs, and permanently rearrange the flow of blood through his heart. Then he'd pop to the surface, naked and screaming, wide-eyed with amazement and anxiety at the new world he'd been cast into. If diving and childbirth were identical processes, Jacques Cousteau might never have gotten into the water.

A fetus waiting to be born is so different from a newborn baby, let alone a panicky scuba diver, that it might as well be another species. Let's start with the placenta, the remarkable organ that acts as both fetal oxygen tank and blood sac.

A healthy full term placenta is disk-shaped and the color of dark blood, about seven inches across and an inch and a half thick. Though the placenta is an incredibly complex organ, in basic terms it's divided into three layers: an inner *basal plate* (the maternal side that clings to the wall of the uterus); an outer *chorionic plate* (the fetal side where the umbilical cord attaches); and an in-between layer filled with maternal blood known as the *intervillous space.*

Throughout pregnancy a mother pumps her blood through the uterine wall and basal plate into the intervillous space. There, fingerlike *villi* filled with fetal blood vessels project from the chorionic plate into the maternal blood "like the fronds of a sea anemone wafting in the seawater of a rock pool," as one obstetrics textbook puts it in an uncharacteristic burst of near poetry. This close contact of maternal blood and fetal villi allows the exchange of necessary chemicals between mother and fetus. Close though that contact is, the separation between mother and fetus is complete; their blood supplies never mix.

Among its myriad jobs, the placenta allows water and molecular nutrients—proteins, fats, sugars, vitamins, minerals, and such—to pass from a mother to her growing fetus, even as fetal waste products are transferred back into the maternal blood for eventual disposal in her urine. The placenta forms a nearly impermeable barrier to germs while providing the fetus with a steady supply of protective maternal antibodies for use after birth. It makes hormones, neutralizes acids, and delivers an uninterrupted supply of oxygen from the early days of pregnancy right up to the moment of birth. And then, when its job is completed, it lets go of the womb and follows the fetus into the light of day.

The oxygen that fuels a fetus's growth starts its journey with a mother's breath. As she inhales, air rushes down her windpipe into millions of tiny lung sacs called *alveoli.* The tissue walls of the alveoli are so microscopically thin that oxygen molecules simply pass through them, jumping from the inhaled air in the alveoli into red blood cells passing by in tiny blood vessels called *capillaries.* The oxygen-rich blood then exits her lungs and travels through the heart to the aorta, the large artery that carries blood to the body's many oxygen-hungry organs.

One of the hungriest organs in a near term woman is the uterus.

Nearly one-fifth of all the blood pumped by her heart is bound for the uterus—fifty times the amount of blood that flowed through the uterine artery before she became pregnant. The placenta, clinging to the inside wall of the uterus, gets the lion's share of that increase. Once maternal blood reaches the intervillous space, oxygen molecules easily pass into the fetal blood vessels in the villi, just as they did into the mother's lung alveoli only moments before. With delivery now complete, the oxygen-depleted maternal blood drains from the intervillous space and travels back to her lungs for another load of oxygen. The placenta has fulfilled the role of fetal lung—or diver's air tank. It's up to the fetus to take it from there.

The umbilical cord comes next, originating in the placenta's chorionic plate, and here more imperfect analogies arise—geographical ones this time—inspired by the umbilical cord's unique role in fetal life. Most texts describe the cord as the bridge between mother and child, or the interstate highway system that links the two, or even the Panama Canal of the womb: the sole path by which food, water, and oxygen move from placenta to fetus. I lean toward astronomical analogies myself. Tethered to the placenta by the umbilical cord, the fetus looks to me like a 1960s spacewalking astronaut, the kind of man I idolized as an elementary school science buff.

Walter Cronkite, the avuncular CBS newsman who covered the 1960s space race, cemented that image in my mind when I was twelve years old. During a live broadcast of history's first space walk, he described the fragile-looking tubing that ran from the capsule to the front of astronaut Ed White's suit as his "umbilical cord." Not knowing much about childbirth in those days—this being the tail end of my babies-found-in-cabbage-patches era—I wasn't entirely sure what he meant. An astronaut with an umbilical cord was simply one more of life's many mysteries. But I worshipped Walter Cronkite, and if he had called that thing the world's longest piece of spaghetti, I'd be writing pasta analogies now.

But even Cronkitean analogies fail to capture the essence of the umbilical cord, because he got the astronaut's relationship to his place in space precisely backward. To be truly fetal, the astronaut and his "umbilical cord" would be safely tucked away *inside* the space capsule (the "mother ship," if you will), not wandering around in space, exposed and defenseless, waiting for a meteor to hit him. Then again, to a fetus the womb may well represent the entire universe, so maybe Cronkite got it right after all.

Stripped of the poorly crafted analogies, an umbilical cord is a foot and a half of rubbery hose connecting the fetus to the placenta. The bulk of the cord, the stuff inside that gives it its characteristic rubberiness, is called "Wharton's jelly," named after the seventeenth-century London physician who first described it.* Deep inside the protective jelly, three blood vessels run the length of the cord. A large umbilical vein carries oxygen-rich blood from the placenta to the fetus while twin umbilical arteries spiral around the vein, returning spent blood from the fetus to the placenta. The cord connects to the fetus at the *umbilical ring*—the future "innie" or "outie"—and it's here that things start to get strange, at least in comparison to the way an adult body works.

It's hard to believe, gazing at it now, that my navel was once critically important to my existence. It hasn't had much to do since the moment my mother's obstetrician caught me in his lap, tied off my umbilical cord with a string, and sliced it in two with a scalpel. At that moment, my umbilical ring began its rapid fall from grace, plunging from its zenith as an essential fetal lifeline (or Panama Canal, etc.), through a brief phase as a shriveling raisin stuck to my newborn tummy, to its nadir as the brunt of a million jokes: a belly button. With the exception of a brief period when my young children used it as a repository for beans and beads and whatever else they cared to drop into it (it's a very deep innie), it's just been there collecting lint ever since. But there was a time when it was the center

---

*In addition to his umbilical cord work, Thomas Wharton (1614–1673) was the first physician to explain the role of saliva in chewing and digestion, and to consider the functions of the thyroid gland, chief among which he believed was "to fill the neck and make it more shapely." Wharton's jelly isn't his only anatomical legacy; you've got a pair of salivary Wharton's ducts on the floor of your mouth, directly beneath the tip of your tongue.

of my world, the sole port through which every molecule of food and oxygen that went into making me arrived.

Like any modern harbor (more analogies—forgive me!), the fetus has its own unique infrastructure to speed the delivery of goods from port to consumer. On entering the fetus's body through the ring, the umbilical vein parts company with the umbilical arteries. The vein (now called the *ductus venosus*) veers sharply upward, aiming straight for the fetal heart. It joins with the inferior vena cava, the large vein that returns blood to the heart from the lower half of the fetus, to speed its fresh, oxygen-rich blood directly into the heart. Mission accomplished—the voyage of those oxygen molecules, from a mother's breath to her growing fetus's heart, takes only a few seconds.

It's here inside the heart that the ingenuity of fetal design really shines. Once we're born, oxygen-poor blood pumped from the body is sent by the heart's right ventricle through the pulmonary artery to the lungs to pick up an oxygen load. The oxygen-rich blood then returns to the left ventricle, from where it is pumped into the aorta and out to the various organs and tissues. Then it's back to the right side of the heart and the lungs in a never-ending loop.

In the fetus, however, pumping blood to the lungs would be a pointless exercise. After all, the lungs are filled with amniotic fluid, not air, and the blood flowing into the heart from the placenta already has all the oxygen a fetus needs. A trip to those sodden lungs would be a waste of fetal time and energy. The solution? A heart-lung bypass system known as right-to-left shunting.

The fetal heart is marvelously designed for right-to-left shunting. A one-way flap of tissue called the *foramen ovale*—literally, the "oval opening"—allows about half of the blood arriving in the right side of the heart to jet directly across to the left side. The other half of the incoming blood follows the usual course and heads out the pulmonary artery toward the lungs. But long before reaching the lungs, most of that blood shunts directly from the pulmonary artery to the aorta through the *ductus arteriosus,* a fetus-only connection between the two. In all, 90 percent of the blood arriving from the placenta never gets to the lungs; the 10 percent that does is just enough to nourish the growing lung tissue.

Whether it gets to the left side of the fetal heart via the foramen ovale or the ductus arteriosus, the oxygen-rich blood then speeds its way down the aorta and out to the body, where it fuels the growth and development of the trillions of cells that will become an Amy Lincoln. Once oxygen delivery is complete, the spent blood finds its way back to the umbilical arteries in the cord, and then on to the placenta for another load of fuel.

That's the setup as labor begins. Fetal blood circulates to the placenta and back, picking up oxygen from maternal blood and delivering it to the fetal tissues. The lungs are simply along for the ride, growing and developing like the kidneys, the brain, and the rest of the organs. The lung bypass channels are open and running. The fetus is warm and cozy, and life is good. Time to wake that kid up.

No one knows for sure what a baby's first clue is that she's about to be born, but it may very well be the sensation of a subtle shift in her blood flow. As labor commences, the uterus begins the long series of contractions that will eventually result in birth. The main purpose of those contractions—pushing the baby out—is intuitively obvious. But another, equally critical event is happening at the same time. Bit by bit, contraction by contraction, the nearly born fetus is being transfused with its own blood.

A full term placenta holds about six ounces of fetal blood, or roughly half of a newborn's total blood volume. That would be like a grown man walking around with—pardon the visual—a three-quart bag of blood hanging from his belly button. Carrying that much blood outside the body would be a bad idea for an adult, but a fetus gets along just fine with this arrangement because very little blood goes to the developing lungs, liver, and kidneys—big blood reservoirs in the child and adult. Instead, the blood that would be found in those organs is carried in the placenta. And by the time of birth, that blood has to be transfused back into the baby.

How? The uterus shrinks in size as it contracts, which puts a squeeze on the placenta. Blood flows from the collapsing placenta down the umbilical vein and into the fetus, kind of like air rushing from a bagpipe when it's played, minus the ungodly noise. The fetal heart continues to pump blood back to the placenta through the umbilical arteries, but because there is less and less space to fit the blood in the shrinking placenta, the in-and-out balance begins to shift. The blood volume inside the fetus grows.

As the fetal blood volume increases, some of it begins to push its way into the blood vessels within the lungs. The force of a uterine contraction—roughly equivalent to the blood pressure of a small adult—is exactly that needed to force open the capillaries that surround the liquid-filled alveoli. Amniotic fluid begins to drain out of the fetal alveoli and into the newly filled capillaries. All that's needed now is a good rafter-rattling first cry to fill the lungs with air and complete the process.

But what makes a newborn baby take that first big breath? The obvious answer—she has to breathe or die—doesn't really begin to explain a baby's first cries. It's not as if Amy had a lot of breathing practice before she was born. A late term fetus makes uncoordinated little gasps that do nothing more than move a little amniotic fluid up and down the windpipe. They're nowhere near the full-chested Tarzan yells she'll be expected to make at the moment of birth. So what starts a baby up?

Theories abound. Cold, light, noise, and pain have all been implicated as the primary breath starter. Gravity, too—a baby's response to being suddenly sprung from the supporting confines of the womb. Some researchers think it's purely a chemical thing, that feeling of panic caused by rising carbon dioxide levels when you hold your breath too long.

It's probably a combination of all of those things. Call it the Ice Bucket Effect. Next time your beloved spouse or partner steps out of a hot, steamy shower, douse him unexpectedly with a bucketful of ice water. First, he'll suck in a deep breath. Second, he'll yell at the top of his lungs. That combination of cold, wetness, and surprise will make any adult cry out, so it isn't surprising that the same combination of factors might rev up a newborn baby.

But when Amy Lincoln took those first breaths she faced one major obstacle that an ice-water-soaked loved one doesn't. Her lungs were still filled with amniotic fluid. Until she emptied them, all the crying in the world wasn't going to do her any good.

How did she do it? Back in my 1970s medical school days, I was taught that most of the amniotic fluid in the lungs is forced into the bloodstream or out of the mouth as the chest is squeezed in the birth canal. One major theoretical flaw: if that were the case, it would be hard to explain how a cesarean section baby, who never travels through the birth canal, could survive. It turns out that what I learned is mostly wrong. All that birth canal squeezing doesn't really accomplish much—it just clears amniotic fluid from the mouth and upper windpipe. The lungs are still pretty wet when a baby pops out of its mother. And that's actually a good thing.

Time for an experiment. Take a couple of never-blown-up balloons, the cheap kind found on the birthday party shelf in any grocery store. Try blowing up the first one. It's not easy—you'll end up with a red, puffy face from forcing air into that collapsed, sticky-on-the-inside piece of latex. Now put a few drops of water into the second balloon and try again. (Amniotic fluid is a complicated chemical stew, but since it might be hard to find any at your local Safeway, plain old tap water makes an adequate stand-in.) It's a lot easier this time.

If the trip through the birth canal really did empty the lungs of all their fluid, the newborn would be faced with a dry-balloon dilemma: the sticky-sided, collapsed alveoli would require tremendous force to open, probably more than the baby could generate with even its most impassioned cry. But wise nature makes sure that all the fluid *doesn't* get squeezed out ahead of time.

Here, then, is the final wet-to-dry sequence of events:

The Ice Bucket Effect jolts the newborn into making that first cry. With each deep breath that follows, more and more wet-balloon alveoli pop open. Since there's a lot more oxygen in air than in maternal blood, the oxygen level in a newborn's bloodstream rises quickly as she cries. That sudden increase in oxygen in turn signals the lung's arteries and capillaries to relax and open up. Blood flow to the lungs increases dramatically; billions of red blood cells race to the newly opened alveoli to absorb the oxygen now pouring into the lungs from the outside world.

The fetus-only bypasses, which served Amy so well in the womb, now begin to close. Cutting the cord ends the flow of blood through the umbilical ring and the ductus venosus leading to the heart. The easy flow of blood to the now inflated lungs causes the blood pressure in the right side of the heart to drop. This forces the foramen ovale, the opening between the right and left sides of the heart that has been held open through fetal life by the high right heart blood pressure, to slam shut forever. Increasing blood oxygen levels trigger a cascade of chemical events that begin the closure of the ductus arteriosus, the artery that allowed blood to bypass the fetal lungs. By five minutes of age, the transition is essentially complete. Her scuba diving days over, Amy's now a full-fledged, air-breathing human being.

Despite nearly strangling on her umbilical cord, I could see as soon as Amy was born that she never came close to any real harm. Her full-chested roar was the tip-off. That and the way she held her body tightly flexed, mimicking her in utero position of the last few months. I assumed that her heart rate was back to normal; no need for a stethoscope with a baby *that* loud. The midwife raised an eyebrow in my direction as soon as Amy was out—did I want to have a look at her? I shook my head. The best place for a lustily crying newborn is at her mother's breast, not stretched out on an examination table. I could see what I needed to see from my unobtrusive perch in the corner.

I watched awhile longer, just to make sure that there were no lingering effects from Amy's noose of a cord. Relatives flocked around Beth and her baby—a pair of new grandmothers, an aunt, and a no longer queasy grandpa who'd spent the last half hour sitting in the hall. Then I made a quick note in Amy's very first hospital chart: "Apgars 8 and 9. No resuscitation required."

I caught Jack's teary eye. He waved, opened his mouth, and then shrugged, dumbstruck. "Congratulations," I called to him. "She's beautiful." Then I circled behind the happy crowd and slipped out the door. There was nothing else for me to do.

Amy Lincoln's relatively easy womb-to-world transition is typical of most modern births. The rarity of things going haywire is striking, given the complexity of the changes at birth. Over 95 percent of newborns make the transition without a hitch, needing little help from those in attendance.

But occasionally it isn't that easy. For every worrisome delivery I'm called to in which I simply watch and wait and then ride off unnoticed into the hospital sunset, there's another that puts me at the center of intense, hair-graying action. Amy's textbook transition went smoothly, but it just as easily might have gone wrong. As the cord tightened around Amy's neck with each contraction, less and less oxygen made its way from the placenta to her body. Had the cord been a bit tighter, or the delivery a few minutes longer, the lack of oxygen might have damaged Amy's brain and heart, changing that sweet moment of new-family bonding into a blur of monitors, catheters, and all the other tools of modern newborn resuscitation.

Amy's rapid transformation from a near strangling victim to a pink cherub cuddled in her mother's arms illustrates a truism about fetuses and babies—they're a lot tougher than we think. But there are limits to what they can take. Whether a just born baby ends up snuggled at her mother's breast or struggling for life in an intensive care nursery is determined by one critical thing: a steady flow of oxygen. Take the case of Sean O'Connor, the baby whose birth I attended a few hours after Amy's.

Sean's mother, Wendy, was one of the fittest pregnant women I have ever known. A gymnast and rock climber in her school days, she had matured into a competitive triathlete and swimmer. Her pregnancy was uneventful. She exercised vigorously right up to a few days before delivery, and took a long hike with her husband, Bill, the morning before Sean was born. When a week before her due date I saw Wendy in my pediatric office with Michael, her fearless but injury-prone toddler, I wished her luck. Not that I thought she'd need it.

Wendy's due date came and went without so much as a contraction. She wasn't overly worried—Michael had been a week late, too. Her obstetrician was optimistic at Wendy's final prenatal visit. Everything was going well.

Then early on the morning of Sean's birth, Wendy, now nearly two weeks overdue, awoke with a sharp, stabbing pain in her lower abdomen. She knew from experience that these weren't normal labor pains. Bill woke quickly. He called the next-door neighbors to come and stay with Michael, then packed Wendy into their brand-new van and sped the three miles to the emergency room, rolling through every stop sign along the way.

Wendy arrived on the maternity ward in a wheelchair pushed by a sprinting emergency room orderly. Bill trailed behind, a suitcase tucked under each arm, still wearing his bedroom slippers. Wendy's pains were worse now; blood stained her nightgown and dripped onto the floor.

As a nurse transferred Wendy to a hospital bed and strapped a fetal heart monitor to her belly, the obstetrician came running. She took quick stock of the situation and made her diagnosis: Wendy was having a placental abruption. Her placenta, well past its forty-week life span programmed by nature, had begun to deteriorate and separate from the wall of the uterus with Sean still inside. With no time to lose, a "code C"—an emergency cesarean section—was called. I was across the hall in the intensive care nursery, just arrived from home, when my pager went off.

An emergency cesarean section is a gown-and-mask whirl of doctors, nurses, and frightened parents-to-be. There is no time for birthing plans or breathing exercises or anything else that would delay the birth. After a quick kiss from Bill, Wendy was whisked into the operating room. Her belly was painted with a brown antiseptic solution and covered with a blue surgical drape, and as quickly and gently as possible she was put to sleep.

The obstetrician worked rapidly, cutting through Wendy's abdomen to her uterus in less than half the time it would have taken her in a less urgent cesarean. Five nerve-racking minutes after the first incision, Sean was delivered. The obstetrician placed Sean in the sterile towel I held out to her. I carried him the few feet to the newborn resuscitation table in the corner of the room.

Sean looked okay at first, all things considered. Though his muscle tone was weak and his skin color was a dusky, still-in-the-womb blue, his pulse was strong and he was breathing on his own. The nurse and I dried him off, kept him crying to clear the amniotic fluid from his lungs, and waited for his color to change. She blew oxygen in Sean's face from a thin plastic tube hooked to a nozzle that hung down from the ceiling. Five minutes passed. His cry grew stronger and his grip tightened on my finger, but despite a river of oxygen flowing into his lungs, Sean's respiratory rate increased and he refused to "pink up"—ominous signs of respiratory distress.

We wrapped Sean in a warm blanket and rushed him to the intensive care nursery, negotiating a small crowd of newly arrived relatives and friends in the hallway outside the operating room. I called to Bill to follow us into the ICN. The rest of the family would have to wait outside for now.

In the ICN came another whirl, this one focused on Sean: IV fluids, X-rays, blood tests, antibiotics, and oxygen, always more oxygen. I snaked a thin catheter through his umbilical artery into the aorta, his body's largest artery. Saline solution and then an emergency blood transfusion went in through the catheter, followed by dopamine, a medication to help raise his blood pressure. None of it helped. Sean's chest and abdomen seesawed up and down as he struggled to breathe. His color worsened; his blood oxygen level was frighteningly low.

Sean needed specialized equipment and treatments that a smaller hospital like ours doesn't usually have. I called the hospital in San Francisco that takes our sickest newborns, talked over Sean's case with the neonatologist on call, and arranged for a transport. Now came the nervous-making part—it would be at least a couple of hours, depending on the traffic, before they arrived.

My bag of therapeutic tricks was nearly exhausted. So was Sean, who was growing too tired to breathe on his own. I opened his mouth, and using a laryngoscope I slid an endotracheal tube—a high-tech soda straw, more or less—into his windpipe. While I held the tube in place, the nurse connected it to a ventilator—a machine to do Sean's breathing for him. Next came a dose of morphine to relieve any pain he might be feeling, and another medicine to temporarily paralyze him so that he wouldn't struggle against the ventilator and rupture a lung. Sean's body soon relaxed, his chest rising and falling in time with the soft puffing of the ventilator.

Three tense up-and-down hours later, the ambulance arrived. The transport team packed Sean and his tubes and monitors into an incubator, then wheeled him to the OR recovery room so that Wendy could have a quick first look at her son. Bill helped Wendy reach in through one of the incubator's portholes and touch Sean's hands, and then his face. She murmured something I couldn't hear.

The lead nurse on the transport team quietly described the nursery where Sean would be going and told them the names of the staff who would be caring for him. She answered Wendy's questions and then handed Bill a map and a list of phone numbers. With that, the team rolled the incubator to a freight elevator just outside the recovery room. I stayed with them until Sean was loaded into an ambulance waiting by the emergency room doors.

An hour later Sean was speeding across the Golden Gate Bridge, still blue but holding his own.

As soon as Sean left I went back to the recovery room. Bill stood by Wendy, who was still coming around from her anesthesia. She was frightened and confused, too woozy at first to follow most of what I was saying. She had seen Sean only briefly, and the sight of his tiny body surrounded by so much medical equipment had been over-whelming. I sat on the chair next to her bed and explained as best I could what had happened and what might happen next.

I started with the positives: Sean was very sick, but underlying it all he was a normal baby. He had all his fingers and toes. From the X-rays and other tests I knew that his heart, lungs, and other organs were perfectly developed. If the doctors in San Francisco could get him through these next few days, I said, there was every reason to believe that he'd recover completely.

From the look on Wendy's face I could see that she wasn't buy-ing it. She talked between sobs, while Bill stroked her hair and dabbed at her tears with a tissue. "He's *not* normal," she said. "He was all blue." She reached for Bill's hand. "What's wrong with him?"

I grabbed a piece of paper and a pencil from the table next to Wendy's bed and sketched an artless diagram: two squares, side by side, one marked "Fetus" and the other "Newborn." On each square I penciled in the basics—a heart and lungs, with blood ves-sels connecting the two to each other and the rest of the body. The main difference between the drawings—and it was a critical one in Sean's case—was that the "Fetus" drawing included a placenta, while the "Newborn" didn't. "What's wrong," I said, tapping the drawings with the tip of the pencil, "is that Sean still thinks he's a fetus." Wendy blinked. Ed shook his head. "I don't get it," he said.

I kept the discussion as simple as I could, given that I was sure that Sean had Persistent Pulmonary Hypertension of the Newborn (PPHN), one of the most difficult-to-explain problems a sick baby can have. I started at the moment of the abruption, when part of the placenta tore away from the wall of Wendy's uterus and the blood that should have been bringing oxygen to Sean began to trickle out of her body.

The decreased blood flow to the maternal side of the placenta had caused Sean's oxygen level to drop sharply. That too-low level of oxygen in Sean's bloodstream, known as *hypoxemia,* had prevented the arteries and capillaries in his lungs from relaxing and opening up as they normally would after birth. The resulting lack of blood flow to his lungs kept Sean hypoxemic, which in turn kept the lung blood vessels constricted. PPHN was once called *persistent fetal circulation,* an apt description of Sean's dilemma: born into an air-breathing world, his heart and lungs were behaving as if he was still in the womb.

I had hoped the medications, IV fluids, and blood transfusion I'd given him would break that pattern, but they hadn't. Sean's lungs were still getting less than half the blood they should have received. The job of the doctors and nurses in San Francisco, I told Wendy and Bill, would be to convince Sean that it was time to let go of his fetal circulation and start using his lungs. And that could take days, even weeks.

Amy Lincoln passed her fetus-to-newborn test with flying colors. She opened her lungs, closed her bypasses, and moved on to the rest of her life. Sean's transition was a miserable failure, nearly killing him before the obstetrician pulled him from Wendy's uterus. What happened?

Sean's transition fell apart before it began, since Wendy wasn't even in labor when the stabbing pain in her abdomen woke her that morning. There's no way to know whether Sean felt anything when the abruption started, but if he did, it might have been the queasy light-headedness a person often feels just before fainting. This was much more than a simple fainting spell, though—once the abruption started, Sean was steadily slipping into shock.

At every stage of life, the human body responds to hemorrhage, and the sudden decrease in oxygen that accompanies it, by shifting blood away from organs less essential for immediate survival, such as the skin and bowel, and toward those organs that are critical for short-term survival. In children and adults, this means that blood is shifted to the lungs and then on to the besieged brain and heart to keep them supplied with oxygen. Things are different in the fetus, though. The diverted blood is sent to the placenta for more oxygen, not the lungs, since the lungs aren't involved in delivering oxygen until after birth.

In Sean's case, the diversion of blood to a hemorrhaging placenta set a vicious cycle in motion. With the placenta failing, less and less oxygen returned to Sean's body. Yet in a frantic attempt to compensate, his body diverted even more blood to the placenta, his only potential source of oxygen. A cycle like that can only go on so long; the emergency cesarean section came just in time to save Sean's life.

Unfortunately, Sean's vicious cycle kept right on going after he was safely delivered. Though the placenta was gone, delivered a couple of minutes after Sean was already out, his body stubbornly refused to send blood to his lungs. Why? Just as I had described to Bill O'Connor, Sean was stuck in fetal mode.

In a normal transition, the arteries leading from the heart to the lungs relax as the blood oxygen level rises with a baby's first cries. The relaxing arteries allow more blood to flow into the lungs; normal out-of-the-womb breathing is established. In Sean's case, though, the lung blood vessels were so tightly clamped down from the lack of oxygen in utero that they couldn't relax, and so most of the oxygen we pumped into Sean's lungs—with so little blood reaching his lungs to absorb it—flowed right back out of his body as he exhaled. His body was caught in a trap, ignoring the lungs that could give him the oxygen he so critically needed while vainly pumping blood to a placenta that was no longer there.

• • •

Back in the recovery room, Wendy moved in and out of sleep as the combination of anesthesia and exhaustion overtook her. Nurses came and went, checking her incision and her IV fluids, offering their encouragement in lowered voices. Bill listened without saying much. His attention soon shifted from me and my explanations to Wendy. He fluffed her pillow and held her head while she took sips of ice water from a plastic cup. A minute later she was softly snoring.

"I think I get it now," he said. "Underneath all this . . . whatever"— he pointed at my drawing—"he's a normal baby, right?" I nodded. "No heart problems, no birth defects, right?" I nodded again. Bill rubbed his eyes and sighed. "So then," he said, "we just wait?" I thought of the other babies I had sent away in ambulances over the years. Most of them had recovered fully. Some had not.

"Yes," I said. "We just wait."

Just after midnight I phoned the ICN in San Francisco. The on-call neonatologist gave me a quick update. He confirmed that Sean, now eighteen hours old, had severe PPHN and was in critical condition. They had placed Sean on a special ventilator that gave him an incredible six hundred tiny breaths a minute, allowing a steady stream of oxygen to flow into his lungs with a minimum amount of trauma to his delicate tissues. It seemed to be helping; his blood oxygen level had risen a bit, a sure sign that more blood was reaching his lungs. He still had a long way to go, but the fact that the treatment was making a difference was encouraging news.

I stopped by Wendy's room to tell her and Bill the news. Wendy was fully awake now, propped up in her hospital bed, talking to someone on the telephone. IV tubing sprouted from both of her arms; thin wires ran from patches on her chest to a cardiac monitor hanging from a pole next to the bed. Her face was puffy from crying and lack of sleep. Traces of mascara lay smeared in the hollows under her eyes.

When she saw me, Wendy handed the phone to Bill, who hung

it up without so much as a good-bye to the person on the other end. "What did they tell you?" she asked, her voice hoarse and cracking. She tried to sit up, but fell back on the bed with a grimace of pain. "Is he any better?"

I sat down next to Bill on the edge of the foldout cot the hospital issued to stay-over relatives. He was rumpled, still dressed in the clothes he had been wearing when he drove Wendy to the hospital early that morning. A pair of thick glasses—he usually wore contact lenses—slid down his nose as he spoke. "This is so awful," he said, wearily jabbing at his glasses with his finger. Then his voice trailed away.

I reached across the bed and closed my hand around Wendy's. I described my conversation with the doctors in San Francisco, emphasizing the little bit of good news they had given me. Wendy began to cry. "When can I get out of here?" she sobbed. She waved her free hand around the room, the IV tubing trailing behind like a leash. "I need to be with my baby!"

The on-call obstetrician had told me a short while before that Wendy's blood pressure was elevated, though it wasn't clear whether this was from stress or a complication of her surgery. At any rate, she was in no condition to travel to San Francisco. "Not tonight," I said, pointing to the blood pressure monitor next to the bed. "You have to heal up a bit first."

We talked awhile about how hard it was for her to be separated from her sick baby. A breast pump sat at the foot of the bed, unused. "You need to start pumping," I said. "What do you expect Sean to eat when he gets better?" I fished a Post-it note from my scrubs pocket and handed it to Wendy. "The nurse taking care of Sean said to tell you to call anytime," I said. Wendy squinted at the name and number on the note, then picked up the phone on the nightstand next to her bed and dialed. I shook Bill's hand and went back to my hospital rounds.

The next day and night were hard for Wendy. Bill left at dawn to be with Sean in San Francisco. Visitors to her room—friends, relatives, coworkers—came and went in an awkward parade. Michael came by with his grandparents and stayed for a couple of hours, huddled next to his mother in bed. Wendy did her best to be up-beat for him, but his repeated questions ("Baby?" he asked over and over, pointing to her bandaged belly. "Baby?") finally wore her down. With promises of unlimited cartoons and an ice cream dinner, his grandparents lured Michael back to their home.

My usual duties—newborn exams, emergency room calls, going to worrisome deliveries—soon closed in. When I had time, I'd stop by and see how Wendy was doing. Mostly she was on the phone, first to Bill in San Francisco for updates, then to her parents, then to a couple of close friends. She was restless, her sleep disturbed by pain and bad dreams. The waiting was killing her, she said.

I called San Francisco myself a couple of times that day so I could clarify Bill's version of what he was being told. Sean was in the up-and-down pattern typical of babies with PPHN: steady improvement followed by a quick nosedive, then a slow return. Overall, though, he was improving. Not quite out of the woods, but at least the trees were thinning.

I stopped by Wendy's room that evening on my way home. She looked more like her old self. She was walking now, and a shower and fresh nightgown had done her a world of good. She smiled as I entered her room, the first time I had seen her smile since Sean's birth.

"I'm getting out of here tomorrow," she announced, "even if I have to tie bedsheets together and go down the wall." I pointed out that the unopenable hospital windows might toss a wrench into her plan. "Do me a favor, then," she said. "Bring a hammer with you tomorrow, just in case I'm still here."

The next morning Wendy's bed was empty and the window was still in one piece. I was late getting to the ward; a call to the emergency room had kept me tied up till almost ten. A nurse told me that Wendy's blood pressure was back to normal, and the minute she was cleared for discharge, she and Bill had headed to San Francisco. They left a note behind for me: my two-box drawing, with a circle and slash drawn through the "Fetus" side in red Magic Marker. "He's getting better!" Bill had written underneath. "Gotta go . . ."

The ward clerk handed me another note, this one a phone message from San Francisco: "Doctor says O'Connor baby improving." I looked from one note to the other and smiled, relieved.

"Hey!" A booming voice from down the hall snapped me back into the moment. "Are you ever going to come and talk to us again?" It was Jack Lincoln, freshly showered, pushing Amy ahead of him in her clear plastic bassinet. "We're going home this morning," he said as he passed me at a half-trot. "You'd better come say hi to Beth."

A half hour and one delivery later, I met with Jack and Beth in their hospital room. Beth looked tired but excited. She was out of her hospital gown and into a set of comfortable maternity clothes. Flowers and balloons lined the room, nearly blocking the sunlight that streamed in through the window. Three suitcases were packed and lined up by the door.

Amy was asleep in Beth's arms, wrapped tightly in a pink and gold receiving blanket her grandmother had crocheted for her. I sat down on the edge of the bed and slowly unwrapped her for a going-home examination. Beth and Jack took turns asking questions. Jack's were more long-term in nature: When would Amy run? When could she catch a ball?

Beth focused on the practical. She asked about lotions for Amy's peeling skin, whether she should worry about Amy's noisy nighttime breathing, and what foods she should avoid while breastfeeding. We talked about Amy's vision and hearing, the tiny birthmark on her thigh, and the importance of having visitors wash their hands before touching her. "That'll be a first for a lot of my buddies," said Jack, staring down at his own permanently grease-stained palms.

I closed with a quick review of newborn safety—car seats and smoke detectors in particular. "And no throwing any baseballs at her," I warned Jack. "At least not till she can throw them back." Jack smiled, crushed my hand, and grabbed the suitcases. "No worries, doc," he said. "I'm a rugby man, anyway."

I helped Beth into the wheelchair that would carry her down the elevator and out to the car. She held Amy in her arms, still a little awkward in that first-time-mother way. "Thanks for everything," she said as the elevator doors closed. "See you in a couple of weeks."

I made a final call to San Francisco that night before leaving the hospital. Sean's condition had deteriorated again. The neonatology staff had tried several maneuvers to coax his lungs back open, but none had worked. It looked as if he was headed for *extracorporeal membrane oxygenation,* or ECMO, a risky lung bypass that acts almost literally as an artificial placenta. Fortunately, just as ECMO loomed, a then experimental medication now commonly associated with a more "adult" problem saved the day.

It's here that my story takes what I hope will be its only R-rated detour. Nitric oxide, the medication that came to Sean's rescue in San Francisco, works on a newborn's lungs in exactly the same way that Viagra and its competitors work on a mature malfunctioning penis. When a man suffering from erectile dysfunction takes Viagra, nitric oxide production is stimulated in the penile blood vessels, causing them to relax and allow blood to flow into his previously flaccid organ. Voilà! An erection follows.

Similarly, when a tiny amount of nitric oxide gas was added to the oxygen Sean received through the endotracheal tube, those clamped-down arteries leading to his lungs slowly began to relax. Bit by bit, more blood flowed to the lungs and picked up oxygen before returning to his heart. As his blood oxygen level gradually rose, Sean's body got the message: there's more to life than searching for a long-gone placenta.

Still, Sean wasn't out of the woods for several more days. The lungs of babies with PPHN are notoriously labile, or "twitchy," as they're called in the business. Recovery is slow and fraught with setbacks. The smallest things—a minor decrease in blood pressure, or a too rapid weaning from the oxygen supplied by the ventilator—can wipe out a day's gains in just a few seconds. Sean suffered a couple of these setbacks, but all in all, his recovery was fairly smooth. He was weaned off the ventilator by his sixth day of life. It took him another week to recover the strength to breast-feed.

On the morning that Beth and Jack brought Amy to see me for her first well-baby checkup, a two-car parade headed north across the Golden Gate Bridge. Wendy's and Bill's parents shared the lead car, with Michael happily working his way through a bag of fruit snacks. In the trailing van, Bill drove while Wendy sat in the seat behind him, her arm draped over the car seat buckled next to her. A soft snoring rose and fell from deep within the seat. Sean O'Connor was going home at last. Two and a half weeks old as he left San Francisco in that caravan of relatives, Sean had finally accomplished the transition that most babies make in the first five minutes.

Chapter 3

An Alternate Route:
Cesarean Birth

I keep a photograph on my writing desk that I took at the cesarean section birth of my second child, John, on New Year's Eve 1991. John is center stage in the picture, his few-seconds-old body brightly lit by a bank of overhead lights that casts the circle of birth attendants surrounding him in half-shadow. Slippery with blood and amniotic fluid and still attached to his mother by his umbilical cord, John seems stunned by his sudden change in circumstance: mouth agape and eyes scrunched shut, his arms are flung skyward, the fingers on both hands spread wide.

Elisabeth is wide awake behind a lowered surgical drape, her head supported by the anesthesiologist. Her eyes are riveted on John. She is oblivious to the gaping wound in her abdomen that, mercifully, is a bit off-camera. To her left, a pediatrician stands with towel in hand, waiting to receive John from the obstetrician. At Elisabeth's feet, with her back turned to the camera, a scrub nurse sorts surgical equipment. Everything is going smoothly. It's all quite routine, just one of several cesareans that would take place in that operating room on the last day of the year.

Some who look at the photo can't get past the gore, but my eyes see the birth of an angel. Put a stubby pair of wings on John's back and you've got a cherub worthy of Michelangelo. Add a bow and arrow and he's a perfect little Cupid.

John's cesarean was scheduled well ahead of time because Elisabeth's pregnancy was complicated by *placenta previa*. We discovered this during a scary bleeding episode in her second trimester, when an ultrasound showed that the placenta lay abnormally low in her uterus, blocking the birth canal. A vaginal birth would have been too risky—John would have had to push his way through the placenta en route to being born, triggering hemorrhage that could have been life-threatening to both of them. Weeks ahead of time, then, we knew this moment would come.

I felt some stomach butterflies when we arrived at the hospital that morning, but more than anything I was relieved. I had run a gamut of emotions in the months leading up to John's delivery. Early on it was the fear that Elisabeth would miscarry or suddenly hemorrhage, or that John would be born prematurely. The last couple of weeks brought the excitement of knowing that things were probably going to be all right—though until we got there, that "probably" still loomed large in my mind.

And so, as Elisabeth was wheeled into the operating room, I relaxed. I knew in my heart that, barring some rare catastrophe, she and John were safe. I even allowed myself a few father-and-son fantasies, like fishing and ball throwing and such. At no point during the cesarean did I fear for their lives.

The ordinariness of John's surgical delivery is a very recent development in the history of human childbirth, as was my presence in the operating room that morning. Had John been born fifty years earlier, there would have been no photograph to record the event. Elisabeth would have missed the whole thing, anesthetized and unconscious during surgery, while I paced the floor in some far-off hospital waiting room. I'd have gotten my first glimpse of John through the window of the newborn nursery, tapping my finger on the glass at the pink face in the wrapped bundle of whiteness that was my son.

A century before that, I would have been waiting out the operation in a nearby church, desperately praying for at least one of them to survive an operation that killed many more mothers and babies than it saved.

And two hundred years ago, in my ancestral Irish village, I'd have been faced with disaster: Elisabeth would likely have bled to death from her ruptured placenta, taking John with her. A cesarean, if it was done at all, would have been performed only as Elisabeth and John lay near death, so that John could be baptized while still barely alive, and the two of them buried in separate graves.

In the span of less than two centuries, cesarean section has transformed from a grisly last rite into a surgery so successful that its arrival gave me a sense of relief rather than horror. The loss of mother or child, once a terrifyingly common event, has become shockingly rare. This is the story of that transformation, and of the people who made it happen.

Zeus invented the cesarean section, or so the story goes. It was a spur-of-the-moment thing, born of that Olympian alpha male's legendary inability to rein in his plus-sized libido. Ingenious though Zeus's obstetric approach was, his technique was a bit over the top, even by the operatic standards of Greek mythology.

The story: Among his innumerable crushes, Zeus once fell in love with Semele, the granddaughter of his brother Poseidon—and, what with incest being a way of life on Mount Olympus, he eventually bedded her. By the time Zeus's long-suffering wife, Hera, got wind of the affair, Semele was already pregnant. Bent on revenge, Hera tricked Zeus into letting loose a really first-class thunderbolt, which, unhappily, blew up his bedchamber and incinerated the unfortunate Semele.

The quick-thinking Zeus pulled Semele's fetus from the resulting inferno and, in a breathtaking display of obstetrical derring-do, sewed it directly into his thigh. At the end of this peculiar pregnancy, Zeus cut the stitches and out popped Dionysus, the god of wine. Father and child both recovered nicely.

At least, that's the Greek version of events. Many other ancient cultures can lay similar claim to the discovery of operative birth. References to cesarean-like deliveries pop up in Roman, Egyptian, and Chinese folklore as well as that of many other lands. But for sheer variety and manic inventiveness in alternative childbirthing, there's no place on earth that can touch India.

Consider that Buddha is said to have been born from his mother's side. Or that the twins Satyavati and Matsya, characters in an epic Sanskrit poem, were delivered from the cut-open belly of a fish. Or the story of Queen Gandhari who, fed up with a miserable two-year pregnancy, removed her fetus from her own womb, divided it into a hundred tiny pieces, and then raised the mini-embryos in pots of melted butter. (They grew up to be the hundred evil enemies of the story's hero.) Or the tale of the sage Aurva, whose mother, fearing an attack on her unborn child by warriors from a rival clan, evicted him from her womb, and—shades of Zeus!—sewed him into her thigh for safekeeping.

Eons later, in my Catholic high school days, when any mention of human reproduction outside the hushed confines of biology lab was a sure ticket to hell or detention, I learned in my Origins of Western Civilization class that Julius Caesar had been the world's first cesarean section baby, and so the operation had been named for him. I carried that belief well into adulthood, when I found out that like a lot of other things I was taught back then—the direct link between "self-abuse" and nearsightedness, for example—it wasn't true.

Not that a "Caesarean cesarean" would have been impossible.* Roman law dealt with the subject as far back as the eighth century B.C. In the *Digesta,* a compilation of old Roman laws commissioned during the reign of Justinian (A.D. 527–565), cesarean birth is ad-

---

*Note the dropped *a.* British and Australian writers still use the "caesarean" spelling; Americans, averse to the "ae" combination (as in the original spellings of "paediatrics" and "gynaecology"), chose the shorter "cesarean." And since I'm in a clarifying mood, the word "cesarean" and "section" both refer to the same thing— the act of cutting. I will avoid that particular redundancy from here on out by using the terms "cesarean delivery" or "cesarean birth," either of which will make the world's etymologists much happier.

dressed in a section titled "On Burying the Dead and Building a Tomb": "The law of the kings forbids burial of a woman who died pregnant until her offspring has been excised from her body; anyone who does otherwise is held to have destroyed the prospects of the offspring being alive when he buried the pregnant mother."

At the time of Julius Caesar's birth, then, a cesarean delivery was performed as a last-ditch attempt to rescue a fledgling Roman citizen. The mother was considered a lost cause; no attempt was made to save her life. The fact that Caesar's mother survived his birth—she lived long enough to correspond with him during his military campaigns—makes it highly unlikely that the future ruler of the then known world had anything but a very ordinary vaginal birth. The term "cesarean" and the association of the operation with Caesar's name more likely originated with the Latin verb *caedare* (to cut). Roman babies born in such a manner, living or dead, were referred to as *caesones*.

The first written record of a mother and child both surviving a cesarean delivery comes from Switzerland in 1500. Jacob Nufer, a pig gelder by trade, is said to have performed the operation on his wife after several days of labor and the unsuccessful ministrations of thirteen midwives. Nufer had some working anatomical knowledge—he had delivered piglets operatively—and after gaining permission from local authorities and his desperate wife, he set to work with a sharp knife and soon delivered a healthy baby boy. Much celebration of Jacob's miraculous feat ensued, though Mrs. Nufer's take on her kitchen table operation somehow escaped the historical record. But she did more than simply survive her ordeal. She went on to give birth to five more children—all vaginally, thank goodness—including twins, and died at the age of seventy-seven.

The story is best taken with a very large grain of salt, since it wasn't recorded until eighty-two years after the fact, when everyone who had been there was long dead. But the oft-told tale of Jacob Nufer's success gave midwives and physicians of the day some degree of hope, and served as the inspiration for further surgical experimentation.

Still, almost no progress in operative childbirth was made for another three hundred years. And with all due respect to Jacob Nufer's pigs, Zeus's stitched-up thigh, and those Indian twins sprouting from the belly of a fish, the story of modern cesarean birth begins in earnest with the dawn of the nineteenth century.

It took a man with a much stronger stomach than mine to be a physician in the nineteenth century. A doctor's bag in those days was a toolbox for a man engaged in human carpentry: chopping, cutting, and slicing away at the afflictions of humankind. One look at the assorted hammers, saws, clamps, and chisels a doctor carried with him on his rounds, and I'd have taken off at a sprint for a career as a teacher, a banker, or maybe even a priest—any profession whose job description didn't include hacking gangrenous limbs from fully conscious human beings.

Rural doctors led a particularly harsh professional life. Out in the countryside, calling for the doctor was usually a last resort, something to be tried when traditional remedies failed to stop an infection, or when someone had suffered a particularly grievous injury. Or, as often happened, when a baby got stuck on its way to being born.

The man called to attend an obstructed labor—and they were almost all men—was often ill prepared for the job. His knowledge of human childbirth was limited to the relatively few cases with which he had been directly involved, since most uncomplicated births were attended solely by midwives, and perhaps a smattering of reading he'd done on the subject. By the time the doctor arrived on horseback, the mother-to-be was already exhausted and perhaps near death from hemorrhage or infection. The doctor was then faced with a slim repertoire of therapeutic choices, all of them risky and grim: obstetrical forceps, craniotomy, and, as a last desperate measure, cesarean delivery.

Obstetrical forceps, invented by the medical Chamberlen clan in Britain around 1600, represented the lone significant improvement in obstetric care in the three centuries between Jacob Nufer's barnyard triumph and the first half of the nineteenth century. The Chamberlens themselves, though, were not exactly humanitarian types. Lining their pockets with the proceeds from their invention, they did nothing for the advancement of obstetric science, successfully guarding their design from competitors for more than a century. This was easier than it sounds. The delivery of a baby by a male attendant was usually accomplished under the cover of a mound of modesty-preserving blankets, allowing the instrument to be kept well hidden from prying eyes. As a final cornering-the-market touch, the Chamberlens insisted that the mother and her attendants be blindfolded until after the delivery.

More or less a set of heavy iron salad tongs that were clamped onto the fetus's head and then pulled, forceps allowed for the relatively safe removal of a fetus from the otherwise normal birth canal of an exhausted or ill mother. But forceps were of no help in the case of a woman whose pelvis was naturally too small to allow the fetus to pass, or one deformed by illness or injury, or, as in the case of a mother overwhelmed by infection early in labor, when the fetus was still lodged high in the pelvis. The choice then literally became one of life or death for mother and child.

In many such cases the parents decided, in consultation with the doctor and perhaps a clergyman, to sacrifice the baby in order to save the mother's life. Craniotomy ensued, a gruesome procedure that involved the collapse of the infant's skull followed by the removal of its body in pieces. The specialized crotchets and forceps that the job required were part of a doctor's standard equipment. As grisly as it was, craniotomy offered the mother a reasonable chance of survival. The fetus, obviously, was a lost cause.

The final available option, cesarean delivery, had remained largely unchanged since Jacob Nufer's time. It was still performed only on a dead or dying mother as a last-ditch attempt to salvage a live baby from a dreadful situation. Mortality rates were astronomical; according to one account, not a single woman survived a cesarean delivery in Paris between 1787 and 1876. The few women in other parts of Europe and America who did manage to survive the operation were often left incapacitated for the rest of their lives by severe pelvic and abdominal injuries. But once in a great while a report of a successful cesarean delivery—with both mother and child surviving—made the medical rounds, buoying the hopes of beleaguered European and American physicians.

The first well-documented, successful cesarean in the English-speaking world occurred on July 25, 1826, in Cape Town, South Africa. The patient was Mrs. Thomas Munnik, the young wife of a prominent snuff merchant. The operator was Dr. James Miranda Stuart Barry, a thirty-year-old surgeon who was both a British Army officer and a physically peculiar specimen.

James Barry stood out like a cub among bears in the testosterone-drenched world of the British Army. Red-haired and beardless, barely five feet tall, he spoke in a high-pitched voice described as "shrill" when it rose in anger, which seems to have happened quite often. To compensate for his diminutive stature he wore elevator shoes, padded his uniform shoulders—giving rise to the behind-the-back nickname of "Kapok Doctor," after the mattress stuffing—and carried an oversized cavalry sword wherever he went. Barry had a mania for privacy and traveled with a Jamaican manservant and a poodle named Psyche.

Barry was a well-known, if not well-loved, member of the army medical community. He was a zealous and cantankerous reformer in a military world wedded to the status quo, and his battles with superiors over the physical and mental welfare of soldiers, prisoners, lunatics, and lepers led to a cycle of promotion, demotion, house arrest, and transfer that took him to nearly every corner of the British Empire. He fought at least one pistol duel over a question of honor and threatened to slice the ears off a judge who tried to jail him for defaming a colleague. When he was transferred from Corfu to Crimea in 1853, Corfu's senior medical officer wrote ahead to his Crimean counterpart to warn him of Barry's imminent arrival: "I may as well warn you that you are to have a visit from the renowned Dr. Barry. . . . [He is] an intolerable bore. . . . He will expect you to listen to every quarrel he has had since coming into the service. You probably know that there are not a few."

It was in Crimea that Barry crossed paths with Florence Nightingale, the founding mother of modern nursing and a passionate reformer in her own right. They clashed openly and often. Barry sought her out for one particularly public dressing-down over a disputed report to the Crimean Sanitation Commission, which Nightingale recalled years later: "I never had such a [berating] in all my life—I who have had more than any woman—than from this Barry sitting on his horse, while I was crossing the Hospital Square with only my cap in the sun. He kept me standing in the midst of quite a crowd of soldiers, Commissariat, servants, camp followers, etc., etc., every one of whom behaved like a gentleman while he behaved like a brute."

But Barry's career was headed for a premature finish even as he roasted Florence Nightingale in the Crimean sun. He suffered from poor health throughout his career, and in 1857 was forced into retirement by chronic bronchitis. His last years were spent in London and Jamaica, desperately and unsuccessfully angling for reinstatement as an army surgeon. James Barry died of cholera in London on July 25, 1865—the thirty-ninth anniversary of his milestone cesarean delivery.

One month later an astonished *Manchester Guardian* reporter filed this story:

An incident is just now being discussed in military circles so extraordinary that were not the truth capable of being vouched for by the official authority, the narration would be deemed absolutely incredible. Our officers quartered at the Cape between 15 and 20 years ago may remember a certain Dr. Barry [who had] a reputation for considerable skill in his profession, especially for firmness, decision and rapidity in difficult operations. . . . He died about a month ago, and upon his death was discovered to be a woman. . . . [T]hus it stands as an indisputable fact, that a woman was for 40 years an officer in the British service, and fought one duel and sought many more, had pursued a legitimate medical education, and received a regular diploma, and had acquired almost a celebrity for skill as a surgical operator. It was a supreme deception.

The reporter ended on a bewildered note, neatly summing up the feelings of many Britons: "How could it happen?"

However she managed to pull off her forty-year masquerade, the fact remains: in the virtually all-male world of early-nineteenth-century Western medicine, the first man to perform a successful cesarean delivery was a woman.

The final word on Barry's life belongs to Florence Nightingale: "After he was dead I was told that he was a woman. . . . I should say that he was one of the most hardened creatures I have ever met."

If James Barry had been present in 1991 at my son John's birth, she would have recognized very little of what went on as the operating team prepared for surgery. Most surprising to her, after she'd grown accustomed to the bright lights, rows of gleaming instruments, and strange lack of urgency, might have been the near absence of men. Of the eight people present when John was born, six of them—the obstetrician, pediatrician, surgical assistant, scrub nurse, circulating nurse, and newborn nursery nurse—were women. If the anesthesiologist, the husband of an old college friend of Elisabeth's, hadn't traded cases with the woman scheduled to be at the delivery, I would have been the lone man in the room.

It might have taken Barry a while to figure out that these strangely dressed people were in fact women, and not just smallish men. She would have envied them their disguises: the gowns, gloves, hats, and masks that obscured everything but their eyes, so much lighter than the hot, heavy military garb she'd worn to her own operations. And what better way to hide one's sex from overly curious colleagues, she might have thought; was that the point of this strange clothing?

Dr. Andrea Bialek, the obstetrician who delivered John, is a woman of Barryesque proportions, though not partial to elevator shoes or shoulder pads. Just before starting the cesarean that morning, she stood with her gloved hands folded in front of her, calmly surveying Elisabeth's belly while the scrub nurse made a final equipment check. Though the trappings of cesarean birth had changed almost beyond recognition since the early nineteenth century, the challenge was still the same: there was a baby to be retrieved from its mother's womb, and the trick was to do it with as little trauma as possible to mother and child.

Dr. Bialek chose a scalpel from the instrument tray and started to work. She made a quick six-inch incision that followed a skin fold low on Elisabeth's abdomen. Beads of blood popped up in the scalpel's wake, oozing from the numerous small veins it severed, and . . .

Time for a small confession. I would like to say that I calmly watched the rest of the operation right alongside Dr. Bialek and her assistants, dispassionately taking notes for the book I would someday write about childbirth in all its variety. But no. This was my dear wife, after all, and my second child on the verge of being born. I hunkered down with Elisabeth behind the surgical drape through the whole thing, squeezing her hand and chattering away in my best *everything's-fine-in-the-cockpit* airline pilot's voice. I've seen enough cesareans, though, to be able to describe what usually happens on the other side of the drape.

A modern cesarean usually begins with a Pfannenstiel skin incision, a transverse cut across the lower abdomen that follows the "bikini line"—the skin crease just above the upper margin of a woman's pubic hair. The Pfannenstiel has grown in obstetric popularity over the years, gradually displacing the midline incision, which leaves a woman with a vertical belly-button-to-pubic-bone scar. The change was prompted partly by medical issues—the Pfannenstiel incision is generally less painful in recovery than the midline, and tends to heal with fewer complications—and partly by cosmetic concerns. In this day of fashionably bared midriffs, it's a lot easier to hide the scar.

Once the skin and the fatty tissue that lies beneath it have been incised and pulled aside with metal retractors, the obstetrician goes to work on the *fascia,* a layer of tough connective tissue that anchors muscles and adds protection to the abdomen. She cuts through the fascia with a pair of blunt-tipped bandage scissors, exposing the long *rectus abdominis* muscles—the "six-pack" abs of a woman's prepregnancy workout days, now barely recognizable thanks to the stretch placed on them by the bulging last trimester uterus. The obstetrician frees the rectus muscles from the surrounding tissue with her fingers or a blunt tool. Her assistant then spreads them widely apart with the retractors.

Beneath the rectus muscles lies the *peritoneum,* a thin double layer of tissue that wraps the abdominal cavity itself and separates its contents—the intestines, organs, bladder, and uterus—from the muscles and fascia that lie above. The obstetrician makes a quick incision through the peritoneum and there's the target: the uterus, gleaming and pink, filling the surgical opening. For safety's sake, the bladder, lying in front of the lower end of the uterus, is pulled down and away from the uterus with a tool called a bladder blade, though it's more of a curved metal spatula than anything sharp.

At this point in the surgery, things slow down. There's now less than an inch of uterine muscle separating scalpel and fetus. The obstetrician slices her way through the lower uterine wall with a series of cautious transverse cuts, each one drawing a little closer to whatever part of the fetus lies beneath. She breaks through the final layer of tissue with her fingers or a blunt probe, and there, visible through the now open uterus, is a first glimpse of baby: a head, a shoulder, perhaps a set of tiny fingers. The obstetrician then signals that she's about to deliver the baby with a curt "Everything out!"

Once "everything" is pulled out of the abdomen—the metal retractors, gauze sponges, towels, and any other tools used on the way in—she reaches her hand into the open uterus, feels for the baby's head, and pulls it toward the incision. Next comes what obstetrics textbooks euphemistically describe as "moderate fundal pressure," which is moderate only in comparison to a boa constrictor's embrace. While the obstetrician works on guiding the head through the uterine opening, the surgical assistant puts pressure on the upper part of the uterus by pressing her forearms down hard on the woman's lower chest and upper abdomen in what looks like an especially clumsy round of CPR.

It can take a surprising amount of physical effort to deliver a cesarean baby. This is because the uterine incision is purposely kept as small as possible, to allow for quicker healing and fewer complications. As a result, a vacuum apparatus is often attached to the fetus's scalp to gently guide the head and, though they're rarely used, a pair of Simpson forceps is kept on hand in case more leverage is needed.

The pulling from below and the pushing from above go on until the fetus's head finally pokes out from the uterus. Then the obstetrician pulls on the head until the shoulders emerge, one at a time, just as they do in a vaginal birth.

Once the shoulders clear the uterine incision, the rest of the body follows quickly. The baby cries, the cord is clamped and cut, and—in a moment captured in my snapshot of John—the obstetrician holds him high for his parents to see. Then she hands the newborn to the waiting pediatrician, who takes him to a nearby table for a quick checkup and a get-acquainted visit with his beaming dad. A short while later, when the baby is brought to his still-awake mother, the placenta has already been delivered through the incision. Now the obstetrician turns her attention to putting everything back together.

Repairing a first-time, or "primary," cesarean is a fairly straightforward process: the uterus is closed with a series of overlapping and interlocking dissolvable sutures, the peritoneum is left to heal on its own, the bladder and rectus muscles slide back into place, the fascia is stitched up, and finally the skin is closed with a row of staples. The whole operation takes less than an hour. Dr. Bialek made her first incision at ten-thirty. John was born seven minutes later, and Elisabeth was on her way to the recovery room shortly after eleven o'clock.

Elisabeth's surgery went smoothly, as it usually does in a scheduled primary cesarean. It was early in the day, the OR crew was well rested, and any unusual challenges—in Elisabeth's case, the abnormally located placenta—were well known. I've watched so many primary cesareans unfold that if the obstetrician ever keeled over in the middle of the operation, I could probably step in and do a halfway decent job of finishing things up.

But it's not always so straightforward. Maternal diseases such as hypertension, diabetes, and infection commonly complicate surgery. An obstetrician has to be prepared for rarer conditions, too, such as maternal cancers, old trauma, and bleeding problems. A mother's physical characteristics—obesity, uterine malformations, or the scars from a previous cesarean, for instance—and prematurity or the presence of multiple fetuses can make a cesarean a dauntingly complex operation.

Things are very different in an emergency, too, in which speed is critical. When pressed, an obstetrician can deliver a baby in a minute, which allows the pediatrician to get to work on a sick baby as quickly as possible. But such speed increases the risk of injury to a mother's abdominal organs and tissues, which can complicate the repair. Still, in my experience, the vast majority of cesarean births—both routine and emergency—end with a healthy mother and child.

An operation by a team of women would have been flabbergasting enough to James Barry, but a cesarean *planned ahead of time*? The idea of Elisabeth and I sitting down with Dr. Bialek a week beforehand and choosing our son's birthday—that would have been simply too much.

There was no such thing as a scheduled cesarean in 1826. The operation was still an act of desperation, as it had been since Zeus's time, and even the bravest of surgeons must have dreaded it. The odds that mother or child would survive the surgery were less than slim; mortality rates were nearly 100 percent. Unfortunately, Barry left no written record of her thoughts that historic morning. Did she have any inkling that either Mrs. Munnik or her baby would live—let alone both of them?

In every surgery she performed, Barry faced three monumental obstacles: pain, hemorrhage, and infection. Every laboring woman struggles with these same three obstacles, but in a vaginal birth the human body has devised some ingenious ways of dealing with them. A stew of hormones lessens the pain of childbirth, aided and abetted these days by everything from herbs to epidurals. The uterus controls its own bleeding as it contracts and shrinks after birth, compressing and sealing the uterine blood vessels in the process. And in a remarkable juggling act, a mother's immune system stays on guard throughout her pregnancy for normal vaginal bacteria that can infect damaged tissues of the uterus and birth canal, while simultaneously dumbing down other parts of its defenses so that the fetus—which is half dad, after all—isn't rejected like a mismatched blood transfusion or a transplanted kidney.

But nothing in human evolution could have prepared Mrs. Munnik's body for a cesarean birth. The pain of the surgery was much worse than that of a normal vaginal birth, the expected bleeding much greater, and infection all but unavoidable. By the time Barry decided that a cesarean was Mrs. Munnik's only hope, though, a normal vaginal birth had long since become an impossibility.

Pain was Barry's most immediate concern, because in the days before adequate pain control, it could turn the operation into a wrestling match between patient and surgical team. Barry's pain relief options that morning were starkly limited.

The invention of inhaled ether anesthesia was still two decades away. As a result, a surgeon's skill in 1826 was measured in large part by how fast he could amputate a limb, suture a laceration, or, in the case of obstetrical surgery, pull a baby from the womb. Battlefield anesthesia consisted of administering morphine or, as morphine was often in short supply, getting the patient stupendously drunk. A soldier with a shattered limb was given a whopping dose of cheap whiskey, then a phalanx of strong men held him down for the surgeon and—zip—off came the leg. The challenge was to finish the operation before the patient slipped into shock, or roared back to life and socked the surgeon in the jaw for his efforts.

Things weren't any better when performing a cesarean. On the battlefield, alcohol was used mainly to make a patient easier to pin down than for any real anesthetic properties, and since it often caused vomiting, it was out of the question for abdominal surgery like a cesarean. A surgeon considering a cesarean shied away from morphine, too, rightly fearing that it would prevent the uterus from contracting and thus worsen internal bleeding. With no other viable alternative, Mrs. Munnik's cesarean was probably done without any anesthesia at all.

The need to work quickly also meant a surgeon had little time to make certain the many arteries and veins sliced through en route to the uterus, known as "bleeders," had all stopped oozing blood by the time he closed the abdominal incision. Which brings us to the second obstacle Barry faced: hemorrhage.

Blood loss plagued cesarean birth until the early twentieth century. The expected bleeding from the skin incision could be stopped with clamps, sutures, and direct pressure, but the uterus itself presented a special problem. The uterine contractions that help stem postpartum bleeding in a normal vaginal birth are no match for the damage caused by a surgical incision. While a modern obstetrician solves this problem by simply closing the uterus with a type of suture that is gradually absorbed by the healing tissue, Barry didn't have that option. The sutures available to her weren't absorbable; their permanent presence in the uterine wall would only have worsened internal bleeding after the surgery was over.

Barry's only real option to control uterine bleeding would have been to apply direct pressure to the open uterus for as long as she could. If that failed, as it often did, massive bleeding would follow, and without access to modern tools such as intravenous fluids and blood transfusions, Mrs. Munnik would have died from hemorrhagic shock. Barry most likely followed standard surgical practice and left the uterine incision open, hoping that it would eventually heal on its own.

Whatever Barry did, it obviously worked. Mrs. Munnik lived through the surgery, though whether from Barry's skill, sheer luck, or a combination of the two it is impossible to say. Though we know she ultimately recovered, her condition would have been touch-and-go for some time, because infection—the third of Barry's obstacles—complicated virtually every cesarean, no matter how successfully bleeding was managed.

Cesarean deliveries are far more infection-prone than vaginal births, a fact as true today as it was in 1826. The tissues damaged by Barry's quick incisions—skin, fat, fascia, and the uterus itself—were, and are, perfect breeding grounds for bacteria. Even today, with the benefit of sterile instruments and modern antibiotics, about one in twenty postcesarean women contracts an infection. Death or serious harm is rare now, but in Barry's time, when surgical hygiene was primitive at best, life-threatening infection was an almost insurmountable challenge, and it would remain so for another half century. Mrs. Munnik was a very fortunate woman.*

The quest to end postcesarean infection began with the struggle to conquer *puerperal fever,* the dreaded complication that once followed many otherwise normal deliveries. Puerperal fever, now known as *postpartum endometritis,* is an infection of the *endometrium,* or inner surface of the uterus. It occurs when normal vaginal bacteria invade the tissues of the uterus and birth canal injured during childbirth; from there the infection can spread through the bloodstream to other parts of the body, a process known as *septicemia.* In the preantibiotic era the disease was often fatal; as late as the 1930s nearly one-fourth of all American and European women who contracted puerperal fever died of the disease.

Puerperal fever was no respecter of wealth or class: among its

*Mrs. Munnik was so grateful to Barry that she named her child James Barry Munnik. He in turn became the godfather of James Barry Munnik Hertzog, prime minister of South Africa from 1924 to 1939. The name lives on: a cricket player named James Barry Munnik lives in South Africa today.

many high- and low-born victims were the early feminist Mary Wollstonecraft, who died in 1797 after giving birth to Mary Shelley, the author of *Frankenstein;* Gabrielle-Émilie Le Tonnelier de Breteuil, Marquise du Châtelet, who, given a proper education by her father only because he thought she was too tall to marry, became Voltaire's lover and Isaac Newton's translator; and Isabella Mary Beeton, the wildly popular nineteenth-century British cook and writer who has been described as "the original Martha Stewart."

Most famously, puerperal fever killed two of Henry VIII's six wives. Jane Seymour, Henry's third wife, died on October 24, 1537, twelve agonizing days after giving birth to Henry's eagerly awaited heir, Edward VI. Catherine Parr, his sixth and final spouse, had the good fortune to outlive Henry, only to perish from puerperal fever after marrying Thomas Seymour—ironically, Jane Seymour's brother.

Whether afflicting rich or poor women, puerperal fever was a relatively uncommon and largely isolated tragedy before the Industrial Revolution. The human immune system had long ago evolved fairly effective ways of checking the spread of vaginal bacteria, and with most babies being born on farms or in private homes, childbirth was a relatively hygienic event. It took the establishment of "lying-in" maternity hospitals in the seventeenth century to set the stage for puerperal fever epidemics, which at their deadliest killed as many as six out of every ten hospitalized mothers.

Ironically, lying-in hospitals were founded with the best of intentions. As peasants from the countryside flooded into large European cities in search of factory work, municipal officials were shocked by the high death rates of poor women who gave birth in tenements and workhouses. In response, lying-in hospitals were built in London, Dublin, and other large cities so that "wives of poor industrious Tradesmen or distressed House-keepers" could be attended through their labors by trained midwives.

Despite their humane beginnings, lying-in hospitals were soon overwhelmed by waves of new arrivals. The appalling conditions that resulted are difficult to imagine in this day of private, well-furnished birthing suites. Wards were huge and barnlike: drafty, filthy, poorly staffed, and grossly overcrowded. Two or three women often labored in a single bed on unwashed sheets. Doctors and nurses grouped sicker patients together and performed vaginal examinations on woman after woman without washing their hands. Epidemics of puerperal fever raged. Their source—the lack of even basic hygiene—seems obvious today, but doctors remained baffled for nearly two centuries.

By the middle of the nineteenth century, scientists suspected a connection between microorganisms and infection. Prominent among them was Louis Pasteur, the famed microbiologist who proved over the course of his long career that bacteria and viruses were the culprits in everything from wine spoilage to potato blight, rabies to anthrax.

Physicians, on the other hand, were still heavily invested in the "miasmic" theory of disease, the belief that illness was spread directly by foul air from swamps, cesspools, and garbage. Despite growing evidence in support of germ theory, doctors remained unaware, or stubbornly in denial, of their own role in the spread of puerperal fever.

In the late 1830s, Dr. Oliver Wendell Holmes made that connection—if only his colleagues had listened. A Harvard medical professor (and father of future Supreme Court justice Oliver Wendell Holmes, Jr.), Holmes's investigation of a case in which a doctor died of infection after performing an autopsy on a puerperal fever victim led him to conclude that physicians themselves were spreading the disease from woman to woman. In his classic essay, "The Contagiousness of Puerperal Fever," Holmes arrived at an unsettling conclusion. "There is . . . no voice loud enough for warning," he wrote. *"The disease known as Puerperal Fever is so far contagious as to be frequently carried from patient to patient by physicians and nurses."* The italics are his.

After making his case, Holmes spelled out eight rules of puerperal fever prevention for obstetricians. Frequent hand washing and changes of clothing were critical, as was not performing autopsies while also caring for live, laboring patients. To break the spread of the disease once it had started, he recommended that physicians associated with more than one case of puerperal fever in a short period of time refrain from delivering babies for up to a month.

Amazingly, his well-researched findings and recommendations were ridiculed by his peers. Their reaction is best summed up by Charles Delucina Meigs, the influential chair of obstetrics at Philadelphia's Jefferson College of Medicine. "Doctors are gentlemen," Meigs proclaimed, "and gentlemen's hands are clean."

No major medical journal would publish Holmes's beyond-the-pale theorizing. "The Contagiousness of Puerperal Fever" finally appeared in 1843 in *The New England Quarterly of Medicine,* a little-known publication that went bankrupt a few months later. Holmes's paper didn't reach a wider medical audience until 1855, when it was reprinted in the journal *Medical Essays.*

In 1844, Dr. Ignaz Semmelweis, an assistant lecturer in the First Obstetric Division of the Vienna Lying-in Hospital, began to make the same connection. Semmelweis noticed that women who gave birth in his First Division, which was staffed by doctors and medical students, had eight times the risk of contracting puerperal fever than those who were delivered by midwives in a distant part of the hospital. Of the many differences in patient care between the two divisions, Semmelweis saw one that stood out. Doctors did autopsies on women who had died of puerperal fever. Midwives did not.

With no access to Holmes's still obscure paper, it took three years and a number of failed hypotheses for Semmelweis to put it all together. The final piece of the puzzle fell into place when, like Holmes, he was struck by the similarities between puerperal fever and the death of a colleague from an infection incurred during an autopsy. "Suddenly a thought crossed my mind," he wrote. "The fingers and hands of students and doctors, soiled by recent dissections, carry those death-dealing cadavers' poisons into the genital organs of women in childbirth."

Semmelweis immediately ordered all doctors and students in the First Division to wash their hands in a chlorinated lime solution before attending to patients. The results were startling: mortality rates from puerperal fever fell from 18 percent in the first half of 1847 to less than 3 percent by that November. But like Holmes's in America, Semmelweis's breakthrough was dismissed by his colleagues, including Friedrich Scanzoni, the most prominent obstetrician in Vienna.

Semmelweis's discovery ultimately led to the ruin of his own career and health. He was dismissed from the Vienna Lying-in Hospital in 1849, in large part because of his increasingly strident arguments with colleagues. Despondent, he spent a few unproductive years at a hospital in his native Hungary before returning to Vienna. There he wrote articles and letters blasting his former colleagues. He even accused them of murder, calling them, among other things, "medical Neros" for ignoring his advice while women died. Disabled by severe depression, Semmelweis died in a mental hospital in 1865—ironically, from an infection that started in a cut on his finger.

Another decade passed before the work of Semmelweis and Holmes began to gain acceptance. It entered the surgical community when the concept of *antisepsis*—the reduction of operative wound infection risks—was introduced by Dr. Joseph Lister of Glasgow in the 1860s.* Lister, a general surgeon on the marvelously named Male Accident Ward at the Royal Glasgow Infirmary, discovered that treating amputation wounds with carbolic acid led to a sharp decrease in deaths from gangrene. Hedging his bets in a medical world still wedded to miasmic theory, Lister had carbolic acid sprayed in the air in his operating room during surgery, too—which must have made for some interesting surgical scenarios, given carbolic acid's tendency to cause distorted perception and hallucinations.

---

* Joseph Lister was the namesake, though not the inventor, of Listerine, which started its commercial life as a surgical antiseptic. When the nation became obsessed with oral health in the late nineteenth century, the inventors—two of Lister's students—tweaked the formula to a more mouth-friendly solution, and the world's first mouthwash was born.

Like Holmes and Semmelweis before him, Lister found his work was met with indifference and hostility. It wasn't until the Franco-Prussian War of 1870, when German surgeons adopted Lister's antiseptic methods and demonstrated their clear benefit in combat, that other surgeons began to adopt the practice. That same year, carbolic acid was introduced into obstetrics by the Swiss obstetrician Johann Bischoff. Within weeks Bischoff saw a steep decline in deaths from puerperal fever in his practice.

By the close of the nineteenth century, Lister's antiseptic techniques had been replaced by *asepsis*—the removal of bacteria from the operating field by means of preoperative cleansing, hand washing, face masks, and the introduction of rubber gloves. Though postcesarean infection remained a significant threat in Europe and America until the introduction of antibiotics in the 1930s, deaths became increasingly rare. The disease had been tamed, if not completely conquered. Cesarean birth moved into its modern phase.

My son John was one of more than nine hundred thousand American babies born by cesarean delivery in 1991. That figure astounded me the first time I saw it—only 165 years after James Barry's harrowing success, cesarean birth had become so commonplace it could even be planned ahead of time, almost like family vacation.

Cesarean deliveries accounted for 22 percent of all American births in 1991, a proportion thought to be a high-water mark at the time. The cesarean rate had hovered at that level since the mid-1980s, and with the trend toward *vaginal birth after cesarean* (VBAC) gaining steam, most physicians figured that rates would gradually drift down to the 10 to 15 percent of all births endorsed by the World Health Organization. That didn't happen. After a modest decline in the 1990s, the 2000s have seen dramatic increases in cesarean deliveries. In 2003, 26.1 percent of all births were cesareans; by 2006, 31.1 percent of all American babies—more than 1.2 million of them—were born in operating rooms. It's a trend that shows no sign of letting up.

If that sounds like an awful lot of surgery, it is. Cesareans are now the most common hospital-based operation performed in the United States. And if it sounds as though it happened awfully fast, it did. In 1971, the year I graduated from high school, only 6 percent of American births were cesareans.

We're far from alone. Cesarean rates in such far-flung places as Turkey, England, and Hong Kong have skyrocketed since the 1980s. South Korea's rates quadrupled between 1984 and 1994; New Zealand's doubled in the same period. With the notable exception of parts of the developing world—particularly sub-Saharan Africa, where obstetricians and operating rooms are in short supply and an increase in cesareans would be a *good* thing—the trend is nearly universal. More women are undergoing cesarean deliveries every year. What in the world is going on?

Cesarean birth's twentieth-century rise to prominence started slowly. Anesthesia and asepsis had made things much safer by the late 1800s, but it was still a dangerous surgery, and one that was performed infrequently. Well into the 1920s, cesareans accounted for fewer than one in a hundred live births.

Medical progress led to two cesarean "boomlets" in the first half of the century. In the 1910s, *hysterectomy*—the removal of the uterus itself—was still often the only way to stop out-of-control bleeding during surgery. That changed dramatically in the 1920s, when improved surgical techniques and newly introduced blood transfusions greatly reduced deaths from severe hemorrhage. Operative births soon rose. The Chicago Lying-in Hospital, for example, saw a fivefold increase—from 0.6 percent to 3 percent of all births—between 1910 and 1928.

The second jump followed the introduction of antibiotics into obstetric care in 1937. As maternal death and disability from infection plummeted, cesarean birth became less risky. Doctors opted for surgery earlier in labor, before a mother was already in serious trouble from exhaustion, bleeding, or uncontrolled infection. Even so, American cesarean rates remained modest, not reaching the 5 percent mark nationwide until the late 1960s.

Cesarean's first "golden age," if you will, began in earnest in the mid-1970s, just as I was starting medical school. The reasons are many and complex, and the usual suspects—doctors, lawyers, politicians, and insurance companies—all have their thumbs in this particular pie. But other, unexpected players appeared at the table as well, from the changing demographics of American motherhood to the sometimes unrealistic expectations of an increasingly lawsuit-happy society.

There will always be problem pregnancies, abnormal labors, and deliveries that suddenly go wrong. A cesarean can be a lifesaving tool, but when to use that tool isn't always clear. At one end of the obstetrics spectrum is Elisabeth's placenta previa, a condition for which a cesarean delivery is an absolute necessity. At the other end lie the majority of pregnancies, for which a vaginal birth is the safest and best. It's that very large middle ground of women with not quite straightforward pregnancies—women with a previous cesarean, diabetes, high blood pressure, or any number of pregnancy-related complications—who keep obstetricians up at night, constantly weighing the pros and cons of surgical intervention.

Ninety percent of the meteoric rise in cesarean birth rates in the 1970s and '80s boiled down to three related factors. An increase in the diagnosis of *dystocia,* a catchall term for a labor that refuses to progress normally, and *fetal distress,* both of which became much easier to detect with the introduction of continuous electronic fetal heart monitoring, led to a rise in primary cesareans. Within a few years, with common medical wisdom declaring that vaginal birth after a cesarean was unsafe, the increase in primary operations inevitably led to an explosion of *repeat cesareans.*

My early career spanned that first boom. The cesareans I attended during my residency and first few years in practice tended to fall into two broad categories: elective cesareans and true emergencies. The elective, scheduled cesareans were often women with medical conditions of their own that made labor and a vaginal birth unsafe. I remember a mother with severe congenital heart disease, another who had badly fractured her hip falling down a flight of stairs just days before her due date, and a newly immigrated Salvadoran woman with a pelvis shrunken and deformed by the one-two punch of rickets and polio. These were women, I knew, who would likely have died in childbirth just a few decades earlier.

The true emergencies came out of the blue, fetuses abruptly in peril for unexpected reasons: a previously healthy woman suddenly comatose from a blood clot in her lung; another with uncontrollable seizures; still another severely beaten by her husband. These cesareans were the stuff of TV medical shows—a mad dash of doctors and nurses, a blur of gowns and masks and scalpels, and suddenly there I stood with a very sick baby in my hands, more or less tossed to me by an obstetrician in the heat of surgery.

Then, as fetal monitoring became standard practice, cesarean birth became a form of preventive medicine. More of the cesareans I attended were uneventful from my perspective, performed at a semileisurely pace. This was a good thing, I remember thinking; we all felt that way. Imagine the lives saved, the babies born undamaged thanks to a monitor that could detect a fetus in distress early on, before real trouble set in.

On the plus side, that beeping monitor at the bedside allowed labor and delivery staff to monitor the fetus's condition on a minute-by-minute basis and to reassure everyone that all was well. But such intense in utero scrutiny also caused a lot of nervousness when a fetus showed even minor difficulties, leading to cesarean deliveries of babies who might well have been born vaginally if they'd been given the chance to straighten things out on their own as in premonitoring times.

The increased detection of dystocia and fetal distress came at the same time that obstetricians were moving away from *operative vaginal deliveries*—the use of forceps, for example. By the 1980s operative vaginal deliveries, with the exception of vacuum-assisted vaginal births, had largely been replaced by ever safer cesarean deliveries.

Societal changes contributed to cesarean birth's sudden 1970s rise, too. Family size shrank as the 1950s gave way to the '60s.

Women put off having babies much longer than their mothers had; as a result, the average age of new motherhood jumped dramatically. In 1970, only 6 percent of first-time mothers were more than thirty years old; by 1990, the proportion had risen to 25 percent. As infertility treatments improved, the concept of "too old to have a baby" changed, too. More than twice as many women over forty gave birth in 1990 than in 1970. These older mothers are more prone to complications of pregnancy than their younger counterparts, and so are at higher risk for a cesarean.

The middle of the twentieth century also saw the fetus become a patient in its own right. Long gone were the days when the average woman gave birth to eight or ten children in her reproductive lifetime, hoping that at least a few of them would live beyond infancy. The rarity of modern maternal or infant death led to the expectation that every pregnancy would produce a healthy child. It also led to closer watching of fetal monitors in the delivery room, and to more cesareans when things in the womb got even a little bit dicey.

Put them all together—the increase in dystocia, fetal distress monitoring, and repeat cesareans, advancing maternal age, and the expectation of a perfect outcome—and it's not surprising that cesarean rates skyrocketed from 10.4 percent of all American births in 1975 to 22.7 percent in 1985. And there they stayed until the turn of the twenty-first century.

We are now several years into cesarean birth's second "golden age." Three hundred and thirty thousand more American babies were cesarean-born in 2005 than in 2000. This big jump was not a given. Between 1990 and 1999 the number of cesareans actually decreased by 5 percent; in the following six years, however, cesareans have increased by nearly 50 percent. The modest decrease in the 1990s and the explosion of cesareans in the 2000s can nearly all be attributed to the rise and sudden fall of the VBAC, or vaginal birth after cesarean.

Almost as soon as women began surviving cesareans, the question arose among obstetricians: How should subsequent pregnancies be managed? Should a woman be allowed to attempt a vaginal birth the second time around, or was it safer to do a repeat cesarean?

A century ago, both options were fraught with danger. The crude surgical techniques of the time put a mother at risk for uterine rupture—a frightening, life-threatening event in which the force of labor contractions splits the uterus open along the old suture line, triggering massive hemorrhage and a fetus who is essentially "born" through the rupture into the abdominal cavity—if she tried a vaginal birth. As ominous as the prospect of uterine rupture was to an early-twentieth-century obstetrician, the idea of performing a repeat cesarean was nearly as frightening. Scar tissue and poor healing from the first operation made a second cesarean treacherous.

Weighing the research of the time, the influential obstetrician Dr. Edwin Cragin came down firmly on the side of repeat cesareans in 1916, declaring in an address to the Eastern Medical Society of the City of New York that a woman who had undergone a cesarean should never again attempt a vaginal birth. His dictum "Once a cesarean, always a cesarean" still echoed in the nation's labor and delivery units when I was in medical school six decades later.

By the 1980s, though, things had started to change. Many physicians, midwives, and nurses began to question the "once a cesarean" rule, citing improved techniques that allowed the uterus to heal seemingly as good as new after surgery. Uterine rupture during an attempted VBAC, that most dreaded complication of Cragin's time, had become a rarity. When studies appeared in the 1980s and early '90s documenting a 60 to 80 percent VBAC success rate, with uterine rupture occurring in fewer than 1 percent of cases, VBAC seemed like the best available tool for reducing cesarean rates. And for a while, it worked. The peak came in 1996, with over 116,000 successful VBACs; not coincidentally, the cesarean rate in 1996 (20.7 percent) is still the lowest in the last twenty years.

But then the bubble burst. As the mid-'90s dawned, studies found that complications such as uterine rupture and the subsequent need for hysterectomy were twice as common in women with previous cesareans who were allowed to labor than for women who had an elective, scheduled repeat cesarean. Though the absolute numbers were low—less than 1 percent of all attempted VBACs—in 1998 the American College of Obstetricians and Gynecologists (ACOG) recommended attempting a VBAC only in a hospital equipped to do an immediate cesarean. Since the vast majority of hospitals do not have the 24-hour obstetric anesthesia coverage this would require, many obstetricians and their patients began to shy away from VBACs. By 2004, only 45,000 American women had a successful vaginal birth after a previous cesarean, and the number of VBACs continues to fall.

And then, as if the fall in VBACs wasn't enough to ensure a steadily rising cesarean rate, along came Britney Spears. In the fall of 2005, the ex-Mouseketeer turned tabloid star became a kind of poster girl for the small but growing number of women who choose to avoid labor altogether, opting instead for an *elective primary cesarean* (EPC)—in other words, a cesarean without medical need for one.

Spears's rationale for choosing a cesarean was straightforward. In an interview just before she gave birth, she said, "I don't want to go through the pain [of a vaginal birth]." Her fear of labor pain was typical. It's the number one reason women seek EPC, followed in order by fear of an emergency situation, fear of fetal distress, fear of future urinary incontinence or sexual dysfunction, and, lastly, convenience.

As with just about every innovation related to giving birth, EPC has set off a firestorm of controversy. The debate was bound to happen sooner or later, given the steady improvement in cesarean outcomes over the course of the twentieth century. As early as 2000, ACOG's president stated that given the increasing safety and apparent benefits to both mother and child of elective cesarean birth, "the time is coming—if not already here—for 'maternal-choice cesarean.'" That time seems to have arrived. In a 2003 *Obstetrics & Gynecology* editorial, Dr. Ingrid Nygaard wrote that "elective cesarean delivery in healthy women who plan small families is now safe enough to warrant individual consideration of such patient requests." In other words: Britney Spears, come on down.

Natural childbirth and consumer advocates have been quick to counterattack. They accuse obstetricians of "spin doctoring" the research and not fully informing pregnant women of the risks to themselves and their babies of elective surgery versus vaginal birth. (Did Britney Spears's obstetricians make it clear that cesareans hurt quite a bit, too? Did they tell her that third cesareans—she's since had a second—are much riskier than a first, should she want more children?) They also point out the obvious conflict of interest inherent in the nation's leading obstetricians lending support to EPC: cesareans can be substantially more lucrative for physicians than vaginal births.

Yet obstetricians themselves are divided. A recent review of EPC coauthored by the Center for Medical Ethics and Health Policy at Baylor College of Medicine came down strongly against obstetricians encouraging EPC, though the authors added a qualifier: if a healthy woman persists in her request for an EPC, that request should be honored, so long as she truly understands the risks and benefits. On the other side of the fence, the International Federation of Gynecology and Obstetrics (FIGO) concluded unequivocally that "at present . . . performing cesarean section for non-medical reasons is not justified."

FIGO's "at present" looms large, because the EPC debate is far from settled. Some of EPC's touted benefits for women—less urinary incontinence later in life, for example—are already being called into question. The pros and cons will continue to evolve as more research is done, and time will play a role, too. For all we know, the pendulum of public opinion may swing away from EPC. The generation of girls being born today may well find the idea of a voluntary cesarean ludicrous.

Notice that the debate in obstetrics circles tends to revolve, understandably, around maternal issues—the ethics of maternal choice, the safety of the surgery, the reduction in urinary incontinence in older women, and so on. The fetus and baby don't get quite as much attention, and both the pros of EPC for the baby (fewer birth injuries, for example) and its cons (more respiratory difficulties, or unexpected prematurity due to wrongly calculated due dates) tend to be focused on short-term outcomes.

An elective primary cesarean seems pretty safe, babywise, at least as long as the baby is still a baby. But little is known of the long-term effects of cesarean by choice. How will EPC affect bonding between mother and baby, or a mother's willingness or ability to breast-feed? Will there be lasting effects on the mother-child relationship? And what of physical complications? Could that normal-looking six-month-old have EPC-related health problems pop up when he's six years old, or sixteen?

"Nature does nothing in vain," Isaac Newton wrote in 1752. The great British scientist was writing about physics, but his words could apply equally to childbirth. In nine short months a pregnant woman builds a new human being from scratch, sending an endless stream of nutrients, enzymes, and hormones across the placenta. Each of those chemicals has a purpose, from building brain and bone to creating an immune system equipped to protect the body from an incredible variety of stresses, including birth itself.

The birth process is the greatest stress any healthy fetus faces. During labor the uterus contracts with such force that its blood vessels collapse, temporarily reducing oxygen flow to the fetus and putting it through the equivalent of a series of very long breath-holding spells. *Oxygen free radicals* form during these periods of low oxygen, and unless these cell-destroying chemicals are quickly neutralized by the body's defenses, severe damage to fetal tissues, known as *oxidative stress,* can occur.

But nature plans for this. A healthy laboring mother floods her vaginally born fetus with *glutathione,* an antioxidant chemical that counteracts oxidative stress. A baby born by a relatively stress-free elective cesarean receives a much smaller dose of glutathione. At this point it isn't known if the difference in antioxidant delivery between vaginal and elective cesarean birth has any lasting effects, but since oxidative stress causes tissue damage throughout life—it plays a role in atherosclerosis and Alzheimer's disease, among other disorders—perhaps the cascade of chemicals that comes with the onset of labor is important to the fine-tuning of a child's biochemical makeup.

Recent research suggests cesarean-born children, particularly those delivered electively, are at somewhat higher risk for developing asthma—an immune system disorder—than those born vaginally. As of this writing it's not clear how a cesarean birth could trigger asthma years down the road, but it may have to do with labor's "priming" effect on the newborn's immune system, or the well-documented differences in the types of bacteria that colonize in the bowels of children born by elective cesareans versus those who traverse the birth canal, differences that may alter a child's immune response to allergens later in life.

It's too early to tell how strong the cesarean-asthma link is, but if it is significant we may also find that an elective cesarean birth puts a child at risk of other immune system–related disorders—rheumatoid arthritis, for example, or diabetes. And though I know it's hardly scientific to draw conclusions from individual cases, my own family's experience leaves me wondering. My son John, born by a medically necessary elective cesarean, suffered from asthma throughout his early childhood. My vaginally born daughter Claire has never wheezed a day in her life.

I'm speculating, of course, but that's really the basis of my concern—we just don't know what we're getting our children into. Whether EPC puts children at risk of subtle or not so subtle health problems is something only careful studies over long periods of time will tell. But studying apparently healthy children for subtle problems related to elective cesarean birth is difficult and expensive, and still very low on the research totem pole. As of 2007 there have been very few long-term studies of children born by cesareans performed for medical reasons, and none at all on children born by EPC.

Meanwhile, an American woman who is determined to have an EPC will probably find a doctor who will do it, if for no other reason than this: a patient is much less likely to sue her doctor when things go wrong if she gets what she wanted in the first place.

Time to put the lawsuit issue, an understandably touchy one for all involved, squarely on the table. Lurking in the background of any discussion of American cesarean delivery rates is the very real fear an obstetrician carries into every delivery: *if anything goes wrong, I'm going to be sued.* This isn't simple paranoia; an average obstetrician will face a major lawsuit two or three times in his or her career.

Even though the large majority of childbirth-related malpractice cases are decided in favor of the obstetrician, it's an expensive process. As a result, obstetricians pay some of the highest malpractice insurance premiums of any medical specialty. Even a single lost case can devastate a career: in 2002 an Oregon physician saw her annual malpractice premiums jump from $28,000 to $255,000 after she lost a multi-million-dollar court settlement.

Rising malpractice premiums and the likelihood of being sued, deservedly or not, are responsible for another disturbing trend: obstetricians are leaving the delivery room. In 2002, one in five Pennsylvania obstetricians reported having given up delivering babies as a direct result of malpractice-related issues. In 2004, one doctor in seven responding to a nationwide ACOG survey reported having done the same.

Unfortunately, it isn't just the unsafe operators who are quitting; many of the Pennsylvania obstetricians had never been sued. Some rural areas of the country are losing their obstetricians altogether, leading to longer drives and more complications for laboring mothers, and—you guessed it—more cesarean deliveries when they finally do get to a hospital.

The problem of the "disappearing obstetrician" is likely to get worse. American medical students are turning away from careers in obstetrics and gynecology. In 2004, only 65 percent of OB-GYN residency slots were filled by graduates of American medical schools, compared with 86 percent just ten years earlier. Though other factors are likely associated with the decrease—the lure of more money and less night call in specialties like cosmetic plastic surgery, for example—malpractice woes no doubt play a significant part.

Everyone from the U.S. Department of Health and Human Services to the World Health Organization agrees that cesarean rates are too high, though to what extent the problem is actually fixable is a matter of much debate. There is simply no way to put the cesarean genie all the way back into the bottle. As Dr. Richard Depp writes in a recent edition of the textbook Gabbe's *Obstetrics,* "We have entered a cycle that will make major [cesarean] rate reduction difficult."

Part of that cycle is related to how new obstetricians are trained, and to the increase in challenging labors they will confront. Some conditions once routinely delivered vaginally—breech babies, for example—will continue to be an indication for surgical delivery in the future, because a cesarean delivery is generally a safer option, and because newer obstetricians have much less opportunity in their training programs to resolve difficult labors vaginally than their predecessors did. Facing an aging population of pregnant women, many with chronic illnesses, they're more likely to recommend a cesarean when confronted with trouble.

The three main factors in the cesarean cycle—dystocia, fetal distress, and repeat cesareans—are amenable to reduction, at least in theory. Reducing cesareans from dystocia and fetal distress will require changes in the way both normal and problematic labors are managed, more accurate ways to determine when a fetus is truly in distress, and, perhaps most important, a less litigious medical environment, if such a thing is possible anymore.

The "cycle" that Dr. Depp was referring to when I quoted him above is really a series of positive and negative trends that often cancel one another out. All roads seem increasingly to lead to the operating room. Obstetricians who want to reduce cesarean rates are, as an obstetrical colleague once put it, stuck between a rock, a hard place, and a lawyer.

If so, American obstetrics can be described as a victim of its own success. The relative safety of cesarean birth has raised the expectations of the childbearing public so high, and the consequences for failing to meet those expectations are so dire, that there is now no easy way to back away from its use. Here in the early years of the twenty-first century we have reached a point of high medical irony that would not be lost on James Barry: it now can take more courage—or foolhardiness—*not* to do a cesarean than it takes to do one.

One of my first calls on the morning of John's birth was to Sister Carola, a ninety-two-year-old Franciscan nun who lived at St. Mary's Hospital in St. Louis. The retired chief of hospital nutrition, Sister Carola had been a mentor to my aunt, who joined the convent just before I was born. The two of us had become lifelong friends, starting when I was a very young boy.

Whenever we visited my aunt at the convent I'd find my way across the park that separated her quarters from the hospital and spend part of the day hanging around in Sister Carola's office, admiring her collections of glass paperweights and stuffed birds. My favorite was an angry-looking pheasant, frozen in full sprint with its beady green-glass eyeballs on the lookout, forever too late, for hunters.

When Sister was done with her paperwork we'd make the rounds of the hospital kitchens, and inevitably some apricot juice and the odd brownie would turn up in need of eating. I remember mostly her face and hands, which were all I could see of her in her black-and-white habit, and her voice, a gentle, rumbling river that rose with her frequent laughter. She was kind and funny and I loved her very much.

Many years later, when Elisabeth and I had trouble conceiving during the first years of our marriage, Sister Carola began to pray for us. She prayed for Elisabeth to get pregnant and for us to have a healthy baby, and we did—Claire, eighteen months old on the day of John's birth, was back home watching a *Nutcracker* video for the umpteenth time with her very patient grandma Peg. After

Claire's birth, Sister kept on praying for another healthy baby, and that, she was sure, gave us John.

Once John was cleaned up and tucked into a warm bed in the nursery, I dialed the convent in St. Louis. It took a few minutes to track Sister Carola down; she had been helping the "older sisters," most of them much younger than she, with crafts projects. When at last Sister came on the line I told her we had a boy, and that John and Elisabeth were fine.

"Oh, thank God!" she said, her voice breaking. She paused a moment, then told me she'd stepped up her prayers on learning that Elisabeth would have to have a cesarean. "I worried so much about that operation," she said with a long sigh. I thanked her, joking that she could ease up on the praying for a while, since the first baby she'd gotten us still wasn't sleeping through the night. We said our good-byes, and she was off to brag to the other sisters about her success in interceding with the Almighty on our behalf.

It wasn't until I began researching this book eight years after her death that I fully understood Sister Carola's need to pray harder when she learned about "that operation." Sister was born in rural Illinois in 1899, a place and time where a cesarean delivery was still an act of sheer desperation. She entered the convent at the age of fifteen and became a registered nurse in 1918. In the preantibiotic 1910s and '20s, when most of Sister's contemporaries were having their babies, mortality from cesarean deliveries was still relatively high. Sister undoubtedly encountered women and babies who didn't survive the surgery, or who were permanently damaged by it. It was likely those memories that made her worry so much about Elisabeth, even though in the span of her very long life, cesarean delivery had been transformed from a life-threatening drama to a nearly routine alternative to vaginal birth.

I left the hospital a couple of days later with a healthy son and a wife well on the road to recovery. It wasn't until much later that I realized how blessed and truly lucky I had been, given cesarean birth's history, to come home with anyone at all.

PART II
Pain and Politics

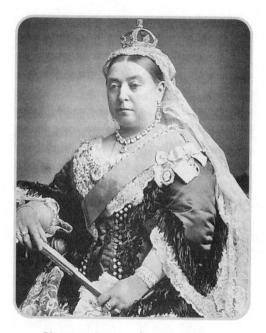

Victoria: Queen of Great Britain,
Defender of the Faith, Obstetric Trailblazer

Chapter 4
B.E. (Before Epidurals)

Take up the battle for painless childbirth[!] Fight not only for yourselves, but fight for your...sex!"
—HANNA RION, feminist and journalist, 1915

Childbirth is ecstasy.
—ALLEN COHEN, poet, midwife, and natural childbirth advocate, 1970

"Give me drugs!"
—NINA SHAPIRO, Slate, 1999

If an alien followed me around on one of my call nights, he might well conclude that the human female sprouts a long, thin plastic tube from her spine just before giving birth. He would reach this conclusion because nearly every woman we popped in on that night would have an epidural catheter in place, one end taped to the skin over her lower back, the other plugged into a pump on a pole at the head of her bed.

There's nothing unusual about my hospital, if you ignore the alien. Most American women—nearly 90 percent in some areas—have their labor pains eased by epidural anesthesia. Epidurals are so ubiquitous in labor rooms today that it's hard for many women to imagine not having one, let alone imagine a time when they weren't available at all.

Yet until very recently the idea of a woman choosing to lessen the pain that comes from forcing a too-big fetus through a too-small opening—and staying conscious through the whole thing—would have astounded the world. Most of that astonishment would have been focused on the fact of a nearly painless birth, of course. But many women, particularly those who gave birth in the middle of the twentieth century, would have been pleasantly shocked at the idea of a woman choosing anything at all about the circumstances of her child's birth.

The search for truly painless childbirth is as long as human history, and nearly as complicated. That search is populated by a wealth of characters, famous and not. Toss together war and peace, suffragettes, "natural" childbirth, self-administered anesthesia, intrepid female reporters, God, hippies, the "science" of eugenics, and, of course, doctors—the evil, the clueless, and some who were pretty darn good—and you've got a story of good intentions and unintended consequences, of pain and, yes, politics. Because overlying a century and a half of scientific advance is a question of control: Who should call the shots in the birthing room?

Childbirth is perhaps the only human condition in which pain is considered by many to be an unqualified good. It's also the only one in which the decision to reduce or eliminate pain is the subject of sometimes ferocious debate. In the past, those on the pro-pain side were often not the same people who actually experienced the pain—the all-male medical experts and religious leaders of nineteenth-century Europe and America, for example—resulting in a "blind-leading-the-pregnant" situation. But in modern times, even among many who have actually borne babies, the "ideal" childbirth is often a tough-it-out, medication-free pain marathon.

The pain of childbirth is natural, of course, and so is the impulse to relieve it. Simple measures such as reassurance, distraction, and belly rubs have no doubt been used since prehistoric times. In second-century Greece, the famed physician Soranus recommended warm-handed massage and the application of cloths soaked in warm oil to a laboring woman's belly. On the more oddly pharmaceutical side of ancient medicine, Pliny the Elder, the Roman military commander and natural philosopher, prescribed drinks that contained ground snails, earthworms, and the dissolved droppings of geese. Other ancient labor pain remedies included belly salves made from viper fat, eel gall, powdered donkey hoof, and the tongues of snakes, chameleons, and rabbits. By the Middle Ages, midwives used a wide variety of herbs, roots, and fungi. The sheer number of remedies testifies both to cultural preference and to the fact that none of them were all that effective.

And not all of them were benign. Henbane (an herb that "taketh away wytte and reason," as described in the thirteenth century), hemlock (whose generic name, *conium,* is derived from the Greek verb *konas,* "to whirl about"), and mandragora (a combination of two Greek words meaning "hurtful to cattle") were particularly dangerous. Mixed into food or drink and given to laboring women, they could produce anything from mild pain relief to seizures, paralysis, coma, and death.

Alcohol, too, played an increasing role as the centuries passed. By the time of Charles Dickens's fictional Sarah Gamp (*Martin Chuzzlewit,* 1844), British midwives were notorious for "helping" their patients through labor by getting them knock-down drunk, even comatose. Not that Victorian-era physicians had a whole lot more to offer their suffering patients. Their favorite remedy was blood-letting—draining blood from a laboring mother's arm until she reached the point of fainting—which presumably kept a woman quiet while the doctor did his work.

Into this nineteenth-century birthing-room bedlam of herbs, alcohol, and hemorrhage came a doctor from the far north of the British Empire, and the very fertile woman who was his queen. With the arrival of James Young Simpson, the management of childbirth pain changed dramatically and forever. But not without a big fight.

• • •

I didn't give much thought to Queen Victoria in my medical school days. My impression to that point, largely unchanged from my high school history class, was that she was a pale, pudgy sourpuss of a sovereign, glowering at her subjects from a blizzard of stamps, currency, and Jubilee portraits.

I remembered reading, too, that Victoria wasn't much of a mother. She hated pregnancy, loathed childbirth, and didn't much care for her children once they arrived, turning her brood of replacement monarchs over to an army of wet nurses and nannies as soon as she could. Not the sort of woman I would have imagined playing a central role in the story of modern human childbirth.

Yet as I researched labor pain years later, Queen Victoria's name repeatedly popped up. She was the first Englishwoman to receive anesthetic medication in childbirth, I read. By taking chloroform over the advice of her own physicians, she single-handedly dragged British obstetrics into the nineteenth century and opened the way to pain-free childbirth for thousands of her pregnant and eternally grateful subjects. Or so the legend goes. As I dug deeper into the story of the queen and her chloroform, I found a more complicated tale peopled with a whole cast of larger-than-life characters.

Victoria, ironically, owed her very existence to a childbirth tragedy. Princess Charlotte, the popular granddaughter of the "mad" King George III and the only legitimate child of his son and successor, King George IV, died while giving birth to a stillborn son in 1817, at the age of twenty-one. Her death set off a race among George III's seven sons, all well into middle age at the time of Charlotte's death, to produce another legitimate heir, something none of them had yet managed to do. The grand prize offered by the king—cancellation of the winner's mountainous gambling debts—set off a series of hastily arranged marriages. With the birth of Victoria on May 24, 1819, Prince Edward, George's fourth son, captured the royal sweepstakes. Edward won by a nose: Victoria's first cousin, George, was born three days later.

Victoria's image as a pregnancy and childbirth crank is based largely on letters she wrote to her eldest child, Princess Victoria, in

1858. The seventeen-year-old princess ("Vicky" to her mother) had married Frederick III, crown prince of Germany, earlier that same year, and promptly became pregnant. She soon wrote glowingly to her mother of her love for the "immortal soul" she carried in her womb.

The queen, who had given birth to her own last child just the year before, wasted no time in sticking a pin into Vicky's bubble: "I think much more of being like a cow or a dog at such moments," she wrote, "when our poor nature becomes so very animal and un-ecstatic." Victoria then went on to catalogue the grim downside of childbearing, with which she had ample firsthand experience: "Aches—and sufferings and miseries and plagues . . . one feels so pinned down—one's wings clipped—in fact, at the best . . . only half oneself. . . . This I call the 'shadow side' [of marriage]. And therefore I think our sex a most unenviable one."

Vicky's reaction to her mother's farm animal analogies, alas, went unrecorded, although she may have seen her mother's point by the end of that pregnancy. She nearly died in childbirth, her labor complicated by breech position and a placental abnormality. Her son, William, was born with a dislocated shoulder that never healed, a birth injury that may have had a profound impact on world history. Driven to prove himself despite his withered arm, William, Vicky's "immortal soul," grew up to be Kaiser Wilhelm II, Germany's spike-helmeted leader during World War I.

But Victoria had not always been so soured on childbirth. Journal entries from her first pregnancy in 1840 show a tenderhearted queen looking forward to Vicky's arrival. After giving birth, Victoria spent so much time with her newborn daughter—painting watercolor portraits of Vicky and showing her off to "the ladies"—that Prince Albert, her husband, worried that the queen was neglecting her royal duties. "[She] interests herself less and less about politics . . . and . . . is a good deal occupied with the Princess Royal."

In order to understand Queen Victoria's transformation from doting new mother at twenty-two to curmudgeonly grandmother-to-be by age thirty-nine, it helps to walk a mile (or a pregnancy or two) in her royal shoes. I was surprised to find that those shoes were quite tiny: Victoria was less than five feet tall. She gave birth to nine children in a little more than sixteen years (November 21, 1840–April 14, 1857) and though newborns were not routinely weighed in those days, her children were typically described as "wonderfully strong and large." With such wonderfully large fetuses crammed into so small a body, Victoria likely spent the last few weeks of each pregnancy in misery, unable to take a deep breath or sleep comfortably, her legs so swollen that even walking became a painful experience.

Victoria particularly dreaded childbirth, which, assuming that her pelvic outlet was in proportion to the rest of her, was more difficult and dangerous than for a larger woman. She undoubtedly faced each confinement with a great deal of fear, both for her physical safety (the fate of her aunt Charlotte could not have been far from her mind) and the safety of her reign itself. Nine times in sixteen years the rules of succession had to be dusted off in the not inconceivable event that Her Majesty might not survive childbirth.

Given the physical discomforts and political worries Victoria suffered with each of her pregnancies, it's no wonder, then, that when the lure of chloroform anesthesia beckoned from north of the border by her eighth pregnancy in 1853, the queen decided, if not in so many words: *the hell with it, give me drugs.*

James Young Simpson, a great mound of a man, was Scotland's preeminent obstetrician in the middle of the nineteenth century. A photograph taken toward the end of his life shows a frail, obese man who nonetheless appears at peace with his life's achievements. Chief among those accomplishments was the introduction of obstetric anesthesia to Great Britain, a feat he gleefully pulled off over the loud protests of London's medical establishment.

Within weeks of the 1846 introduction of inhaled anesthesia to Great Britain for use in surgery, Simpson began using it to treat difficult labors in his Edinburgh practice. He was an immediate convert—the abolition of pain gave him time to relieve many cases of obstructed labor that might previously have killed both mother and child. Galvanized, Simpson soon pushed for its use in routine, uncomplicated childbirth. In a span of a few weeks he anesthetized at least fifty normally laboring women and wrote glowingly of the experience.

Victoria appears to have caught wind of this remarkable development early on. There is evidence she considered chloroform in her sixth pregnancy, in 1848, and Prince Albert is known to have sought the opinion of John Snow, a renowned London physician, during Victoria's seventh pregnancy in 1850. But Sir James Clark, the Royal Physician and no fan of chloroform (or of Simpson), vetoed the idea on both occasions as too risky.*

Most of London's medical community shared Clark's concerns. Opponents fell into several overlapping categories: those who objected on medical grounds, those who did so out of moral concerns, and a much smaller contingent who based their opposition on an age-old scriptural interpretation of a woman's lot in life. A fourth, rather large category consisted of those physicians who simply could not abide the blustering James Simpson.

Simpson loved a good fight. Described as "irresistible when right in argument, and when wrong, formidable," he relished the opportunity to take on those who opposed his use of chloroform. That he was a Scot and most of his naysayers were English likely played a role in his enthusiasm—Edinburgh was the center of European medical training in the first half of the nineteenth century, and Scottish physicians weren't shy about reminding their English counterparts of that fact. Within a month of Simpson's first chloroform-assisted delivery in January 1847, public criticism had started. Simpson's hackles rose; the battle began.

Medical objections to Simpson's use of chloroform centered on

---

*Simpson was Queen Victoria's Royal Physician for Scotland, but as Her Majesty's babies were all born in London, the issue of chloroform use fell under the jurisdiction of her Royal Physician there.

two issues: the usefulness or necessity of a laboring mother's pain, and the riskiness of administering a medication with worrisome toxicity to a woman undergoing an otherwise normal physical process.

Many physicians considered pain to be a useful guide to the progress of a woman's labor. Charles Delucina Meigs, America's premier obstetrician, wrote directly to Simpson of "the needful and useful connection of the pain and the powers of parturition." He also added his concern over the safety of the procedure. Little was known of the effects of chloroform on the body of a pregnant woman, he wrote, let alone the child she carried: "What sufficient motive have I to risk the life of one in a thousand in a questionable attempt to abrogate one of the general health conditions of man?" Meigs concluded that chloroform had no place in the management of a normal process like childbirth, and at any rate was no more effective an anesthetic than alcohol.

Simpson's reply was swift and indignant. Was Meigs suggesting, he wrote, that a physician had no better way of assessing labor's progress than to depend on the "excruciating tortures and writhings, and shrieks of patients?" As to the rising concerns for chloroform's safety, Simpson pointed to the experience of several hospitals throughout Britain, each of which had seen a sharp decrease in mortality when limb amputations were performed under anesthesia. Thus, he declared, chloroform was safe in any medical application, including childbirth. Boggled by Simpson's apples-to-amputations comparison, his ever angrier opponents battled on.

The fight spilled into medical journals and newspapers. By late 1847, only months after Simpson's first case, the argument had turned personal. Robert Barnes, a distinguished London obstetrician, attacked Simpson in *The Lancet,* England's premier medical journal: "The question is not to be decided . . . by inconclusive arguments reared on a few imperfect and doubtful facts . . . by false analogy, bad arithmetic and statistics run wild; however . . . agreeable to the taste of the Edinburgh professor of midwifery." Simpson was, in so many words, a big fat liar, and a Scottish one to boot.

Simpson bided his time. He was, among his many other attri-
butes, a visionary, gifted with the ability to see (and promote) his
own greatness, even if his contemporaries could not.* He was also
a skilled politician with a keen understanding of the value of public relations.

Within weeks of his first use of chloroform, Simpson had widely
publicized his new treatment through pamphlets and reports in
medical journals. Chloroform soon became a subject for spirited
public discussion. Physicians who opposed obstetric anesthesia
were wasting their time, Simpson wrote, because the public clamor
for "pain-free" childbirth would soon carry the day: "The whole
question is, even now [in early 1848], one merely of time."

Simpson's opponents, perhaps fearing that the big-mouthed
Scot was right, counterattacked with moral and religious arguments. Many physicians were taken aback by the behavior they
witnessed in some patients under the influence of chloroform,
likening its effect to drunkenness. Charles Meigs, preeminent
among American physician-moralist prigs, minced no words: "To be
insensible from whiskey, and gin, and brandy, and wine, and beer,
and ether, and chloroform, is to be what in the world is called
Dead-drunk," he wrote in his popular obstetrics textbook. "No
reasoning—no argumentation is strong enough to point out the
millionth part of a split hair's difference between them."†

The moral argument took on a decidedly prurient tone when a
French physician reported the case of a young woman who con-
fessed to having frankly sexual dreams of her husband while giving
birth under the influence of chloroform. The elimination of labor
pain, the doctor cautioned, could unleash an uncontrollable female
sexual frenzy.

---

*Among his many achievements in the field of obstetrics and gynecology, Simp-
son foresaw the rise of radiology and other forms of medical imaging more than
half a century before they came into actual use, and invented the Simpson forceps that are still on hand in most labor and delivery wards.
†Moral objections, in the Victorian sense, referred to physical and emotional self-
control and were separate from religious issues.

Anesthesia opponents nearly trampled one another in their over-heated theorizing. Dr. G. T. Gream of London topped them all when he described the presence of the fetal head in the vagina of a chloroformed woman as behaving more or less like a giant penis, triggering dreams that should "only occur in prostitutes." A wise physician should think twice, he wrote, before anesthetizing up-standing, "less depraved" women. Gream then one-upped the French doctor's warning, concluding that the obliteration of pain not only put a woman at risk of later debauchery and prostitution, but even placed the physician himself in danger of being sexually assaulted by his laboring patient.

In a society whose most popular book for newly wed young women, *Advice to a Wife,* condemned even dancing—particularly while pregnant—and valued "pure blood and pure mind [over] any other earthly possession whatever!" the drunken, erotic ravings of a woman in labor were decidedly unsettling. What upstanding British man would want his wife to behave in such a manner?

And just in case drunkenness and an unleashed female libido weren't compelling enough reasons to convince physicians to for-sake chloroform, Simpson's opponents called God Himself as a witness, by way of the Old Testament.

In Genesis, God returns to the Garden to find that Adam and Eve, with the serpent's help, have ruined Paradise. Furious, he sen-tences Adam to a life of working for his food and then heaps spe-cial woe upon the head of poor Eve: "I will greatly increase your pains in childbearing; with pain you will give birth to your chil-dren." Armed solely with those seventeen words, some physicians and clergy denounced the relief of that pain, even in an obstetric emergency, as frankly blasphemous.

That argument didn't bear up long under the scrutiny of reli-gious leaders. Thomas Chalmers, a prominent nineteenth-century Scottish cleric, made short work of the matter in 1847, calling it a subject fit only for "small theologians." George Rapall Noyes, pro-fessor of biblical literature at Harvard Divinity School, wrote that the application of "agents of nature" in the relief of human pain was an example of man's God-given ingenuity, not blasphemy. And James Simpson himself studied the Hebrew texts, concluding that the original word should have been translated as "labor" or "toil" rather than "pain." Though the biblical "injunction" against childbirth anesthesia remained entrenched for years in parts of England and America, it quickly lost its power to sway most physicians and members of the public.

Victoria, then, had watched the controversy play out over the six years between chloroform's appearance and the onset of her eighth pregnancy. What she thought of all the mudslinging and character assassination flying between London and Edinburgh isn't known, but as the birth of Prince Leopold approached, she and Prince Albert once again consulted with Dr. John Snow.

The royal request was honored this time. On April 7, 1853, Dr. Snow was admitted to the royal chambers, where he administered chloroform to the queen of England:

"At twenty minutes past twelve by a clock in the Queen's apartment I commenced to give a little chloroform with each pain. . . . Her majesty expressed great relief from the application, the pains being trifling during the uterine contractions, and whilst between the periods of contraction there was complete ease. The infant was born at 13 minutes past one by the clock in the room . . . the Queen appeared very cheerful and well, expressing herself much gratified with the effect of the chloroform."

Perhaps anticipating his colleagues' reactions to his treatment, Snow added in his clearest handwriting, and with a fresh pen: "The effect of the chloroform was not at any time carried to the extent of quite removing consciousness."

The response from the medical establishment was indeed harsh and swift. On May 14, the editors of *The Lancet* were so flabbergasted by Snow's account that they went so far as to question whether it was true: "Intense astonishment . . . has been excited throughout the profession by the rumor that her Majesty during her last labor was placed under the influence of chloroform, an agent which has caused instantaneous death in a considerable number of cases. [The dangers of chloroform] being perfectly well known to the medical world, we could not imagine that any one had incurred the awful responsibility of advising the administration of chloroform to her Majesty during a perfectly natural labor. . . ."

The editors concluded, in so many words, that no doctor in his right mind would have taken such a risk with the queen of England, and so in fact none could have—the whole thing must have been a rumor, spread by "officious meddlers about the Court." But, they continued, if by some remote chance the royal physicians *did* use chloroform on Her Majesty, they were to be flatly condemned for doing so, and given that the queen was only thirty-four years old and perhaps not yet done with her royal childbearing duties, they'd better not do it again.

But Snow was back in the royal chambers four years later, on April 14, 1857, for the birth of Princess Beatrice, Victoria's ninth and last child. The queen was two weeks overdue, and her contractions were stronger and more painful than expected. She asked for, and received, more chloroform than she had with Leopold's birth, being rendered unconscious on at least one occasion.

Fortunately for all involved, Beatrice's birth went smoothly. Snow wrote in his case book that evening that "the Queen's recovery was very favorable." A grateful Victoria declared chloroform to be "delightful beyond measure." Perhaps as a result, the response of the medical community was decidedly more subdued than it had been four years previously.

Despite legend to the contrary, Victoria's decision to take chloroform did not lead to an overnight clamor for obstetric anesthesia. No public announcement of her chloroform use was even made until 1859. John Snow, though well known for his work with chloroform, anesthetized only seventy-seven women in his career, and his casebooks show no increase in the demand for his services after he treated Victoria.

What Her Majesty's acceptance of chloroform did accomplish, though, was to make it impossible for anyone again to argue against the relief of labor pains on biblical or moral grounds. What foolhardy soul would dare liken the queen of England—who was also the head of the Church of England and Defender of the Faith—to a drunken prostitute? Victoria's bold choice allowed obstetric anesthesia, especially in cases of obstructed labor, to move ahead with the speed of science.

And James Simpson? The man once dismissed as "the Edinburgh professor of midwifery" ended his career showered with honors for his contributions to obstetrics and gynecology, including honorary doctorates from Dublin and Oxford. He was made a baronet by Queen Victoria in 1866, and was awarded the freedom of the City of Edinburgh in 1869. On his death the following year, his funeral procession was witnessed by tens of thousands of mourners, including, no doubt, many of his obstetric patients and some of his envious old adversaries.

And that should have been that, at least from the perspective of women facing childbirth in 1870. Labor pain had been conquered forever by chloroform, they assumed—an apparently safe, easy to administer drug, one that had been used hundreds of times and had even received the endorsement of the queen of England. What reason could there be *not* to use it?

Unfortunately, chloroform was neither as safe nor as easy to use as Simpson had led the public to believe. His over-the-top enthusiasm for the drug clouded his ability to see any of its shortcomings. Remember that Simpson began using chloroform in childbirth just three weeks after the drug was introduced to England, and that the first of his many influential papers on the subject was based on only five cases. Simpson's body of work was long on assumption and woefully short on statistics, a problem common to much medical literature of the time. His scholarly articles read more like long-winded debates with his opponents than like hard science.

By the early 1860s, Simpson's unshakable faith in chloroform's benefits and his direct-to-consumer marketing genius had created a tidal wave of demand. But even as the public clamored for painless childbirth, experience with Simpson's wonder drug and its sometimes frightening side effects grew. Accounts of sudden maternal death after only a few breaths of chloroform surfaced. Physicians gradually came to realize that chloroform was capable of destroying a mother's liver, too. And the risk wasn't limited to her alone; chloroform freely crosses the placenta, and doctors soon learned through bitter experience that prolonged exposure to the drug could harm or even kill the fetus or newborn.

Part of the danger in using chloroform was that there was neither a standardized dose to be used in labor nor an agreed-upon way to administer it. This led to an era of freelance anesthesia: many doctors followed Simpson's example, using large amounts of chloroform over the entire labor, while other, more cautious physicians used it sparingly, only for the strongest contractions that came at the end of labor. Some physicians gave just enough chloroform to quiet a patient's moans; others kept going until a woman stopped moving entirely. Fatal and near fatal overdoses were not uncommon.

The uncertainties of dosing and administration were made worse by a logistical problem: childbirth and chloroform administration happened at opposite ends of a woman's body, and a doctor couldn't be both places at once. Paying for both a physician and an assistant trained in administering chloroform was beyond the means of all but the wealthiest of families. So when the doctor arrived at the home of a laboring woman, he pressed whoever was available into action as an amateur anesthetist, a group that might include "ignorant nurses, husbands [and] bystanders," according to one physician's account.

Some doctors even had the mother administer her own anesthetic. One physician proudly described his technique: he'd hand the mother a drinking glass filled with chloroform-soaked cotton to hold over her nose, and then tell her to breathe deeply. "When [her hand] become[s] unsteady and the glass falls away," the doctor wrote, he knew she was sufficiently knocked out to go about his business. When she came to, he reloaded the glass with chloroform and handed it back to her. Given the lack of standardized dosing and the jury-rigged way it was administered, it isn't surprising that chloroform's true dangers weren't known for years.

Much of the medical concern about chloroform's effects was lost on the childbearing public. The second half of the nineteenth century was a time of optimism and a nearly unquestioning faith in scientific progress. Pain and suffering, long attributed to a vengeful God or to human failure, were increasingly seen as biological phenomena that could be relieved by human intervention. In medicine, that progress was most evident in the operating room—the field of surgery had been revolutionized by the introduction of anesthetic medications.

Yet even as the public marveled at surgical advances, obstetrical care appeared to be moving backward. Doctors were increasingly reluctant to use chloroform in the birthing room, or at least not as freely as James Simpson had given it. And with no promising new obstetrical anesthetic techniques apparent on the horizon, women became suspicious of doctors' motives in letting them suffer. It was Adam and Eve all over again: charges of medical misogyny were inevitable.

The conflict between physicians and their patients over labor pain control grew steadily in the first decade of the twentieth century, in parallel with the rise of the feminist movement, which saw labor pain relief as one of the prime issues facing modern women, on a par with the right to vote and equal pay for equal work. By the time word of a German obstetrical marvel reached the rest of Europe and America, the stage was set for a dramatic showdown.

In late 1913, just months before the outbreak of World War I would have made the trip impossible, Marguerite Tracy and her companion Constance Leupp journeyed from New York City to Freiburg, a small medieval town on the edge of Germany's Black Forest. Reporters for *McClure's Magazine,* they had been sent to investigate an apparent miracle: doctors in Freiburg had perfected a method of completely painless childbirth they called *Dämmer-*

schlaf, or "Twilight Sleep," as it came to be known in England and America. Were the reports of hundreds of painless Twilight Sleep births true, the *McClure's* editors wanted to know? And if so, why on earth weren't American women sharing in this miracle?

It took the two women about ten days to reach Freiburg by ocean liner and train. Once they had settled into their Freiburg lodgings, Tracy and Leupp turned their attention to the modern, well-equipped building located "just three blocks from the Middle Ages" (as they described central Freiburg): the Frauenklinik, or Women's Clinic, of the State University of Baden. It was here that the reports of safe, completely painless childbirth had originated.

The Frauenklinik was directed by Dr. Bernhardt Kronig and his junior colleague, Dr. Karl Gauss. Tracy and Leupp spent a few days "casing" the clinic from the outside, observing the two doctors walking the clinic grounds, usually deep in conversation. Kronig, with his military bearing and stiffly waxed Kaiser Wilhelm mustache, struck Tracy as "so adequate, in his big white coat, and his hair all pricked up and standing attentively over his original head." The sad-eyed Gauss, with his softer beard, looked "wistful and sympathetic" to the women. As it turned out, the inventors of Twilight Sleep were tough, battle-scarred veterans of many bitter fights with the German medical establishment, and neither was particularly sympathetic to the needs of a pair of eager American reporters.

After a few days the women approached the Frauenklinik office with a request to interview the doctors in charge. To their great surprise, they were flatly refused. Not only would the clinic directors not speak to them, they were barred from interviewing the clinic staff as well, and from access to Kronig's and Gauss's original papers in the university library. No explanations were offered for the rejection, which Tracy later described as "baffling and obstructive to the last degree." Undaunted by the temporary setback—Tracy and Leupp were the kind of women that newspapers of the day would describe as "plucky"—they set out on a three-pronged course of research.

First, they did the next best thing to interviewing Kronig and Gauss: they talked with dozens of local women who had given birth at the Frauenklinik, nearly all of whom spoke glowingly of the experience—the quiet birthing suites, the considerate staff, and the astonishment of waking from a refreshing sleep to find that labor was over, their neatly swaddled babies lying in bedside cradles.

Next, Constance Leupp located copies of both men's research in a Freiburg secondhand bookstore, including a "faded, dust-stained, dog-eared" monograph by Gauss on the administration of *Dämmer-schlaf*. She hired an English instructor from the local Berlitz school to translate it aloud while she painstakingly wrote everything down. It took several weeks to copy the text and to analyze what she had found—her transcription ran to nearly a hundred pages, including graphs and statistical charts—but in the end the women could claim a better understanding of the science of Twilight Sleep than any but a handful of the world's doctors.

Leupp also learned from her read-and-write sessions that Kronig's "original head" had been obsessed with Twilight Sleep for more than a decade, and that his interest in the treatment of labor pain was both scientific and humanitarian. Observing the "army of suffering women" he had attended early in his career, he concluded that the pain of labor, rather than being a necessary part of childbirth, actually interfered with the functioning of the uterus. Much of the complications and tragedy that so often accompanied birth were, in fact, the consequences of untreated pain. Labor pain, he wrote, was "not merely a disagreeable accompaniment of childbirth, but . . . a dangerous and destructive accompaniment."

This was particularly true for the "modern," well-to-do woman, whom Kronig saw as physically and emotionally weaker than her hard-working peasant cousin. "The modern woman," he wrote in 1906, ". . . responds to the stimulus of severe pain more rapidly with nervous exhaustion and paralysis of the will to carry the labor to a conclusion." That "paralysis of the will" set off a vicious cycle: faced with an exhausted, terrified woman pleading for pain relief, obstetricians frequently opted to hasten the delivery with forceps, a technique that too often led to injury, infection, and ultimately more pain.

Severe pain did more than just complicate a woman's labor—it could also produce *neurasthenia,* a debilitating combination of anxiety and depression that could leave a woman bedridden for months after birth, often "embitter[ing] her whole life." Even for those women who were spared neurasthenia, Kronig wrote, the dread of the pain of future labors hung like a dark cloud over their childbearing years. A generation of "modern" women lived in mortal fear of "the terrors of childbearing."

Marguerite Tracy was no stranger to those fears. Though childless herself, she was no doubt aware of the case of a pregnant New York woman who had recently committed suicide rather than face another labor. In her 1915 book, *Painless Childbirth,* she quoted an American doctor—one of the few men who Tracy felt really understood what women were going through—as saying that if he were a woman, he would "hang myself in the first month of pregnancy." As far as Tracy could see, Twilight Sleep, with its promise of both pain relief and complete amnesia of birth's traumas, was a godsend.

Kronig and Gauss's work had built on Dr. Richard von Steinbuchel's earlier obstetrics research with *scopolamine,* a drug long known as a poison—Hamlet's father was killed with henbane, the highly toxic plant from which scopolamine is derived—but one that had gained some acceptance for use in general surgery. Many of Steinbuchel's obstetrics experiments, though, had ended badly. Scopolamine, described by Tracy as a "Dr. Jekyll and Mr. Hyde drug," was tricky to administer. Overdoses were common. Misused, it prolonged labor, increased forceps use, and harmed so many mothers and babies that by the time Kronig and Gauss turned their attention to the drug, the German medical establishment had given up on scopolamine as too dangerous for obstetric use.

But in their research, Kronig and Gauss found that scopolamine, when given carefully with a single small dose of the painkiller morphine, produced a "clouded consciousness, with complete forgetfulness"—Twilight Sleep. Women who gave birth under Twilight Sleep's effects awoke with no memories of the birth whatsoever. With pain and fear removed by the two drugs, they had fewer complications of childbirth than women who gave birth more conventionally, and they recovered far more quickly. Rather than the two weeks a new mother usually spent in bed, Twilight Sleep mothers were typically up and around by the second postpartum day. The Frauenklinik soon had the lowest maternal and neonatal death rates in the state of Baden.

Electrified by their findings, Kronig and Gauss presented a series of papers on Twilight Sleep at a national obstetrics conference in Berlin in 1906. To their dismay, they were met with indifference and open hostility, partly due to the fact that the German obstetricians present saw no reason to revisit such a dangerous drug, and partly to institutional bias: the bigwigs in Berlin were inclined to look down on their country cousins from Freiburg.

Kronig and Gauss persevered, publishing a series of papers over the next couple of years that documented their continued success. Gradually, wealthy German women began to vote with their feet, opting to travel to Freiburg to have their "painless babies." Berlin, forced by the attention to acknowledge that the Frauenklinik doctors might actually be onto something, sent a team of their own doctors to look into Twilight Sleep. Or, more accurately, to destroy it.

The investigation was purposely half-hearted—one of the Berlin doctors spent most of his research time touring the countryside around Freiburg—and a series of poorly designed trials back in Berlin "proved" that Twilight Sleep was indeed dangerous, just as the Berlin establishment had said all along. The investigating doctors dismissed it in their final report as "a poison . . . incalculable in its effects." By the second decade of the 1900s, Tracy wrote, "Germany had heard enough about the subject." Twilight Sleep nearly disappeared. Kronig and Gauss retreated to Freiburg to lick their wounds and quietly continue their work.

The third and final research path the reporters took was the cleverest of all. Refused professional access to the secrets of Twilight Sleep, they pulled off an inside job: Marguerite Tracy enlisted the help of the pregnant feminist Mary Sumner Boyd, who came to Freiburg and gave birth in the Frauenklinik that summer, attended by Karl Gauss himself. Gauss was unaware that this highly satisfied American mother and her chatty friend would soon thrust Bernhardt Kronig and himself into the international limelight. The directors of the Frauenklinik were about to become icons of the burgeoning American women's rights movement.

Tracy's timing was impeccable. Her *McClure's* article ignited a Western world already rattled by an increasingly active, sometimes violent feminist movement. The battle for women's rights was often fought on the fringes: in England, W. L. George, a novelist, playwright, and prominent (male) feminist leader, supported the abolition of marriage and called for an outright "sex war"; with an actual shooting war looming, German feminists clamored to join the army; and in a quest that bemused and baffled many of their compatriots, French feminists fought for a woman's "right" to be guillotined, just like a man.

American feminists took a pass on guillotine rights; their energies were already tied up in a struggle with members of their own sex. Called "anti-feminists" by the press, many wealthy and well-connected women bridled at feminist claims of working for the good of all women. They railed publicly against such "unnatural" feminist demands as equal pay for equal work and a woman's right to vote, seeking to derail a movement that they believed would soon destroy the nation, or at least their privileged corner of it.

The anti-feminists were particularly appalled by the notion of birth control—the idea that a woman should have the right to determine how many, if any, children she wished to bear. The argument was made along both moral and practical lines. Sex for reasons other than procreation was a very bad thing, of course, but embedded in the anti-feminist credo was a streak of racism that revealed an upper class growing increasingly nervous about a changing American demographic.

Mrs. John Martin, writing in *The New York Times Magazine,* singled out elite, college-educated, childless women for particular scorn. If these "fruitless twigs on the tree of life" refused their God-given childbearing duties, she wrote, America would soon have to "find its future Governors and Judges . . . among the dull-faced and semi-civilized who are now landing at Ellis Island." To Mrs. Martin—her own first name never appears in the article—feminists were guilty of "race-suicide," which could only be countered by women of the better classes out-reproducing the masses of unwashed immigrants and slave descendants.

Marguerite Tracy was one of those "fruitless twigs" who so riled Mrs. Martin. Well educated and independent, she never married or had children. When she died in 1939, she was survived only by her sister, the fabulously named Countess Raoul de Roussy de Sales. But the prospect of painless childbirth that she laid out in *McClure's* that spring was an issue that cut across political battle lines, uniting feminists and anti-feminists in a shaky coalition.

Feminists saw Twilight Sleep as their due—medical men had oppressed laboring women quite long enough. Anti-feminists rallied behind the Freiburg method, too, because it promised to make a woman's "God-given duties" less onerous, and thus perhaps induce some upper-class twigs to bear fruit.

American women first read the *McClure's* article in May 1914; by June all hell had broken loose. Buoyed by glowing reports of well-to-do women who had crossed the Atlantic to give birth in Freiburg, newspapers and popular magazines across the country pressed American obstetricians to follow in their German colleagues' more enlightened footsteps and adopt Twilight Sleep as a standard for all laboring women.

The National Twilight Sleep Association was formed when Mary Sumner Boyd—who cowrote the bestselling 1915 book *Painless Childbirth* with Marguerite Tracy, based in part on her own Freiburg experience—was overwhelmed by letters from American women wanting to know more about Twilight Sleep. She turned to such influential friends as Madeleine Astor, widow of John Jacob Astor, the richest man to go down with the *Titanic,* who moved quickly to spread the news of the Freiburg miracle.

Less than six months after Tracy's article appeared, the NTSA's high-profile leaders and patrons already included Rheta Childe Dorr of the Committee on the Industrial Conditions of Women and Children, Mary Ware Dennett of the National Suffrage Association (later the National Birth Control League), and Dr. Bertha Van Hoosen, a crusty Chicago obstetrician who was America's most prominent medical advocate for Twilight Sleep.

Van Hoosen came to her feminism gradually. She was born in 1863 to a rural Michigan family who expected her to follow her mother's and sister's example and become a teacher. Her decision to pursue a career in medicine drove her father to tears, and to cut off her college money. Unmoved, Van Hoosen went it alone, earning her medical school tuition, ironically, by teaching.

She entered the University of Michigan medical school—the first American university to accept women as medical students—in 1885, where the reception she and her female colleagues received was decidedly cool. In her memoir, Van Hoosen recalls professors who forced women students to face away from the podium, or who refused to lecture to them at all, and male students who "made clucking sounds and blew kisses" when the women passed by. Van Hoosen responded by nearly disappearing, spending her days at Michigan dressed in nunlike black clothing and "never raising my eyes from the ground" as she walked between classes.

By the time she helped form the National Twilight Sleep Association, though, Van Hoosen had blossomed into a prominent Chicago obstetrician, famed for her skill at repairing vaginal lacerations and other maternal birth injuries. Just as Gauss had described in Germany, Van Hoosen saw that many birth injuries were the result of poorly managed pain that led to too-early forceps use. Aware of Kronig and Gauss's work, she was struck by their reports of dramatically less forceps use—and thus fewer injuries—in women undergoing Twilight Sleep.

Familiar with scopolamine from its use in surgery, she became convinced that the drug's ability to cut off the conscious mind from the reflex action of the uterus would lead to "a return of more physiological births." In other words, if women weren't aware of what was going on during labor, babies would be born as nature intended: slowly, and with a minimum of injury to mother and baby. Setting up shop at Chicago's Mary Thompson Hospital, Van Hoosen was soon successfully administering Twilight Sleep to a growing number of women.

Van Hoosen, though, had a much larger motive in mind than simply relieving the pain of having a baby, and it was here that she veered into the sometimes bizarre hotbed of sexual politics that surrounded the quest for painless childbirth.

According to Van Hoosen, the pain of childbirth had nothing to do with the fall of Adam and Eve. Having a baby hurt because the human female reproductive organs had too long been used "more frequently for pleasure than for reproduction." Over the centuries such chronic sexual overstimulation had rendered the uterus and vagina "so hypersensitive that the real function [birth], so relatively seldom performed, should have become universally and persistently painful." Van Hoosen's solution was to use anesthesia to break up the link between the brain and the sexual organs, thus "reestablish[ing] the female sexual supremacy of the animal kingdom."

Twilight Sleep, then, was Van Hoosen's ideal tool for "strik[ing] at the root of many of the evils of our civilization." In stark contrast to the opinion of the London antichloroform physician G. T. Gream, who seven decades earlier saw the abolition of labor pain as a sure ticket to debauchery for pregnant women, Van Hoosen predicted that painless childbirth would "[do] away with prostitution, abortions, divorces, unwilling motherhood, sexual excesses in married life, and inability to perform lactation. [Twilight Sleep] would help us control, if not eradicate, venereal diseases, and,

most of all, it would preserve that most beautiful of relations between men and women—the relation of lovers."

Van Hoosen's early embrace of Twilight Sleep wasn't typical of
American doctors, most of whom were caught off guard by the
avalanche of demand for the procedure that followed Tracy's articles. Many reacted angrily, unaccustomed to being scooped by
what they considered a "ladies' magazine." But the speed with
which the nation's doctors backpedaled in the face of the Twilight
Sleep juggernaut is breathtaking.

In the fall 1914 issue of the *New York Medical Journal,* even as
one physician-author decried the attempt to "dragoon" doctors into
"indiscriminate administration" of a procedure that "had already
been tested and found wanting," the *Journal*'s editors deemed it a
"privilege" to trumpet the initial reports of the success of Twilight
Sleep at a local hospital. The push was on to outdo Freiburg: "With
a few more clever American improvements," the editors wrote, "we
shall have [an] anesthetic technique of inestimable value." Faced
with enormous popular pressure, and the potential loss of obstetric
business to physicians who offered the Freiburg childbirth miracle,
doctors and hospitals from New York to San Francisco scrambled
to put together their own Twilight Sleep units.

Despite all of its nationally prominent supporters, it was Mrs.
Francis X. Carmody, the wife of a Brooklyn lawyer, who became the
public face of Twilight Sleep in the United States. Carmody was
the first American woman to have her baby in Freiburg as a direct
result of Marguerite Tracy's article. She had been traumatized by
the extreme pain of her first child's birth, an experience that left her
a bedridden invalid for several months. Deeply depressed at the
prospect of her looming second delivery, Carmody read Tracy's account of Twilight Sleep in *McClure*'s and immediately decided to
travel to Freiburg. Her own obstetrician, intrigued by the prospect
of learning to administer Twilight Sleep himself, went with her.

The delivery, attended by Karl Gauss, was flawless. Carmody
entered the Frauenklinik late in the afternoon of July 13, 1914, and
received her first dose of scopolamine an hour later. "The next

thing I knew," she later told Marguerite Tracy, "I woke up . . . and looked at the clock." It was 7:00 A.M., and she was alone in the room, or so she thought. Figuring she had slept through the night with false labor pains, she rose to get dressed, only to notice that something about her was different: "I felt lighter, and my figure had changed." She refused to believe the baby sleeping quietly in the cradle next to her bed was her own until family members came into the room with Dr. Gauss and confirmed it.

Carmody was euphoric. Rather than the customary two weeks of postpartum bed rest back in the United States, she was up and around a few hours after she awoke, "even [taking] some dance steps" in her room. The next day she took a two-hour automobile ride in the hills outside of town. With the exception of temporarily blurred vision, she suffered no ill effects from the once feared scopolamine. Her husband was mightily pleased, too; this time there was "no deranged nervous system to recuperate," as he delicately put it.

Carmody returned to the States a changed woman. She became an ardent advocate for Twilight Sleep, tirelessly touring New York and New England giving speeches and showing off her "painless baby" to women at huge rallies in churches, town squares, and Gimbels department stores, and from the back of her car to whoever would listen. She ended each speech with the same rallying cry: "If you women want [Twilight Sleep] you will have to fight for it, for the mass of doctors are opposed to it!" Putting her money where her mouth was, Carmody and her husband opened a Twilight Sleep hospital for the women of Brooklyn.

The movement continued to gain strength. By early 1915, as Marguerite Tracy railed against "the stupid brutality" of the dwindling number of Twilight Sleep opponents, mainstream medicine was nearly won over. Bertha Van Hoosen was ecstatic. "Now, after centuries of fulfillment [of God's condemnation of Eve]," she wrote, "this ban is being lifted, both in respect to the painful childbirth and the domination of man over woman; we are about to obtain almost at the same moment a release from both!"

Alas, the euphoria was short-lived. The Twilight Sleep movement crashed abruptly in the summer of 1915, only a little more than a year after its rise. The seeds of its demise were planted early on, and to anyone alive then who was old enough to remember the fall of chloroform, the parallels were inescapable.

The first problem: Twilight Sleep was a tricky thing to do well. The key to Kronig and Gauss's success had been their meticulousness. They stayed with their patients from the first dose of scopolamine until the baby was born, often twenty-four hours or more, increasing or decreasing the amount of medication given based on the woman's level of awareness of her surroundings. They knew that women under the influence of scopolamine were highly susceptible to terrifying disorientation, so they went to great lengths to shield their patients from overstimulation: laboring women slept in special tentlike beds, wore dark glasses, and had their ears plugged with cotton dipped in oil. Even so, not every delivery was a success. The Frauenklinik kept leather restraints on hand to tie disoriented women to their beds, and about one in ten births was completed under general anesthesia. These details didn't find their way into Marguerite Tracy's glowing accounts of Twilight Sleep.

The second problem was one of economics. Kronig and Gauss practiced in a state-supported university hospital, their incomes assured by government stipend no matter how many babies they delivered. An American doctor, particularly one for whom delivering babies was just one part of a busy general practice, didn't have the luxury of spending an entire day or more with one patient, as the Freiburg doctors did. Yet, as had been the case with chloroform sixty years before, a doctor who refused to offer this new, painless childbirth technique to his patients was likely to lose them to someone who would.

As the Twilight Sleep frenzy reached its peak, the waves of women seeking it quickly outstripped the number of doctors trained to provide it. Gauss recommended a three-year course of study to master the technique; he was appalled by physicians who visited the Frauenklinik, observed a few deliveries, and then declared themselves to be Twilight Sleep–trained.

Back home again, these doctors looked for shortcuts in their own busy practices. They abandoned the Frauenklinik doctors' hands-on, individualized approach, instead giving fixed doses of morphine and scopolamine and then turning over the labor to untrained nurses until the time for delivery came. As a result, fewer women achieved a true Freiburg-style birth, and more of them experienced—and remembered—the terror and pain that came with inadequate medication. Things got so bad that neighbors of one New York Twilight Sleep hospital sought to shut it down. The screams that echoed down the street from the hospital at all hours kept them from sleeping.

Then, the final blow: Mrs. Francis X. Carmody, the American face of the Twilight Sleep movement, died while giving birth to her third child, in August 1915. Though her husband and her doctor insisted she died from hemorrhage, not from the effects of Twilight Sleep, the damage was done. Only fifteen months after taking America by storm, demand for the "Freiburg Miracle" virtually disappeared.

Doctors came away from the Twilight Sleep debacle with mixed feelings. They felt justified in their initial reluctance to adopt a treatment they had felt was unproven and perhaps even dangerous, yet they were also embarrassed by the speed with which they had caved in to public demand for it.

But even with its shortcomings, Twilight Sleep helped doctors accomplish something they had sought for a long time: control of the birthing suite. One doctor wrote that Twilight Sleep gave "absolute control over your patient at all stages of the game . . . You are 'boss.'" Twilight Sleep had accelerated the trend toward hospital births; as the 1920s approached, fewer and fewer babies were home-born.

Hospital birth also allowed a doctor to separate his patient from her sometimes meddlesome family members, sending them home at the onset of labor, allegedly so that the hospital staff could focus on delivering her baby. When Twilight Sleep worked well, the family-free doctor was treated to something that he and his professional forebears had rarely encountered in attending childbirth: silence. "I catch up on my reading and writing," wrote one happy physician. "I am never harassed by relatives who want me to tell them things."

Despite the crash of 1915, Twilight Sleep never really disappeared. It just morphed into different forms and other drugs, gradually transforming "painless childbirth" into an assembly line, more or less, a hospital-based program of heavy sedation and amnesia. Well into the 1970s, when, as we'll see, the drive toward conscious childbirth finally ended the practice, most American women had their babies in a haze of anesthetic medications and tranquilizers.

My mother is a midcentury case in point. She gave birth seven times between 1948 and 1961 and slept through every delivery. When I asked her once to tell me about her birth experiences, she smiled and shrugged. "I wish I could," she said. "But you see, I wasn't really there."

Chapter 5
Nowadays: An "Epidural Monoculture"?

I · Epidurals, Mostly

A woman laboring in a typical American hospital today won't be knocked out with chloroform or sedated with scopolamine. She won't have to wear dark glasses or have her ears plugged with oily cotton balls, either. Her family won't be chased away, and the odds are good that she'll be wide awake when her baby is born. That's not to say she won't run into a bit of controversy along the way, though. When it comes to labor pain relief choices, the debate that James Young Simpson started lives on, if in somewhat muted fashion.

That American woman will likely be encouraged to walk the halls and bend or squat to keep herself comfortable early on, techniques that would have been seen as unacceptably primitive by hospital staff only a half century ago. She may also be offered a warm shower, a labor ball to sit on, and bars to grip when her contractions come. But when the pain gets intense her choices will narrow to a very short menu of pharmacologic pain relievers: an opioid, a local anesthetic injection, or an epidural.

Opioids, a large group of chemical compounds that includes morphine, fentanyl, and meperidine (Demerol), are widely used in hospitals and clinics to treat pain of all kinds. Their use in labor, though, is limited by side effects such as maternal drowsiness and nausea, a tendency to cause breathing problems in the newborn if the dose is given too close to delivery, and problems initiating breast-feeding.

Local anesthetic injections can be given in three places as birth nears: around the edge of the cervix during the first stage of labor (a paracervical block); near the nerves that transmit pain sensation from the floor of the pelvis when pushing starts (a pudendal block); or directly into the skin of the perineum as the fetus's emerging head stretches it. These injections are generally safe for mother and fetus, but as with any injected medication, complications— from misdirected needles to allergic reactions—occasionally occur.

It turns out neither opioids nor injected local anesthetics provide great pain relief in labor. Add the fact that the relief they provide is short-lived, and it's not surprising that women don't rate these medications very highly, particularly when compared with an epidural. So the pressing issue for a pregnant American woman is, to paraphrase Hamlet: *Epidural or no epidural?* That is the question.

James Simpson would have loved epidurals. Chloroform administration—holding an anesthetic-soaked rag over a woman's face until she passed out—was a crude procedure at best. The boundary between enough anesthetic and too much was a fuzzy, inexact combination of dose and duration that was frequently crossed, sometimes with disastrous results. The idea of a precisely measurable pain medication, one with low risks and absolutely no potential for turning laboring women into raving sex fiends, would have pleased him greatly.

Epidural blockade, a term that can refer to either epidural *analgesia* (pain relief) or epidural *anesthesia* (the complete loss of sensation), is infinitely more refined than chloroform ever was. Once active labor has begun—usually when the cervix is dilated to three or four centimeters—the anesthesiologist inserts a long needle between two vertebrae in a woman's lower back, then slides a thin, floppy catheter through the needle into the epidural space, which lies just outside the spinal cord. The needle comes out, the catheter stays in, and a novocaine-like local anesthetic medication, and perhaps an opioid as well, is slowly pumped in over the course of labor. The flow of medication can be increased or decreased depending on the needs of the woman giving birth. A safe, adjustable pain relief delivery system sounds perfectly Simpsonian, but as is the case with nearly every aspect of modern hospital childbirth, controversy dogs the procedure.

If James Simpson were alive today, still tormenting his London obstetrical counterparts, he would immediately recognize the "hot button" issues. Is pain itself an important part of childbirth? Does its relief lead to more difficult or complicated births? Do the risks of an epidural to mother and child outweigh its benefits? He would also recognize the overarching question, the same one that drove the painless childbirth controversy of a century and a half ago: Who should control what goes on in the labor room, the doctor or the woman giving birth?

The battle lines are clearly drawn, or so it would seem from a quick survey of childbirth-related Internet websites. On one side stands the laboring mother, wanting nothing more than a natural, intervention-free birth experience. On the other is the doctor, an uncaring, profit-driven, epidural-pushing cold fish. It's a black-and-white morality play: motherhood versus the "medicalization" of childbirth.

But the lines aren't that clear-cut today, just as they weren't in 1848. There are pregnant women on both sides of the pain relief divide; for every woman who insists on a medication-free birth, there are others signing up for an epidural long before labor begins. And obstetricians, more and more of whom are women themselves, come to the delivery room with a wide variety of attitudes toward labor pain relief.

James Simpson would recognize the modern debate because, in a very real way, he started it. Simpson was a pioneer in "direct-to-consumer" marketing; we've grown so accustomed to seeing television commercials for everything from allergy pills to erectile dysfunction treatments that it's hard to remember there was a time when deciding which medicine a patient received was entirely up to the doctor. Simpson's decision to take the chloroform debate public with his pamphlets and forums let the consumer genie out of the bottle. Never again would the debate over labor pain be strictly medical. By the end of the 1850s women were clamoring for pain-free childbirth, and doctors, despite some misgivings, were providing it.

By the 1950s, though, the public's faith in the unbridled good of science and technology was fading. This was true in all of medicine, but particularly so in obstetrics. As women learned that alcoholic drinks and cigarette smoke could have harmful effects on their unborn babies, it was only natural for them to question the medicines given to them during pregnancy and labor. Those fears became much more intense in 1956, when the first of thousands of "thalidomide babies" were born, their limbs severely deformed by a morning sickness treatment marketed to pregnant women in Europe.

Doctors themselves had already begun to question the value of drugs that deeply sedated women and wiped out all memory of childbirth, but those doubts rose more from changes in obstetric practice than concerns about medication side effects. The relationship between Twilight Sleep–type medications and forceps use had long been a self-fulfilling prophecy. The level of sedation required for a Twilight Sleep–style birth made it difficult for a woman to push at the end of her labor; as a result, forceps were often required to pull her baby out. The frequent use of forceps, or the assumption that they would likely be required, led doctors to use higher doses of pain medication—which, of course, made forceps use a necessity.

But forceps-assisted deliveries began a steep decline in the mid-twentieth century, a dramatic change brought on by several factors. As cesarean birth became safer, obstetricians began to choose surgery over forceps for resolving difficult labors. Antibiotic use flourished, decreasing the risk of perinatal infection and allowing doctors to wait longer before intervening. And as we'll see, the natural childbirth movement of the 1950s and beyond played a large role in getting doctors to slow things down and let nature take a bit more of its course.

Attitudes about labor pain were changing, too. Where it had once been lumped with hunger, poverty, and slavery on the list of "pains and sufferings" that progressive nineteenth-century Europeans and Americans sought to conquer, the idea that labor pain might serve a purpose, even a transformative one in a woman's life, grew. As the Twilight Sleep era staggered to a close in the 1970s, doctors didn't have a lot else to turn to, pain-relief-wise. Of all the experimental pain medications and techniques that rose and fell in the first half of the twentieth century, only one remained. The epidural age began.

One thing I figured out early in my medical school obstetrics rotation: I could never truly understand what it feels like to give birth. This basic fact of life put me at a disadvantage with my laboring patients, one that I hadn't faced in my other hospital rotations. I'd suffered enough high school football injuries to relate to the woes of my orthopedic patients, and though I'd never had appendicitis, I could guess what a sharp, stabbing pain in my right lower abdomen might feel like. But the first time a laboring woman tried to describe the feeling of a fetus pushing its way out of her belly through a tiny opening in her bottom, my mouth dropped open like a six-year-old's, and all I could say was, whoa, that's *got* to hurt.

There was nothing in my personal pain experience, not even in my then vivid medical imagination, that came close. I could learn the basics of obstetric care—how to deliver a baby or assist at a cesarean section and such—but the experience of actually giving birth? No one could teach me that.

Not that the obstetrics staff didn't try. Mitch, my resident, took a crack at describing labor pain, but in the end his explanation—that it was kind of like being split open, but not all the way—wasn't very helpful. The final word on the subject came one morning from the chief of obstetrics, during his lecture on labor pain management. After unsuccessfully browbeating the lone female student in the room who'd had a baby to describe what it felt like ("It just . . . *hurts,*" she said, near tears), he drew a baby-sized oval with horizontal stripes on the dilapidated chalkboard at the front of the room. If a man wanted to know what giving birth feels like, he said, jabbing the chalky oval with his finger, he should "try crapping a watermelon."

I don't remember anything else from that lecture. The chief must have gone on to talk about the treatment of labor pain, about opioids and epidurals and such, but that watermelon had made a big impression. I spent the rest of the hour wincing.

How much *does* it hurt to have a baby? I ask this question as an outsider because, of course, I've never actually given birth. But after watching a lot of women have babies over the years I've come to the conclusion that it hurts quite a bit. It turns out that most new mothers agree.

Pain is a very difficult thing to quantify. The International Association for the Study of Pain blandly defines it as "an unpleasant sensory and emotional experience." Historically, pain researchers have focused on the sensory aspect of pain—the transmission of pain sensation along nerve pathways from the point of injury to the brain. Pain was seen first as a mechanical process, later as an electrical one: impulses traveled along nerves like water through a pipe or electricity through a wire, their severity measured objectively by the calculator-like brain. Pharmacologic pain management, from aspirin to morphine, was designed to obliterate the "unpleasant sensory experience." What pain *meant* to the patient, and how his or her "emotional experience" might in turn amplify suffering, was left unaddressed.

One major confounder in measuring pain is that humans experience so many different kinds of it. Which hurts more: the throb of a toothache, the rip of a sprained ankle, or the burn of acid reflux? It's easy enough to rank the severity of pain when the tooth, ankle, and stomach all belong to the same person—he gets all the votes. But it becomes a much more difficult task when other people are involved. Which is worse, my toothache or yours? Your sprained ankle or my stomachache? Add in the intensifying effect of fear and other emotions, and pain measurement becomes incredibly complicated. Does your tooth hurt more than mine because your cavity is bigger or because I'm a tough guy and you're just a wimp?

Forget toothaches. There's an inherent, even bigger problem in assessing something as intense as labor pain: only half the population is at risk of ever experiencing it, meaning that the other half often doesn't "get" it. The pain of childbirth is undoubtedly the most severe gender-specific human pain there is. A swift kick to the testicles is about as bad as it gets for men (and it *is* bad, ladies), but after watching a woman give birth most men would gladly opt for the boot.

Tonya took a stab, so to speak, at quantifying her labor pain with her childbirth-versus-knifing rating scale. It worked for me. I knew instantly from her description that labor was intensely painful for her, the worst pain she had ever felt in a life filled with excruciating experiences, and that the dread of the coming pain seemed to make it worse. Though there was no thermometer-like number I could attach to her pain, and no graph I could chart it on, Tonya's quick comparison told me what I needed to know: this was a bad pain to have. In those days, that was about as far as pain measurement went.

In the years after my medical school days, however, more sensitive tools were devised to help patients communicate the quality and intensity of their pain to those who care for them. In 1981, Dr. Ronald Melzack and his research team were the first to take a try at measuring labor pain. Melzack administered the McGill Pain Questionnaire, originally designed to quantify "phantom limb" pain—the severe, chronic pain that often follows the loss of an arm or a leg—to three groups of subjects: first-time mothers, women having a second (or subsequent) baby, and people being treated for chronic back pain, nonterminal cancer, or phantom limb pain.

Their findings supported Tonya's quick sketch: 59 percent of first-time mothers described their pain as more severe than did the people suffering from cancer or phantom limb pain. One-fourth of all first-time mothers in the survey described their pain as "horrible" or "excruciating." The pain wasn't quite as bad for mothers who had been through labor before, but still, nearly half of those women ranked labor pain as more severe than the pain reported by cancer patients.

Labor pain is actually a combination of two distinct kinds of pain. *Visceral pain* is the dull, crampy, hard-to-point-to ache that originates in the abdominal organs, or viscera. It's familiar to anyone who has ever had menstrual cramps or even a bad case of diarrhea. *Somatic pain,* on the other hand, originates in skin, muscle, bones, joints, or connective tissues, and tends to be sharp and well localized—a pulled muscle, say, or a sliver in your palm.

Early in labor, the pain is mainly visceral: a dull, increasingly severe cramping sensation that results from uterine contractions and the dilation of the cervix. Like other types of visceral pain, it's often felt in the lower back, buttocks, or thighs, too, as well as in the lower abdomen. The second stage of labor, from full cervical dilation to the birth of the baby, is dominated by sharp, well-localized somatic pain caused by the stretching of the pelvic floor, the vagina, and the skin of the perineum as the fetus's head begins to emerge. The two types of pain are carried by different sets of nerves: visceral pain impulses are relayed to the brain through nerves that enter the spinal cord in the middle of the back, while somatic pain sensation travels to the brain via the sacral nerves, which join the cord just above the tailbone.

The pain of labor follows a set pattern, increasing as the cervix dilates and as uterine contractions become more frequent, stronger, and longer. At least that's the textbook version of things I learned in medical school. In reality, the pain a woman experiences in giving birth is highly individualized and influenced by a complex mix of physical, psychosocial, and environmental factors. It doesn't always correlate neatly with the stages of labor.

For starters, some labors are just more painful than others. A fetus who comes down the birth canal in an abnormal position—the most common being the flipped-over "sunny-side up" arrangement—will cause its mother considerable extra pain. A woman with an unusually large fetus, especially if her pelvis is narrower than average, as Queen Victoria's likely was, can have a rougher go of it, too. And women who suffer from dysmenorrhea—extremely painful menstrual cramps—before becoming pregnant will often have stronger, more painful uterine contractions in labor.

Anxiety and fear play a major role, too. Some degree of anxiety is normal with any labor, but excessive anxiety, often brought on by the fear of pain, causes an increase in the body's production of adrenaline and other catecholamines, chemicals that are known to amplify pain signals. Not only does adrenaline increase the perception of pain, it can also directly slow uterine contractions, leading to a vicious cycle of prolonged, complicated, and more painful labor.

Then there is the matter of a woman's previous pain experience. Labor is the first exposure to intense pain for many women. This can be helpful or unhelpful. A young woman with no significant pain history may be well equipped to cope with labor by virtue of her overall good health, or she may be overwhelmed by the unexpected magnitude of her pain. Likewise, a woman who has experienced severe pain in the past from accident or illness may be better or worse prepared to deal with the pain of labor, depending on how well she was able to cope with that previous pain.

A final factor that can strongly affect the intensity of labor pain, and one that is frequently overlooked, is early life trauma. Unresolved physical or sexual abuse, family dysfunction, or the loss of a parent, for example, can lead to increased pain during labor and even post-traumatic stress disorder afterward.

One thing that does *not* appear to be a factor in the intensity of a woman's labor pain is the culture into which she is born. Pick any group of women—white Americans, African Americans, Australians, Bedouins, Kuwaitis, Israelis, Italians, or Palestinians, to name a few—and the degree of pain they report after they've given birth is remarkably similar. Comparable numbers of women in each culture describe the pain they experienced as more painful than, less painful than, or as painful as they thought it would be.

Dr. Nancy Lowe, a midwife and professor of nursing at Ohio State University, describes this highly individualized mix of physical characteristics, emotional makeup, and life history as the "private pain experience" of a woman in childbirth. Lowe argues that American hospitals are too quick to resort to epidurals, too eager to obliterate the sensory aspect of pain while ignoring the emotional underpinnings of that pain.

It is ironic, Lowe writes, that "a society that celebrates individuals who endure great pain and distress in the pursuit of mountain peaks or completion of a marathon race" should be so quick to label labor pain a bad thing. Many women approach labor as a challenge, she notes, and leave it with a profound sense of life-changing accomplishment. Routinely removing that pain may rob women of a fundamental life experience.

Dr. Lowe is right—there is no generic laboring woman any more than there is a generic father-to-be hovering by her side. The one-size-fits-all, epidural-based nature of labor pain control in many American hospitals often ignores the needs of individual women. Like Dr. Lowe, I have known many women who emerged from an epidural-free childbirth with a sense of exhilaration and triumph, and many others who, once the baby arrived, felt that by having an epidural they had missed out on a crucial aspect of the birth of their child.

On the other hand, I often hear new mothers speak of the trauma of labor pain, regardless of how well their pain was managed from a strictly sensory aspect. Like many of their early-twentieth-century counterparts who fought for the right to painless childbirth, they dread the idea of ever giving birth again, and some of them never do. So while we should celebrate the woman who reaches her goal of a medication-free birth and support her in that effort, it's good to remember that not every woman wants to climb Mount Everest.

Say what you will about epidurals, but one thing is indisputable: they work. Every time I attend a cesarean birth I'm convinced all over again. On one side of the surgical drape the mother-to-be chats with her husband; on the other, the obstetrician is hard at work with his scalpel. It's an eerie sight, like watching a magician in the act of sawing a wide-awake woman in half.

Women consistently report a high degree of satisfaction with the pain control an epidural provides during labor, much higher than with morphine or any other analgesic medication. The number of repeat customers attests to that satisfaction; the majority of women who give birth with an epidural plan to do so with their next labor, too. The benefit of having an epidural, then—the relief of most or all of the pain associated with giving birth—is obvious. But what are the risks? How safe is that catheter in the back for mother and child?

Back in 1990, when my wife, Elisabeth, was pregnant with Claire, we joined four other couples in a prepared childbirth class that dealt with labor pain management. The woman who taught the class was up-front about her feelings on the subject. She was "anti" just about anything that came out of a pharmacy, dismissing all pain medications as "drugs." She reserved her harshest criticism for what she called the growing "fad" of epidural pain relief.

"I would be putting my license at risk," she told us in a dramatic, spooky-campfire-story tone of voice, "if I didn't warn you that one out of every thirteen thousand of you who gets an epidural will end up paralyzed for the rest of your life!" I took her warning with a grain of salt. In an earlier class she'd counseled us all to bring condoms to the hospital, because birth was such an "emotional high" that many couples left for home already pregnant again. (The response of a woman in a nearby couple neatly summed up the feelings of the group: "That's like, *ick!*")

I don't know where our instructor got her statistics. The chance of paralysis or other severe permanent nerve damage from an epidural was many times lower than the 1-in-13,000 figure she quoted us in 1990, and it's much lower still today. That's not to say that tragedy never strikes, of course, but it does so rarely that it can be difficult to tell if the epidural caused the injury or if something simply went wrong for a woman who happened to have an epidural. Consider this: childbirth itself is five times more likely than an epidural to produce permanent maternal neurological damage.

Most women seeking an epidural aren't put off by stories of looming paralysis—the numbers are just too minuscule to register as a real risk. But what they sometimes overlook, despite reading and signing a detailed informed consent before the procedure, is just how much an epidural will affect their birth experience.

First, there's the IV. When the epidural pump is switched on and analgesic medication begins to numb the nerves crossing the epidural space on their way to the spinal cord, many women will experience hypotension, or low blood pressure. This in turn can lead to a decrease in the fetal heart rate. The hypotension is usually brief and the dip in fetal heart rate harmless, but it can sometimes be difficult to distinguish from true fetal distress.

To prevent this, an IV catheter is inserted in the mother's arm and a fetal heart monitor lead is strapped to her belly well before the epidural pump is switched on. A liter or so of saline solution is then run in through the IV to boost her blood pressure. If significant hypotension occurs despite the extra fluids, the woman is given ephedrine, or another adrenaline-like medication, which usually raises her blood pressure to a safe level but can also cause her heart to beat rapidly and add to any anxiety she may already be feeling.

Once the epidural medication starts to work, the numbness and muscle weakness that can result mean it's no longer safe for the mother-to-be to walk around, or even move into a common labor position like squatting. This catches many women by surprise and sometimes leaves them feeling trapped in their hospital beds, tied to the IV pole, the fetal monitor, and the epidural pump.

Epidural analgesia can cause other discomforts and complications as well. Headache, nausea, shivering, and itchiness (an opioid side effect) are common, but since these can occur in unmedicated labor, too, it's hard to tell in a given case whether the epidural is the culprit.

Maternal fever (defined as a temperature greater than 100.8 degrees) is common with epidurals, and since it's difficult to separate fevers due to epidurals from those caused by infections that may threaten the fetus and newborn, babies born of mothers with epidurals are somewhat more likely to end up with what's known as a sepsis workup: at minimum a blood test, maybe a urine examination, too. If that doesn't rule out an infection, a spinal tap and a day or more of IV antibiotics in the intensive care nursery may be required to play it safe, because even a brief delay in treating neonatal infections can be catastrophic. Not every baby whose mother has a fever in labor will need a sepsis workup, though. Most experienced neonatologists and pediatricians limit lab tests and antibiotics to babies who appear to be at real risk of infection—those whose mothers have an obvious uterine infection, for example.

Epidurals can make it more difficult for a woman to push, too, thus prolonging the second stage of labor. That second stage delay doesn't appear to increase a woman's chances of a cesarean birth, but it definitely makes an operative vaginal delivery—a birth helped along with a vacuum or, much less often, forceps—more likely. Maternal injuries from an operative vaginal delivery were far more common in the heyday of forceps use—anything from small, easily repaired tears to severe lacerations that could lead to incontinence and other quality-of-life problems decades down the road. The switch from metal forceps to today's soft plastic vacuum cup has greatly decreased the risk of such injuries, but even perfect technique can't eliminate it completely.

It's important to emphasize again that epidurals are safe for the large majority of mothers. Minor side effects are common, but bad outcomes are extremely rare. The chance of permanent neurologic damage following an epidural in labor has recently been estimated at about 1 in 250,000, a figure that includes less serious injuries like isolated numbness or mild muscle weakness. The actual number is no doubt even lower than that—remember that nerve damage can occur in normal, unmedicated vaginal birth, too; determining whether the epidural is to blame in a given case can be difficult, if not impossible.

What about the baby? Do the epidural medications her mother receives—all of which freely cross the placenta and can linger in a newborn's body for many hours—pose a direct threat to the newborn herself? Rarely, at least as far as life-threatening complications go. As I mentioned earlier, opioids can cause breathing difficulties in the newborn, but since the fetus gets his oxygen supply from his mother via the placenta rather than by breathing, this isn't a problem unless the dose is given close to delivery. Anesthesiologists and obstetricians are well aware of that risk, and tend to shy away from opioids as birth approaches. I only rarely see a newborn with respiratory problems caused by epidural medications, and when I do the difficulties are usually minor and temporary.

But epidural medications may cause subtler neonatal problems. Studies of newborn behavior in the early 1980s found differences between babies exposed to relatively high doses of medications and those born to unmedicated mothers—the "medicated" babies tended to be more irritable or sluggish in the hours after birth, and had more sleep difficulties. All the babies recovered completely, but it took some of them several days to do so. Other studies found that epidural-exposed babies had more difficulty with breast-feeding, particularly in the first postpartum day, and that they were weaned to formula at an earlier age than were "unmedicated" babies—perhaps because of lingering effects from those early troubles.

Obstetric anesthesia practice has changed considerably since the 1980s, of course, with technical improvements, lower doses, and new medications. Recent research often finds less neonatal effect from epidural medications, or none at all. Many of those studies have been criticized, though, for using less sensitive newborn assessment tools than was the case in the 1980s. To paraphrase the critics, you can't find subtle problems if you're not really looking for them. The issue of the direct effects of epidural medications on the fetus and newborn—including long-term effects, which remain largely unstudied—is far from settled. Much more research is on the way.

Epidural medications can definitely have indirect effects on the newborn, though. As mentioned above, maternal fever increases the chance of blood tests and antibiotics for the newborn. And, as we've seen, women with epidurals tend to have a somewhat longer second stage of labor, which increases the chance of a vacuum- or forceps-assisted birth. When performed properly, a vacuum is much safer for the baby than forceps, causing little trauma beyond scalp swelling, some minor bruising, or a cephalhematoma—a usually harmless collection of blood trapped between the scalp and the skull. In very rare cases, when more force than usual is needed to get the baby out (typically in a sudden, dire emergency unrelated to epidural use), more serious head injury can occur.

But I want to emphasize again that rare things happen rarely. When all the side effects are tallied, maternal epidural analgesia has proven safe for the vast majority of the tens of millions of babies whose mothers have employed it over the past several decades.

What's on the horizon in the pharmacologic treatment of labor pain? Nothing earth-shattering, it seems. Hospital-based labor pain management will be tied to the epidural for the foreseeable future, and most advances are in the tinkering-around-the-edges range rather than anything revolutionary.

The combined spinal-epidural block (CSE) has been gaining in popularity for several years. In a CSE, the anesthesiologist injects a small amount of an opioid medication directly into the subarachnoid space—the fluid-filled space that lies between the epidural space and the spinal cord—at the same time the epidural catheter is inserted. Pain relief from the opioid injection is immediate, compared with the twenty minutes a traditional epidural can take. And since numbness-inducing local anesthetics aren't pumped into the epidural space until the opioid injection has worn off later in labor, some women have a longer period of mobility, which gives the procedure its nickname: the "walking epidural."

That nickname is misleading. Many women can't walk after a combined spinal-epidural because of low blood pressure, wobbly legs, or hospital medical-legal concerns over potential falls. Anesthesiologists are experimenting with CSE in hopes of finding a combination of medications and techniques that will allow a woman to walk and change positions right up to the time of delivery, but for now the "walking" epidural is usually as nonwalking as a standard epidural.

One promising spin on the epidural is patient-controlled epidural analgesia (PCEA), which allows a woman to use a handheld control to increase or decrease the dose of her medications as her pain relief needs fluctuate throughout labor. PCEA has been shown to decrease the total amount of medication a woman uses (compared to when an anesthesiologist is repeatedly called to adjust the dose), which can help decrease the potential risk of breastfeeding difficulties and newborn behavioral changes. It also gives the laboring woman a sense of control over her pain management, which as we'll see increases her overall satisfaction with the birth experience. PCEA is catching on—about one-fourth of California hospitals offer it today, and the number is growing.

But that's about it. In most American hospitals the pharmacologic pain relief choices will continue to boil down to epidural or no epidural, with some opioids or local blocks tossed in for temporary relief.

Time for the final epidural scorecard. On the plus side of the ledger there's excellent pain relief, usually with little if any harm; on the minus side are the altered birth experience, the common minor discomforts such as shivering and itching, the fever and its implication for the newborn, the increased chance of an operative vaginal birth and potential injury to mother or child, the possible effects on newborn behavior and breast-feeding, and very, very rare tragedies.

My goal here isn't to talk women out of epidurals; rather, it's to open a conversation that will lead to an informed decision about labor pain management. I've been to enough deliveries, seen enough healthy babies, and talked with enough satisfied epidural customers to know that most of the time, women are glad they had one. But I've also heard from a lot of "second-guessers"—women who, after the fact, regretted the trapped-in-bed feeling, the loss of control of their bodies, the rush to ask for an epidural before thinking things through.

So, long before labor begins, a woman would do well to search her soul and ask, *What's most important to me?* Do I want to take on the challenge of climbing a drug-free Mount Everest or to avoid pain at all costs? Or do I want something in between? She should talk to women she trusts, to friends and relatives who've given birth with and without epidurals, and weigh the pros and cons for herself. Lastly, before signing up for an epidural, she should ask her doctor or midwife: *Is that all there is?*

II · Is That All There Is?

If the woman who opened this chapter went into labor while vacationing in Europe or Canada, she would find a more expanded set of pain relief options awaiting her. Hospitals outside the United States offer a broader range of both pharmacologic and nonpharmacologic treatments, and women use them with some success. The difference is philosophical as well as pharmacologic. Here at home the goal of hospital labor pain management is often the complete obliteration of pain; in Europe and elsewhere, particularly in countries like England, where most uncomplicated vaginal deliveries are performed by midwives, the objective is "good enough" pain relief.

"Good enough" labor analgesia is a concept that doesn't get much attention in the United States—most American women have never even heard of the expression—and I think it should. In our drive to eliminate pain we risk overlooking a critical fact: in the typical woman's experience, pain relief is far from the most important thing in determining her overall satisfaction with childbirth.

In fact, pain relief consistently ranks fourth in postpartum satisfaction surveys here and abroad, behind the quality of the relationship a woman has with her doctor or midwife, the support she receives from caregivers, and her involvement in making decisions regarding her care during labor. In other words, a completely pain-free birth can still be an unsatisfying one, a seeming paradox that baffled me early in my career, when I saw childbirth primarily in terms of the pain it so obviously caused. But by focusing too much on pain relief we can miss this age-old point: it's the simple human aspects of childbirth that actually make all the difference.

Epidurals and opioids are commonly used in hospitals in other Western countries, of course, but a woman laboring there will also be offered at least one pharmacologic alternative—inhaled nitrous oxide—and a host of nonpharmacologic interventions from aromatherapy to acupuncture. She's likely to accept one or more of them, too. Sixty-two percent of all British women who labored in 2000 used inhaled nitrous oxide for pain relief, and most used at least one nonpharmacologic pain relief method as well. Many received opioid injections, too, and nearly one-third ended up with epidurals, but compare those numbers to the American experience. Here in the United States, where more than 70 percent of women now give birth with an epidural, fewer than one in a hundred use nitrous oxide.

It's pretty clear that women outside the United States are successfully employing a variety of pain relief medications and treatments not readily available to most of their American counterparts. And in some areas the model of care is moving further away from the American standard—a hospital in London recently did away with opioid injections altogether, for example, using inhaled nitrous oxide as first line pain treatment, and then epidurals if stronger pain relief is needed.

The question, then: Why, in a consumer-choice-driven culture such as ours, are an American woman's labor pain management choices so starkly limited?

Nitrous oxide is an invisible gas with a slightly sweet taste and odor. It was first synthesized in 1775 by Joseph Priestly, the English pastor and chemist who discovered oxygen and carbon dioxide (and later invented the carbonated drink) when he heated a mixture of iron filings and nitric acid as part of his study of "airs," or gases. Unlike many who followed him, though, Priestly didn't experiment with inhaling his invention, known then and now by its more familiar nickname, "laughing gas."

Most Americans, if they encounter nitrous oxide at all, do so at the dentist's office. Nitrous oxide has been a mainstay in the dental bag of pain relief tricks since 1844, when a medical school dropout named Gardner Quincy Colton toured New England, knocking villagers loopy in a series of nitrous oxide "grand exhibitions." The exhibitions showcased both of nitrous's main effects on humans: analgesia and euphoria. Colton banked on the euphoria part. As a poster advertising one such program boasted, "The effect of the Gas is to make those who inhale it either Laugh, Sing, Dance, Speak or Fight, &c. &c."

Dr. Horace Wells, a Connecticut dentist, was so impressed with one of Colton's shows, during which an under-the-influence townsman badly gashed his leg on a chair but didn't notice the wound until the gas wore off, that he decided to put the alleged wonder drug to a very personal test. Shortly afterward, with Colton doing the gassing, Wells had one of his own molars painlessly extracted by another local dentist, and presto!—nitrous oxide's career as a dental painkiller was launched.

I had no such luck with my own childhood dentist. Dr. Wilson is seared in my memory as a tall, kindly man with a passion for ham radios and an unfortunate inability to get the correct tooth numb before drilling on it. He had plenty of opportunity to practice on me; by the time I finished high school I had about twice as many cavities as I had teeth. But more often than not Dr. Wilson's novocaine shot numbed the wrong tooth or paralyzed my lip, and I'd leave his office an hour later in a cold sweat, with an aching jaw and drool running down my chin. If Dr. Wilson ever heard of Horace Wells and his pain-killing gas, he wasn't letting on.

Fast-forward thirty-odd years. My son John, who regrettably inherited his father's soft enamel, love of sweets, and aversion to early childhood dental hygiene, came home from his eight-year-old dental checkup with five cavities. Elisabeth, who has had maybe one teensy cavity in her entire life, implied that this was my fault and nominated me to take John to get them filled.

Parked outside the dentist's office a week later, I tried to prepare John for what was to come: the long needle, the wrong tooth, the drool-stained shirt. I secretly hoped he'd learn the lesson I never did—brush 'em or suffer the consequences. But then a chirpy young dental assistant in Winnie-the-Pooh scrubs nestled John into a comfy recliner, fitted a small mask over his nose, and told him to take a few deep breaths. John sniffed. His eyelids drooped.

"Isn't that relaxing?" the assistant asked. John nodded dreamily. He lay there with a goofy grin on his face through the whole thing: the novocaine shot, the whining of the drill, the shiny fillings that the dentist placed one by one in his happy-to-be-here molars. When we got back to the car I asked him if he'd felt any pain. "A little bit," he said, lost in half-remembered reverie. "Mostly I was just trying not to giggle."

Sobersided Joseph Priestly may have limited his nitrous oxide work to the lab, but the famed British scientist Sir Humphry Davy (1778–1829) did not. Davy, whose accomplishments in the field of electrochemistry were so widely acclaimed that he was permitted to travel to Paris to receive a medal from Napoleon in the midst of war between England and France, apparently divided his time between experimenting with chemicals and eagerly inhaling the results.

Davy was particularly fond of nitrous oxide, which he promoted both as a surgical anesthetic agent and a recreational drug. Though not much of a poet, Davy was moved to pen an ode to his favorite gas: *"Yet are my eyes with sparkling lustre fill'd / Yet is my mouth replete with murmuring sound / Yet are my limbs with inward transports fill'd / And clad with new-born mightiness around."* Davy may well have been under nitrous's influence—sparkly-eyed, talkative, and feeling mighty—when he wrote it.

Nitrous has an impressive historical fan club. Winston Churchill experimented with it, as did Peter Mark Roget, the nineteenth-century author of that indispensable writer's tool, *Roget's Thesaurus*. The American physician and philosopher William James (1842–1910) wrote extensively of nitrous-induced euphoria, sometimes jotting down his impressions while in the act of inhaling it. One under-the-influence journal entry from 1882: "Medical school; divinity school, school! SCHOOL! Oh my God, oh God; oh God!"

The Beat writers of the 1950s—Kerouac, Cassady, Burroughs—were fond of nitrous, too; Allen Ginsberg even wrote a poem titled "Laughing Gas." And, lest we forget, it was nitrous oxide that inspired Uncle Albert to sing "I Love to Laugh" from his dining room ceiling in the 1964 movie version of *Mary Poppins*. This wasn't just a sly sixties drug reference; in P. L. Travers's original 1934 book, chapter 3 is titled "Laughing Gas."

On the more sober side of things, nitrous oxide has long been known as a moderately effective pain reliever, even before Gardner Quincy Colton's traveling exhibitions. Though nitrous has been largely displaced in medicine by more powerful agents, it's the only one of the original three inhaled anesthetic agents—chloroform and ether being the other two—that is still in use.

How nitrous relieves pain isn't exactly clear. The usual biochemical suspects—endorphins, dopamine, and such—are trucked out in any discussion of its effects, but nitrous oxide's ability to induce a "who cares?" attitude about pain may be as important as its analgesic properties. That's the effect John was describing on our drive home from the dentist's office. He felt a little pain as the needle went in, but with his nitrous mask fitted snugly to his nose, he just didn't care.

Nitrous oxide was introduced to obstetrics in 1881, but its popularity soared in the 1930s when the Liverpool anesthetist Ralph Minnitt introduced his "Gas and Air Machine," which allowed laboring women to self-administer a fixed dose of nitrous oxide whenever they felt they needed it. Much safer than the do-it-yourself chloroform dosing of James Simpson's era, nitrous soon became the European labor pain reliever of choice.

The story was the same in the United States, at least for a while. Nitrous was widely used in hospitals that did not have an anesthesiologist readily available to administer the riskier Twilight Sleep–type drugs. But the idea of self-administration didn't really catch on, and the need for a nurse or doctor to hold a mask over the mother's face with each contraction became impractical as the baby boom hit and maternity wards grew ever busier.

Nitrous use declined quickly with the appearance of two newer inhaled anesthetic agents: trichloroethylene (Trilene) in the early 1950s, and methoxyflurane (Penthrane) about a decade later. Both had the advantage of much longer lasting pain relief than nitrous and so didn't require the constant presence of a mask-holding attendant.

But Trilene and Penthrane eventually got into their own trouble. When Trilene was combined with certain general anesthetic agents, such as in an emergency cesarean performed on a woman who had been using Trilene in labor, toxic compounds resulted, including phosgene, better known by its World War I trench warfare nickname: mustard gas. Penthrane was supposed to be the answer to Trilene, but it was soon found to cause kidney problems with prolonged use. And Trilene and Penthrane both easily crossed the placenta, a significant worry at a time when the world was just awakening to the horrors of thalidomide.

The final nail in nitrous oxide's coffin was, of course, the epidural needle in a laboring woman's back. With demand for wide-awake birth increasing as the natural childbirth movement gained steam, women and their physicians increasingly turned away from drowsiness-inducing pain relievers, especially those that could cross the placenta and potentially harm the fetus. With not a whole lot else available in the anesthesiologist's bag of tricks, enthusiasm for epidural analgesia grew. Nitrous, condemned as a "drug" right along with most other "unnatural" pharmacologic interventions, virtually disappeared from hospital maternity wards. By the mid-1980s, only a handful of hospitals in the United States even offered it as an option.

The University of California, San Francisco (UCSF), is one of perhaps two or three hospitals on the West Coast that still offer nitrous oxide to their laboring patients. It is also exactly fifty miles south of my front door, so one late summer day in 2007 I drove down through Marin County and over the Golden Gate Bridge to meet with Dr. Mark Rosen, director of UCSF's obstetric anesthesia department and an unabashed supporter of nitrous oxide use in labor.

I had read several of Rosen's articles on nitrous oxide before our meeting, including a thorough review of the subject published in the *American Journal of Obstetrics & Gynecology* in 2002. Prior to that I had assumed that nitrous was gone from the labor and delivery unit with good reason—toxicity, maybe, or patient dissatisfaction—though its continued popularity in Europe was a bit puzzling to me. Did they know something over there that American doctors didn't, or were Europeans just clinging to an out-of-date therapy from habit?

According to Rosen's review, though, there really didn't seem to be any good explanation for nitrous oxide's disappearance from American labor rooms. It works, after all—it may not be the strongest analgesic around, but nitrous provides many women with "good enough" pain relief to get them through the hardest parts of having a baby. It works quickly, too. When inhaled in a fixed half-and-half mixture of nitrous and oxygen, it takes thirty seconds or so for the pain relief to kick in; when a woman stops inhaling it, the gas is completely gone from her system within a few breaths.

I met Dr. Rosen in the lobby of UCSF's Long Hospital, and together we took the elevator to the labor and delivery unit on the fifteenth floor. A soft-spoken man with a clear passion for his work, Rosen has been an advocate for nitrous oxide use since arriving at UCSF nearly three decades ago. In an unused labor room with a stunning view of downtown San Francisco beyond a grove of eucalyptus trees, he walked me through the use of nitrous oxide in labor.

The equipment seemed almost comically simple, especially when compared with the trappings of an epidural or a cesarean delivery. A small Nitronox machine, no bigger than a half-gallon milk carton, sat on a wheeled pole next to the labor bed. If the machine had been in use that afternoon—no one needed it on what was an unusually quiet day in the unit—it would have been connected to the wall by three supply hoses: one running to a blue socket labeled "nitrous," another to a green one marked "oxygen," and the third to a white "suction" outlet. A length of clear tubing led from the machine to a valve attached to an ordinary plastic face mask.

Here's how it's administered: when a contraction comes, the woman simply holds the mask over her own nose and mouth and breathes in. The force of her inspiration opens the valve and allows the Nitronox-mixed gas to flow to her. When she exhales into the mask, the suction tube "scavenges" the gas so that very little nitrous escapes into the room. In between contractions she can either continue to breathe the nitrous-oxygen mixture or take off the mask, which shuts off the flow of nitrous, and breathe room air until her pain returns. That's all there is to it. In between times she can walk, talk, bathe, change positions, and do whatever else eases her discomfort.

As enthusiastic as UCSF's doctors, midwives, and nurses are about nitrous, it isn't used as often as Rosen would like. He estimates that only about 5 to 10 percent of the women who pass through the labor and delivery unit use the Nitronox machine for their pain. That number would no doubt be much higher if UCSF weren't a tertiary referral center. Many of the mothers who deliver there are considered "high risk"—transferred from other hospitals because of complicated pregnancies or serious maternal or fetal health issues—who have more extensive pain relief needs than nitrous can provide.

Most of the women who do use nitrous at UCSF like it, though, and they often request it in subsequent deliveries. Those who don't like nitrous tend to be the small minority who feel claustrophobic with a face mask or who complain of side effects like dizziness, drowsiness, or the mildly detached "What, me worry?" feeling it can sometimes induce. (UCSF isn't running any Coltonesque "grand exhibitions," by the way; with the fifty-fifty mix of nitrous and oxygen, euphoria, if it occurs at all, is quite mild.)

The occasional dizziness, drowsiness, and such are about the only side effects that come from the use of nitrous oxide in labor. Because it exits the body so quickly in exhaled breath, nitrous doesn't accumulate in maternal tissues. And because a woman is required to administer it herself, there's no danger of an overdose. If she accidentally gives herself too much—shades of the do-it-yourself chloroform days of yore—her hand and the mask fall away. Two or three breaths later she's back to normal. In Rosen's experience even such temporary, harmless overdoses are extremely rare.

Nitrous appears to be safe for the fetus and baby as well. There are no known neonatal complications from its use. Though recent animal research has suggested that all general anesthetic agents, including nitrous oxide, may subtly damage developing brain cells when given in high doses over long periods of time, this seems extremely unlikely to be true of obstetric nitrous oxide use. With low doses and intermittent self-administration, a fetus is exposed to far less medication from maternal nitrous use than from an epidural, let alone general anesthesia. Nitrous doesn't affect a newborn's level of alertness or ability to breast-feed, as can opioids given too close to delivery. After nearly three decades of use at UCSF, Rosen says he has never seen a groggy baby from maternal inhalation of nitrous oxide. It just doesn't happen.

Nitrous is safe for the people who work with it, too. Though older studies had raised occupational health issues—a slightly increased chance of birth defects in pregnant labor and delivery staff—Rosen points out that those studies were badly flawed, and done with obsolete, nonscavenging equipment in labor rooms that lacked the kind of ventilation that's standard in modern hospitals. If those studies were repeated today, he believes, even that tiny risk would disappear. The Occupational Safety and Health Administration (OSHA) and the American Society of Anesthesiologists agree: neither organization feels that routine monitoring of health care personnel who work in properly equipped and ventilated hospital units is necessary.

One nagging issue is nitrous oxide's role in global warming. Nitrous is a potent greenhouse gas, many times more efficient in trapping heat than a comparable amount of carbon dioxide. Its contribution to the problem at present isn't certain—nitrous oxide is estimated to account for anywhere from a tenth of a percent of all greenhouse gases in the atmosphere to as much as 6 percent—and the vast majority of that comes from natural sources.

The primary man-made sources of atmospheric nitrous oxide are fossil fuel combustion (mainly at power plants), sewage treatment, nitrogen-containing fertilizers, and slash-and-burn agriculture. Less important but still significant sources include such varied human activities as worm farming, drag racing (it's a fuel booster for "nitro-burning funny cars," among other hot rods), and whipped cream squirting—nitrous is a commonly used propellant in the processed food industry. Obstetrical nitrous is clearly a very tiny part of the problem, and gas-scrubbing technology already in the works will likely eliminate even that small contribution in the not too distant future.

UCSF's highly positive nitrous experience is similar to that seen in European studies. In addition to the British experience I mentioned earlier, nearly half the women in Finland, Sweden, and Canada inhale nitrous oxide during labor as well, and over 80 percent of them feel that it was at least somewhat helpful. Though it is often not the only pharmacologic pain relief medication they choose—many also receive opioids and, ultimately, epidurals—the large majority rate nitrous favorably, and like their San Francisco counterparts, most want it for their next delivery, too.

So then why isn't nitrous more widely available in the United States? As we've seen, it's a moderately effective pain reliever, easy to administer, inexpensive, safe for mother and baby, and all the rage in most of the rest of the Western world. So why not here?

Some nitrous backers see a conspiracy of profit-hungry, epidural-pushing anesthesiologists behind nitrous oxide's baffling absence from the American childbirthing scene, but the real reason is probably much less sinister. Dr. Donald Caton, the dean of obstetric anesthesia historians, puts it this way: as epidurals muscled their way past inhaled analgesics onto the nation's maternity wards, nitrous oxide more or less got lost along the way.

It's high time to bring it back. But how? With no financial incentive—there is rarely a push from pharmaceutical companies to revive a dirt-cheap medication—and lacking any pregnant "A-list" celebrities to tout its wonders, resuscitating nitrous oxide in the United States sounds like a tough task. But it just may happen.

Enter Judith Rooks, midwife, epidemiologist, teacher, author, and the leader of a growing movement to restore nitrous oxide to the American way of birth. In a 2007 editorial published in the journal *Birth,* Rooks challenged U.S. midwives and midwifery instructors to educate themselves about nitrous and advocate for its return. She likened nitrous to other, older "orphan" drugs—"little known . . . lacking 'pizazz,' " as she described it, "with no companies or professional groups that stand to profit by its greater use." Hence the need for a push from within the profession itself.

Rooks extends her challenge to natural childbirth advocates, too, calling on them to reconsider their reluctance to endorse drugs of any kind. Nitrous isn't a narcotic, she points out, and it's the only pharmacologic choice for labor pain relief that allows a woman complete control of how and when it's used. Nitrous offers the woman who wants a drug-free birth an alternative—should the intensity of her pain lead her to the point of asking for a pharmacologic pain reliever—to what Rooks calls the "evolving epidural monoculture" of American hospital birth.

Rooks has a keen sense of irony. Here in a country that prides itself on autonomy and informed choice, she notes, and even as the obstetrical world debates the "ethical imperative" of a woman's right to choose a cesarean birth without medical need for one, American women lack the basic ability to choose something as obviously helpful and harmless as nitrous oxide. Stay tuned.

Time for the flip side of things. If 70 percent of American women give birth with the help of an epidural, then by definition 30 percent—over a million women a year—do not. Many of these women get temporary relief with injected opioids or local anesthetic injections, but many others choose to give birth with no pharmacologic help at all. What, then, is available in the United States for the woman who wants a completely drug-and-epidural-free birth? How is a woman in that steadily shrinking demographic supposed to cope with her labor pain?

Drug-free pain relief methods and techniques come in a bewildering variety. Popular methods (and this list is by no means exhaustive) include acupuncture, acupressure, hydrotherapy, hypnosis, massage or "healing touch," maternal movement and repositioning, music therapy, aromatherapy, mind-body techniques, herbal treatments, homeopathic preparations, hot and cold therapy, chiropractic adjustments, electrical stimulation, flower remedies, reflexology, water birth, and yoga. Then there are the natural childbirth methods, which, though not necessarily focused on pain relief per se, often incorporate one or more nonpharmacologic analgesic methods. These methods are usually named for their founders, some of them more familiar than others: Dick-Read, Lamaze, Bradley, Leboyer, Gamper, Odent, Kitzinger, and others.

The availability of any of these "alternative" labor pain treatments is limited both by where a laboring woman lives and where she chooses to have her baby. It's no doubt easier to find a labor hypnotist in a large city than in an isolated rural area, for example, and a midwife who performs a home birth is more likely to offer alternative pain relief options than one who works under the direct supervision of an obstetrician in a busy hospital. And it bears repeating that most nonpharmacologic labor pain relief methods are far more readily available in Europe and Canada than they are in the United States.

Each of these methods and techniques has been the subject of rapturous books, pamphlets, and websites, generating a stream of enthusiastic anecdotes from mothers and practitioners but precious little hard research. Proponents passionately swear by their method of choice, and often rage in disbelief that the medical world refuses to adopt them as standard practice. Doctors, for their part, want to see some evidence before they recommend nonpharmacologic treatments to their patients. So which ones have been shown to actually work?

Penny Simkin, a physical therapist and renowned childbirth educator, and Dr. MaryAnn O'Hara, a professor of family medicine at the University of Washington, surveyed the nonpharmacologic research landscape in an article that appeared in 2002 in the *American Journal of Obstetrics & Gynecology*—the same issue in which Mark Rosen's nitrous oxide paper appeared. They reviewed dozens of research articles on the five best-studied methods: baths, touch and massage, maternal movement and repositioning, intradermal water injections, and continuous labor support. Their findings: all five of the methods seemed to help reduce pain, some more clearly than others. Their review also showed how difficult it can be to study pain relief methods, especially those that don't involve a measured dose of medicine.

The randomized controlled trial, or RCT, is the "gold standard" in medical research. In an RCT, patients are randomly placed in either a "treatment" or a "control" group. The treatment group then receives a new medication or other intervention for the condition under study—high blood pressure, say, or perhaps how quickly an infection resolves—while the control group may receive the current standard practice, a placebo treatment (the proverbial "sugar pill"), or no treatment at all. Ideally, the study is "double-blinded"— neither the patients nor the researchers know who's in which group, which helps eliminate bias and conflicts of interest. At the end of the study period the blinders come off and the patients in the treatment group are compared to those in the control group in terms of how well the intervention worked.

There are several obstacles to performing RCTs on labor pain treatments, not the least of which is the highly subjective nature of labor pain. Still, studying a pharmacologic treatment like epidural analgesia is made easier by the fact that one major variable is controlled: the medication dose can be precisely measured. Although the response to the medication may vary from woman to woman, researchers know exactly how much of which drug was injected, and given a large enough study, its effectiveness can be fairly well determined.

Compare that with trying to study an alternative, nonpharmacologic method like touch. Simkin and O'Hara found three surveys of touch and massage (sometimes referred to as "healing touch") that involved a total of only 230 women, and one small, nonblinded RCT. It's easy to understand why researchers would have a hard time assessing the effectiveness of touch. A woman in labor is touched by any number of people, from nurses, doctors, and midwives to family and friends. The types of touch, and the meaning of those touches, can be almost infinitely variable.

A true RCT would assign one group of women to receive a certain type of touch or massage, presumably administered by a trained therapist to eliminate variability in "dose," while a control group would receive whatever touch came their way in the course of giving birth. It would no doubt take a very large study to clearly demonstrate the pain reduction benefits of a specific form of touch or massage, and a research team would have to decide whether confirming what seems to be common sense is really worth the time and energy. Most women I've observed in labor actively seek out touch from loved ones, and it usually seems to help.

The one RCT in Simkin and O'Hara's review that looked at the issue found that women who were massaged by their partners "had significant emotional and physical relief, as reported by the women themselves, and assessed by their partners and a blinded observer." Given that gentle touch and massage have no conceivable side effects—the risk of an accidental strangling seems pretty remote—isn't that enough?

Intradermal water injections, on the other hand, have been shown in well-designed RCTs to reduce back pain during labor. The technique is simple: one-tenth of a milliliter of sterile water is injected into a woman's skin at several sites on her lower back. Women report noticeable reduction in back pain for up to two hours afterward and there are no side effects, except for the thirty seconds or so of stinging that follow injection.

How sterile water injections actually work isn't known, but they may block transmission of pain signals to the brain from deeper tissues in the lower back, or cause beta-endorphins, the body's natural painkillers, to be released near the spinal cord. Whatever the case, since the injections don't do much for abdominal pain from uterine contractions, the studies showed no decrease in overall use of other pain medication. Still, for women with back pain in labor, sterile water injections can provide significant temporary relief.

The idea of seeking relief in a tub of warm water during labor makes intuitive sense—a bath is a traditional remedy for aches and pains of all kinds. In the studies that Simkin and O'Hara reviewed, many women reported baths to be soothing and relaxing, in addition to providing them with a sense of personal control and at least some pain relief. A bath is low tech, highly satisfying, and easily administered. What could possibly go wrong?

Plenty, it turns out, but fortunately the side effects associated with labor baths are easily avoidable. Women who take baths in early labor, for instance, may actually slow down their uterine contractions and prolong labor. This effect can be chalked up to a simple fact of obstetrical physics: pregnant bellies float.

When a laboring woman climbs into a bath, the refreshing buoyancy she feels sets off a chain of physical and hormonal events. As her muscles relax, her catecholamine levels—the "fight or flight" hormones that rise in labor—decrease. This can actually help her labor progress, as excessive levels of catecholamines are known to slow down uterine contractions.

But countering that lowered-catecholamine labor boost is the effect that water pressure has on other maternal hormones. When a mother sinks deep into a tub, the weight of the water on her body forces fluid contained in her tissues into her bloodstream, thus increasing her blood volume. Sounds like a good idea—increased blood volume means increased cardiac output and oxygen-carrying capacity, and oxygen is a good thing to have coursing through your arteries when you're trying to have a baby.

But the weight of the water on a woman's body also causes a "pooling" effect in the blood vessels inside her chest, because the rib cage protects the lungs from the water-pressure squeeze exerted on the softer tissues of the limbs and abdomen. Over time this leads to a complicated hormonal chain reaction that results in decreased secretion of oxytocin, the uterine-contraction hormone, from the pituitary gland within the brain. With less oxytocin circulating than before she climbed in the tub, a woman's labor can slow down significantly.

The labor-slowing effect of taking a bath seems to be a problem only if the bath is taken early in labor, though. Once a woman is in active labor, the oxytocin surges are strong enough that no bath in the world can derail them. The exact stage of labor at which this happens isn't clear from current research, but it seems prudent to hold off on baths until the cervix has dilated to about five centimeters.

Other concerns about labor baths have been satisfactorily addressed. Baths do not increase the risk of infection for mother or child, and so long as the water is kept at or slightly below body temperature, there's no risk of overheating either mother or fetus.

But does a bath really relieve pain? The short answer—yes, but not for long—seems to agree with most people's experience with the effects of warm water on their own sore muscles. Three well-designed studies using "one-to-ten" pain scales found that women experienced temporary pain relief during the bath, but the effect subsided quickly once the bath was over. A fourth study found no difference in the overall use of epidurals and other pharmacologic pain relievers, though whether or not a woman ended up with an epidural is a pretty crude measure of how soothing a short bath may have been several hours before.

There's still research needed on such arcana as the proper depth and temperature of the water and the optimal frequency and length of baths, but it seems clear that baths should be available to laboring women as one component of pain management.

Back in the opening chapter I told the story of George Engelmann, the nineteenth-century St. Louis obstetrician who, puzzling over the wisdom of having women lie flat on their backs to give birth, did the first extensive cross-cultural study of "optimal" labor positions. In the end he gave up, concluding that whatever position a woman chose was probably the best one for her. Later research showed that upright positions, particularly squatting, enlarged the birth canal significantly and helped labor progress more quickly.

So changing positions helps labor to progress, but does it directly relieve labor pain? Once again, Simkin and O'Hara reviewed every research study available on the subject and found, like Engelmann, that women in labor like to walk, move, and change positions frequently. Unlike Engelmann's observations, however, in the modern studies only a small number of women actually chose either to walk or to assume an upright position. This difference speaks more to the impact of cultural conditioning than actual preferences. Staff routines and the central location of the bed in the delivery room can send a strong message to laboring women: stay put. But in other studies, in which women were encouraged to get up and move, and there was plenty of room to do so and a variety of furniture in the room, they willingly walked and assumed a number of positions.

Assessing what women did during labor is one thing; whether all that movement actually decreased their pain is quite another. When all was said and done, Simkin and O'Hara wrote, "it is difficult to interpret the results." Reading the details of the studies, it's not hard to see why. In some of them, women were expected to stay in one position for long periods; in others they were told to change positions on a rigid schedule. It didn't work. Ninety percent of the women assigned to specific positions in one study took a *the-hell-with-that!* approach and dropped out, opting for more comfortable positions than the researchers had planned for them.

Observers who assessed pain intensity revealed their own biases, too—one nurse-observer rated every woman studied as having "very high" comfort levels throughout all stages of labor, no matter what position she was in. And constantly asking for pain reassessments might actually have worsened the pain for some women, since distraction techniques and focusing on something other than the pain—hard to do with a pesky researcher in your face—are frequently employed coping techniques.

Much as George Engelmann did a century and a half before them, Simkin and O'Hara found that movement and position changes during labor "do not seem to lend themselves to regulation and rigorous scientific inquiry." The issue of labor position and overall pain relief remains unresolved, at least from a research point of view. But with no evidence that lying flat on the back is beneficial to labor, nor that moving around causes any harm, Simkin and O'Hara concluded that women should be allowed to labor in positions they find most comfortable.

The last of the five nonpharmacologic methods that Simkin and O'Hara examined is continuous labor support, defined as continuous nonmedical care of the laboring woman: providing physical and emotional support, giving nonmedical advice and explanations of the birth process, and facilitating communication with the medical staff.

Continuous labor support is nothing new. Prior to the twentieth century, when the "medicalization" of childbirth drove nonmedical personnel from the labor room, women were attended not only by midwives or doctors, but by supportive, experienced female companions as well. The companion was usually a family member or friend who focused on the laboring woman's immediate needs: fluffing her pillows, fetching cool drinks, holding her hand, and such.

Continuous labor support is a simple concept—the support person stays with the woman throughout labor, and usually for some time after birth as well—and it is strikingly effective. In several North American studies, continuous labor support was associated with a decreased need for pain medications, including epidurals, and has never been shown to cause any harm. Because its benefits extend well beyond the issue of pain relief, I'll discuss continuous labor support and the history of birth attendance at greater length in chapter 7.

Other nonpharmacologic methods have been studied, too, though with less clear results. Some of them show promise, including acupuncture, hypnosis, and transcutaneous electrical nerve stimulation (TENS), which involves the use of mild, continuous electrical current to block labor pain sensation, but they haven't been studied enough to be sure how beneficial they really are. The currently available scientific literature on the pain relief benefits of acupressure, aromatherapy, relaxation and breathing, hot and cold therapy, childbirth education, and music therapy is either too sketchy or the findings are too variable to draw conclusions.

Acupuncture is a good case in point, again showing the difficulty of doing labor pain research. In traditional Chinese medicine, pain is thought to be caused by a stagnation of *Qi*, or life energy. Acupuncture, which involves penetration of the skin with very thin needles at specific points on the body, alleviates pain by manipulation of the needles to produce a sensation of tingling, numbness, or heaviness known as *de qi*.

Acupuncture is widely used during labor in Europe—more than half of the Swedish midwives responding to a survey of labor pain management practices in 2006 said they routinely used acupuncture and felt that it was invaluable. However, when the investigators looked at *how* the midwives were giving acupuncture, they found most of them weren't doing it right.

A key tenet of acupuncture is that the needles must be manipulated, either by twirling, by burning herbs on the end of the needle, or, in modern times, by sending an electrical current through the needle, in order to stimulate *de qi*. Many of the midwives in the Swedish survey simply inserted the needles and then left them alone. Yet, in testimony heard time and again with just about anything that has been used to help alleviate labor pain, most of the women who delivered with such quasi-acupuncture felt it really helped.

The bottom line: pain is in the eye, or body, of the pained. If a woman says that a bath, a massage, or badly done acupuncture gives her relief during labor, then it does. In absence of any real side effects, it makes sense to provide women with a wide variety of nonpharmacologic therapies to choose from.

"What would you do if this were your own child?" That's a question familiar to any pediatrician. It often comes up in my own practice in the course of discussing vaccines or antibiotics, say, or whether to go ahead with an elective operation. After I've laid out the science and added up the pros and cons of the treatment for parents, it's sometimes the deciding question: What would I do with my own kid?

So, fair enough: What would I tell Claire about all this? What advice would I give her about pain relief, about epidurals and baths and such, when she approaches her first labor?

First of all, I hope the discussion is a few years off, since Claire is still in high school as I write this. By the time she gets around to starting a family, things could be quite different in the world of labor pain relief. Maybe someone will invent a highly specific analgesic pill between now and then, one that targets only the nerves that transmit labor pain impulses to the brain and doesn't block the ones that keep your legs from going all noodly. Or an as yet undiscovered rainforest herb will turn up to do the trick. Or maybe by then men will be giving birth themselves and Claire and I can just skip the whole thing.

Most likely the pain relief options available to Claire will be pretty much what they are now. Doctors will tend to recommend epidurals, midwives will push for more natural, less invasive alternatives, and everyone from homeopaths to hypnotists will try to make their voices heard in the swirling debate over the "best" way to handle a pain that is so subjective and individualized that it will forever defy one-size-fits-all treatment. What's a young woman facing the most intense day of her life to do?

A lot depends on where Claire is in her life at that point. To date she's been pretty lucky, painwise. No surgeries, no major accidents, not even any cuts bad enough to need stitches. (Her brother, John, is the family crash-and-burn specialist.) With the exception of some nasty migraines and a headfirst collision with the side of our neighbor's pool years ago—lots of blood, not much actual injury—Claire's personal experience with pain is fairly limited. It's safe to say that, barring any unwelcome changes, labor will be the biggest pain challenge of her life.

So my first bit of fatherly advice to Claire will be to learn all she can about what's coming. She'll probably beat me to the punch; Claire has been intensely curious about childbirth since she was very young. (At age four she had an *Aha!* moment: "I get it! The mommy's bottom opens up like a butterfly net and—boom!—the baby falls out!") She'll probably start hitting the childbirthing books as soon as she sees the little pink plus sign on her pregnancy test strip.

I'll suggest, too, that she read up on every kind of pain relief treatment, pharmacologic and not, from epidurals and nitrous oxide to warm baths and acupuncture. I'll want her to go with what makes sense to her, to find out what's available in the place where she lives and talk both to the people who provide those treatments and to the women who've used them.

I'll want her to visit the hospitals and birthing centers near her, to find a midwife or obstetrician who makes her feel completely comfortable, and who in turn is comfortable with Claire's plans for her delivery. Her relationship with the person who will deliver her baby will be, as we've seen, a key to a satisfying birth experience.

Which brings me to another hard-earned bit of advice I'll give her: be flexible. Nothing ever goes exactly as planned in childbirth. Labors go faster or slower than expected, for example, and fetuses can be bigger than anticipated or come down the birth canal in awkward positions. And in the end, having a baby may simply hurt a lot more (or less) than Claire expects. Labor pain is a dynamic process, waxing and waning, changing in character, building to an intense peak and then, finally, ending. Rigid plans work best if you're building a skyscraper; with something as mysteriously human as giving birth, it's best, both literally and figuratively, to keep your knees bent.

Finally, and most important of all, I will tell Claire—and any other woman approaching the birth of her child—to gather the people she loves around her. Because when all is said and done, when the pushing and pulling are over, when the massages have ended and the epidural or acupuncture needles are put away, she will find it was the people there with her during labor—and those who waited by the phone for news—who were her biggest source of comfort. And unlike other labor pain relievers she may choose, their benefits will last the rest of her life.

PART III
Significant Others

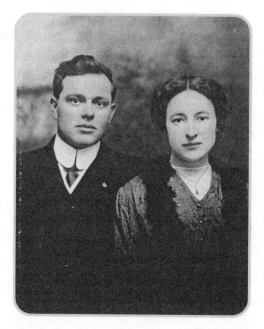

My paternal grandparents, John Henry Sloan and
Ellen Drusilla Colgan, wedding photograph, 1914

Chapter 6
Daddies

My grandfather Sloan was a farmer. He didn't have much in common with the Rockefeller and Roosevelt men of his time, but there was this: none of them was ever expected to be a labor coach.

Like most American men who had their children prior to the 1970s, my grandfather's knowledge of human childbirth was sketchy, and in his case extrapolated from observations of barnyard animals. He really didn't need to know any more than that. When birthing time came, my grandmother sent him into town to fetch the midwife and then shooed him back out to the fields, just like any other day. Sooner or later, while he was planting or harvesting, the baby arrived. That, in sum, was my grandfather's childbirth experience.

My father, Barney Sloan, confirms this by way of explaining his own inexperience with the birthing of babies. He remembers clearly the 1927 arrival of his baby sister, Mary Ellen, when he was eight years old. On a blustery March morning, the town midwife—a tiny, neat German woman with the ethnically improbable name of Auntie Beauregard—stepped down from my grandfather's sputtering Model T and promptly took over the house. She sent my grandfather back to the farm work, and then pointed Dad and his twelve-year-old brother, Nick, to the kitchen table. They were to sit and wait for orders, she said, and there was to be no talking or noisemaking. My grandmother had already retired to the small bedroom adjacent to the kitchen, the room in which she gave birth to all of her children and where, a half century later, she would die.

Auntie Beauregard bustled between kitchen and bedroom with practiced, almost military precision. She boiled pots of water on the coal-burning stove, hauling them into the bedroom past the two wide-eyed boys. "I didn't know what she was doing in there," my father recalls of those long hours of waiting. "But whatever it was, it needed steam."

The house was silent except for the crackling fire and bubbling pots. Auntie spoke only when something was needed—a terse order for more water, or corncob kindling for the fire—and the boys nearly trampled each other in complying, grateful for something to do.

From time to time the screen door swung open. Grandpa would pull up a chair across from Dad and Nick, then fold his hands and close his eyes. Seeing him there on one of her kitchen excursions, Auntie Beauregard would beckon him into the living room—never the bedroom—for a progress report. Then Grandpa would emerge, his jaw set, and with a quick nod to his sons head out the door and back to the endless chores of the farm. "Be helpful," he admonished the boys.

Late in the afternoon Auntie's routine broke. She made straight for the kitchen table and pulled Nick up by the arm. "Go get your father," she said in a stern voice. "Tell him it is almost time." Nick sprinted out the kitchen door, down the front steps, and across the yard to the horse barn. A minute later he was back, trotting behind his long-striding father.

Grandpa followed Auntie into the living room. The door closed. When he returned to the kitchen his face was tense; this time he didn't go back outside. A silent hour passed. My grandfather sat straight in his chair, eyes closed, arms folded across his chest. When at last the sound of a baby's cry came from the bedroom, he smiled and clapped his hands, just once, then recrossed his arms and waited. Soon Auntie Beauregard called him into the bedroom to see his daughter. A while later the boys were allowed a peek at their new sister. A half hour after that my grandfather was out in the fields again, this time with his sons in tow. "And for years that's how I thought you had babies," my father says today, nicely summing up the male childbirth experience for most of recorded history. "You boiled water and you waited."

Dad went on to have seven kids of his own, five of them in the 1950s. A sire-to-be's job description hadn't changed much in the three decades since he and Nick had watched Auntie Beauregard go about her mysterious work. The scene was different—Dad was a city dweller by the time I arrived, and most babies were born in hospitals by then—but fathers still operated on childbirth's fringes. "My job was to fetch your mother's orange Popsicles and Grape-Nuts"—her food cravings—"and make sure that she got to the hospital on time," he recalls. His responsibilities ended at the hospital door, and that was fine with him. "I wouldn't have had any idea what to do after that," he says, with the wide-eyed look of a man who has narrowly avoided a gruesome traffic accident.

I was born in Dubuque, Iowa, on March 18, 1953. My parents lived high on a hill in a rented half of an old stucco mansion, just a few blocks from the Mississippi River. It was a spooky place. Bats nested in the attic, and Dad kept a tennis racket handy to whack any that flapped into the living quarters. Over the north side of the hill was downtown Dubuque, and Rooster Mills, the feed grain plant where Dad worked. On the south side, one steep block down, was Mercy Hospital.

My mother's pregnancy was not going well. She had endured her usual three months of morning sickness, and by the end she was suffering from high blood pressure. The worst part was the severe swelling that came with her condition. "I was swollen everywhere you could be swollen," she remembers. She switched from shoes to slippers a couple of weeks before my birth.

My grandmother Sloan had come to Dubuque from the farm a couple of weeks before my expected arrival to help wrestle my older brothers—three-year-old Bernard and seventeen-month-old Steve—into bath and bed while Mom rested her ever puffier legs.

My grandfather, consistent to the end, stayed home and worked the farm. The go-and-fetch position was already ably filled by Dad, he must have figured. What was there for another man to do?

Two days before I was born, Dad packed Mom and her suitcase into the Pontiac and took the half-minute drive down to Mercy. Her blood pressure had gotten out of control. The doctor had called my parents that morning: if Mom's labor didn't start after a couple of days of bed rest, he said, he'd give her some medicine and start it for her.

Dad parked in front of Mercy's front door, fetched a wheelchair from inside, and carted Mom to the admitting desk. An immaculate white-uniformed nurse took over from there. Dad kissed my mother good-bye, watched her disappear around a corner, and then climbed back into the Pontiac. He drove up the hill to his bat-filled half-mansion where Gram waited with the boys. Two days later he was back at Mercy, holding a card that said "Sloan" up to the nursery window, waiting for a nurse to notice him and bring me around for a first look. Dad's childbirthing work was done.

Even if my father had wanted to attend my birth, everything in 1950s America conspired against him. Childbirth had become fully "medicalized" by the middle of the twentieth century. Maternity wards were sterile steel-and-chrome monuments to a kind of progress that had no room for gawking dads. A phalanx of starchy, hard-bitten nurses guarded the gates. There'd be no men in their kingdom, except for the doctors, of course, who were the real kings. Births were planned to fit into the royal schedule. My mother's induction was originally intended for March 17, and what a glorious birthday that would have been in my Irish Catholic family. But my birth was put off a day because the obstetrician—Dr. Storck, no less—had a social engagement he did not want to miss.

Even if Dad had been of a mind to force his way into the labor room, what would he have done there? Whom could he have turned to as a role model? Certainly not his own father, busily slopping the hogs back home. Not his brother Nick, whose own wife was midway through a gaggle of six children, born in military hospitals around the world while he moved up the ranks in a distinguished army career. Not a single man my father knew—none of his relatives, neighbors, or old army buddies—ever attended the birth of his own child. Popular culture, the movies, and nascent television programs were no help. The prevailing image of new fatherhood in 1950s America wasn't that of an attentive labor coach. It was Ricky Ricardo going nuts.

Two months before I was born, CBS aired an episode of *I Love Lucy* titled "Lucy Goes to the Hospital." The show ran live, and the plot paralleled real life for Lucille Ball and Desi Arnaz: their son, Desi Junior, was born a few hours after the broadcast ended.

The action begins in the Ricardos' New York apartment, where a dreamy Lucy announces to Ricky that "it" is about to happen. The show ends with Ricky, dressed in blackface, fangs, and a voodoo fright wig, passed out on the nursery floor. In between there's a snooty nurse, a fainting spell, a conga number, and a cop with a gun. Ah, the miracle of midcentury childbirth.

That scene—minus the gun, the cop, the fainting, and the voodoo makeup—was my father's experience at my birth, too. And it was his father's, and maybe that of all the fathers in my direct ancestral line back to Cro-Magnon times and beyond. In hospitals, farmhouses, caves, and jungle clearings, Sloan men did what a father was supposed to do: they hauled the water, fetched the Popsicles, and stayed the hell out of the way.

Thirty-seven years later, it was my turn. After five years of trying for a baby of our own, Elisabeth sat me down the day after the 1989 San Francisco earthquake and said, "Look, if you think yesterday was a jolt . . ." And just like that I was launched onto the path so well trodden by millions of men before me. I was going to be a father. A pleasant fuzzy-headed sensation descended, mixed with just a whiff of panic. I had dreamed of that moment for a long time, but I hadn't given a lot of thought to what came next. Reality hit quickly as we held hands and talked: What was I supposed to do now?

The role of the American father-to-be had changed radically since the day my father coasted down the hill to Mercy Hospital with my mother and the unborn me on board. Anthropologist William Kunst-Wilson hit the nail on the head when he wrote in 1981 that in one short generation a father's role had morphed from "an unnecessary source of infection, to an essential source of affection, for both mother and newborn." In a blink of biological time, fathers had come in from their wheat fields and waiting rooms and entered that most female of sanctuaries: the birthing room. Attendance was expected—nearly required by the time fatherhood rolled around for me—but what was expected of a father while he attended the birth of his child was still a bit murky.

It was an awkward, often difficult transition. Role models were still scarce. There weren't many books written for expectant fathers in the 1970s and '80s, and the printed advice that was available tended to echo the role of the father from ages past. Be supportive. Rub her back. Stay the hell out of the way.

I had been a pediatrician for a decade when Elisabeth gave me the news that morning. Observing scores of fathers in action had given me pause to think about what kind of labor room dad I wanted to be. I considered and rejected such roles as the Fascist Dad ("Push, dammit!"), the Why-Am-I-Here? Dad ("You'd think for what we're paying we'd at least get a TV with a remote"), and the Clueless Dad (the unfortunate fellow who, when his wife asked for pain medication, clapped his hand over her mouth and said, "We've already decided this. You know it doesn't hurt that bad." Her reply, once she had ripped his hand away: "How the hell would *you* know?!" He spent the rest of the delivery huddled in a chair, deflated).

There were many other men whose labor room shoes I did not want to fill. I most especially did not want to end up like the legendary Running Dad, a first-time expectant father who lived in Chicago in the mid-1970s. When the call came that his wife was in labor, he leaped up from his office desk and sprinted the mile to the hospital. He burst onto the maternity ward with a bellow, then slipped on the newly waxed floor, skidded face-first past a knot of startled nurses, and crashed into the side of a medicine cart, splitting open his forehead and knocking himself unconscious. He awoke in the emergency room, only to learn that his wife and child weren't there. He had run to the wrong hospital. The man was reunited with his wife and new son later that afternoon in the right maternity ward, where he became the butt of a thousand jokes for everyone involved in the delivery of babies.

I was a medical student during the Running Dad's brief period of notoriety, completing the same two-month obstetrics rotation that had unceremoniously introduced me to Tonya and the wonders of childbirth. I didn't know the Running Dad's real name, and neither did any of the staff I worked with that summer. When pressed, they'd admit that they weren't sure whether the man's wrong-way run had happened this year or last, nor which hospitals were actually involved. And the details of the story varied with the teller. In one version the man fainted in front of the hospital, clad only in his underwear. In another he'd run to the right hospital but burst onto the wrong ward, passing out in front of a surprised operating room team in the middle of an appendectomy.

I laughed right along with the obstetrics staff with each telling of the Running Dad's cross-town sprint. Like all medical students, I was beginning to absorb the tough-as-nails, seen-it-all mannerisms of new doctors everywhere. Had I heard the one about the dad who chained himself to his wife's bed so they couldn't make him leave? How about the guy who wanted morphine for his *own* labor pains? *Oh, yeah*, I'd snicker with the practiced cynicism of the truly inexperienced. *What a bunch of nuts!*

By the end of my rotation the Running Dad had passed into the realm of urban legend. And like most urban legends—the alligators lurking in the sewer systems of every large American city, for example—there was just enough about the story to make it believable. New father, wrong hospital, general new-dad goofiness—if it didn't happen then and there, it no doubt did happen somewhere else, some other time, with some other baby.

By the time I became an expectant father myself, though, I saw the Running Dad in a different, more sympathetic light. I'd watched enough men go through that particular passage to realize how hard a job it really is, freighted with tension, fear, and often unrealistic expectations.

I was determined to be a Perfect Dad, a Helpmate Dad, the kind of Dad who wouldn't draw too much attention from the nurses or blaze any new urban legend trails. I would read up on labor coaching. I'd attend every prenatal class, maybe twice. I vowed to fetch Elisabeth's Popsicles and Grape-Nuts, or whatever she needed, and get her to the hospital—the right one—at the right time. And I would definitely be on the lookout for newly waxed floors.

Every expectant father goes a bit nuts. This is particularly true of first-time dads. It may be as subtle as a quaver in his voice or as operatic as a mid-delivery swoon, but anyone watching a brand-new father-to-be in a maternity ward can tell at a glance: the boy's not right.

The transformation starts early. From the moment a man learns of his partner's pregnancy he can feel his old, comfortable world slipping away. Just a year ago, he and his bride were sipping champagne in a Honolulu honeymoon suite. Now she's either walking around in a dreamy daze or throwing up in the sink. What happened to their perfect world, he wonders? Where did his love go?

If he gets the feeling that some strange and alien force has carried his wife away, he's not far off the mark. Before he's even aware of the tiny third party now intruding on his love life, she's already a goner. The monthly hormonal ebbs and flows he has more or less learned to anticipate have been hijacked. She is now in the service of the little being growing inside her, a mini-tyrant who hijacks food and oxygen, makes her nauseous for weeks on end, and steals the lion's share of the attention that she once showered on him.

And it just gets worse. There are doctor appointments and baby showers to come, and avalanches of books and "helpful" advice from friends, relatives, and total strangers. Not to mention those ten thousand baby names to sift through, only one of which will be the right one, and it's probably not either of his first choices, Bambi and Thor.

His whole world has been turned on its head, and no matter how much he may be looking forward to little Thor's arrival, it's not surprising that he feels a bit out of sorts. What *is* surprising is the explanation for that feeling: just like his wife, our soon-to-be dad is a victim of runaway hormones.

Men know all about women and hormones, or at least they think they do. The basics are laid out in junior high science class—there's estrogen and there's progesterone, two hormones locked in a monthly up-and-down duel that ends with a period or, if everyone isn't careful about things, a baby. Boy hormones are much simpler. Good old testosterone takes off at adolescence and rockets through a man's veins till the end of his days. Straightforward stuff; none of this bleeding and cycling business. Why can't women be more like men, a young (male) student might ask? Biology tests would be a lot easier.

Men acquire a working knowledge of the behavioral effects of female hormones from a lifetime of living among women—mothers and sisters at first, later girlfriends and spouses. A man in a committed relationship might learn that at certain times of the month he is the most desirable of mates, a true gem of a human being. At others he'd be better off freezing on the north slope of Everest, far from a mate in the throes of plummeting estrogen levels. It is a monthly cycle that becomes predictable, if not necessarily comprehensible.

But by the time a man finds out that he's going to be a daddy, those cycles are already over. His beloved and her hormones have been overrun. Under the direction of the ever more demanding fetus, levels of progesterone, a hormone key to a pregnancy's early survival, rise nearly twentyfold. Estrogen and its hormonal relatives rise even more dramatically: blood estriol concentrations rise by a factor of a thousand. Not satisfied with simply jacking up existing hormone production, the fetus (and placenta) produce completely new hormones, chemicals that the mother's body has never before seen.

The primary reason for this hormone hijacking is to ensure that a mother's body becomes a safe, nourishing, fetus-friendly environment. By the end of pregnancy, this roiling hormonal stew will produce an astounding variety of effects, from altering a woman's sense of smell to stimulating her appetite, from blunting her response to stress to decreasing the pain of labor and delivery. A pregnant woman owes her larger breasts, extra fat, and those puffy last trimester ankles to hormones. Morning sickness? That second trimester "glow"? An immune system that can't seem to decide whether to fight infections or surrender to them? It's all in the hormones.

A secondary change is taking place as well, less obvious perhaps than a bulging tummy but just as important to a newborn's survival. The hormonal surges that prepare a mother's body for birth and breast-feeding also bathe her brain, subtly altering her behavior in ways that prepare her to take on the role of mother. Those changes in a mother-to-be's behavior that we take for granted—the sudden interest in all things baby, for instance, or the nest-building behavior at the end of pregnancy—are hormonal in origin. Just as surely as hormones turn a woman's body into a perfect environment for fetal growth, they transform her emotions, too. By the end of her pregnancy she will put the needs of her baby above all else, including her own needs and those of her sometimes forlorn mate.

This all makes perfect biological sense, of course. It is in a fetus's best interests to exert influence on a mother's body early on, and a growing fetus exerts influence like a backroom politician. Or, as hormone researcher John A. Russell put it, "The fetus and placenta certainly make a loud, orchestrated [hormonal] statement that they have arrived and intend to stay."

So if a new father-to-be soon feels as if his partner has been carried off to Babyland, he's right. The little dictator in the womb is making sure that he or she will be safe and healthy at birth, and that his mama will be there for him till he's old enough to fend for himself. What our new dad doesn't realize is that his baby-to-be's hormonal manipulations don't end with his mother.

A brief recap of guy hormones: your junior high biology teacher got it pretty much right. A fetus's testicles begin production of testosterone in the seventh week of pregnancy and, long story short, they never stop. There is a surge of testosterone at birth—no one understands the reason; the baby girls certainly don't seem impressed—and then production slows down until things go wild at the onset of adolescence.

Testosterone production reaches its peak in midpuberty, right about the time a boy's voice begins to crack, and continues pretty much unchanged until around age forty. From there, testosterone secretion slowly decreases but never completely stops. A healthy octogenarian may have testosterone levels in the low normal range for a much younger man.

Testosterone makes the man, quite literally. It is the hormone responsible for growth and maturation of the penis, testicles, and scrotum; for sperm production; for mustache, beard, and body hair growth; for thickening the vocal cords and lowering the pitch of the voice; for increased height and muscle mass, particularly in the shoulders and chest; and for an increase in blood volume. It is also responsible for a man's libido and sexual potency. Nearly every physical characteristic we think of as "manly" is produced by the effects of this single hormone (or its lesser cousin, dihydrotestosterone). Women are right: men are simple. Know testosterone, know Tarzan; no testosterone, no Tarzan.

Given that testosterone production is so central to male reproductive success, it's not surprising that it takes a significant physical whack to slow it down. Chronic illnesses of the kidneys, liver, heart, or any other major organ system can do it. So can prolonged infection, trauma, or cancer and its treatments. Alcohol and drug abuse can lead to decreased testosterone production and atrophy of the testicles. In every one of these cases a serious bodily malfunction sends a message to the testicles that there are more important things to attend to at the moment than making babies.

Energy is diverted away from things reproductive and toward healing the stresses afflicting the body.

But there is one testosterone-diminishing condition that has nothing to do with illness or injury. It often occurs during a man's peak years of fitness, and you won't find it listed in most endocrinology textbooks. As a matter of fact, it has almost nothing to do with a man's health at all. It's pregnancy.

Research on expectant fathers has lagged behind that dedicated to pregnant women for one good and obvious reason: men don't have babies. No man has ever experienced a vaginal birth or a cesarean section. None have died in labor. There's not even a single reported case of a new father with pregnancy-related varicose veins. What's to study?

Interest in the internal workings of fathers-to-be has picked up in the last decade or two, though, as an offshoot of research into the effects of hormones on maternal behavior. The big question: How does a man become a daddy? What changes him from a guy who never even noticed babies into a big sentimental lug with a wallet full of kid photos? If hormones are largely responsible for the changes in a woman's behavior as she moves through her pregnancy, might the same thing be happening in her mate's brain?

Biologists Sandra Berg and Katherine Wynne-Edwards at Queen's University in Ontario began exploring this largely uncharted territory in the late 1990s. Animal research earlier in the decade had suggested that hormonal changes may in fact induce "paternal" behavior in a wide variety of creatures. The logical next question they posed: If that's the case in other animals, what about humans?

In 1999, Berg and Wynne-Edwards followed a volunteer group of thirty-four expectant Canadian fathers in Kingston, Ontario, from their first prenatal class until three months after the births of their babies. They also recruited fourteen nonfathers from the general population to act as a comparison group. They measured testosterone and two other hormones—estradiol, that traditionally "female" hormone, and cortisol, a hormone released during times of stress—from weekly saliva collections.

Their findings were a bit unsettling for the kind of guy who sees himself as a walking ad for manliness: all of the fathers-to-be had lower testosterone levels than the nonfather control subjects. This held true even after Berg and Wynne-Edwards took into account the men's ages, the time of year, and other factors that might have skewed the results. Even more startling, the expectant fathers also had significantly higher levels of estradiol, one of the main hormones associated with pregnancy in women. Though the levels didn't approach those seen in pregnant women, the overall hormone profile for this group of Canadian men was unmistakable—they were becoming "feminized" as their mates' pregnancies rolled on.

Another Canadian study published in 1999 agreed with Berg and Wynne-Edwards's findings, and then some. The dads-to-be in the study not only had lower testosterone and higher estradiol levels than the nondads, they also had higher levels of prolactin—the hormone intimately associated with breast-feeding and maternal behavior. In other words, the same chemicals that prepare a woman's body and emotions for motherhood run wild in her mate's bloodstream as well.

There are limitations to these studies, and the authors are quick to point them out. These were all volunteer Canadian men from a stratum of society that believes in the importance of childbirth education, as evidenced by their willingness to pay for it. The hormone profiles of richer or poorer Canadian men (or those who wouldn't be caught dead at a prenatal class) may well prove to be different from those of this small, homogeneous group of research subjects. And no one has any idea what new-dad hormones are doing in the deserts of Saudi Arabia, say, or the rainforests of the Amazon.

Still, it's hard to ignore the findings, particularly in light of the evidence from extensive animal studies. If it's any consolation to those hormonally altered Canadian dads, they're far from alone among their fellow mammals. Pregnancy-related hormone changes have been found in a variety of species in which fathers help care for their offspring, including hamsters and marmosets, prairie voles and mice, and a cute little South American monkey called the cotton-top tamarin. But in species with no tendency toward paternal care there's no measurable difference in hormone levels between expectant dads and nondads. Why the disparity?

The main determinant of paternal hormone levels in mammals seems to be a male's proximity to a pregnant mate. As delivery approaches, there is a fairly straight-line relationship between the amount of time a male spends with his pregnant mate and his hormone levels. And those hormone changes in turn are directly related to how involved a male will be with his babies.

Take hamsters, for example. At one end of the paternal-care spectrum is the Djungarian hamster father-to-be, who participates extensively in newborn care. His testosterone levels drop sharply during his mate's pregnancy. At the other extreme is the closely related Siberian hamster male, who ignores his mate and his offspring. His testosterone level doesn't change at all, presumably leaving him free to pursue his hamster-about-town ways with the ladies. How can two closely related species differ so much in their parenting styles and hormone levels? As with so many other biological puzzles, the answer can be found at Charles Darwin's doorstep.

Every successful species evolves its own reproductive strategies to ensure a next generation of its kind. For many animals, some degree of paternal involvement after birth is essential to that success, whether to help with food gathering, protection from predators, or the teaching of survival skills to its offspring. The Djungarian hamster father's payback for his devotion to his mate and kids is "paternity assurance," a term that will surface again in a later chapter. His close proximity to the mother during mating and her subsequent pregnancy means that he is most likely the father of her young. His attentiveness after birth helps to ensure the survival of his progeny, making him an evolutionary success. The Siberian hamster father, though, takes a different tack. He mates with more females than does his Djungarian cousin, and some of his many offspring are bound to survive, even without his help. Voilà! His genes pass on to the next generation. He, too, is a Darwinian success story.

That's all well and good for hamsters, but what about humans?

There are a couple of possible reasons for this "feminization" of an expectant human male's hormones. The first, and most obvious: as childbirth became complicated by our tendency toward big-headed, helpless babies, a woman's chance of survival was improved by having a man around. An involved dad meant a steady source of food and protection from predators at a very vulnerable time in her life. Doting dadhood was a good deal for the man as well. A father invested in the care of his children was more likely to see them survive and carry on his genetic line. That's a win-win evolutionary situation.

The second, not so obvious reason for the taming of the father-beast is rooted in a dark fact of mammalian life: infanticide. In species with a male-dominated social hierarchy, including such varied creatures as the lion, the gerbil, and those primates most closely related to humans, dominant males often kill the offspring of vanquished rivals. Though it sounds heartless to us, this makes evolutionary sense—the fittest male has taken over the pack or pride, and he isn't inclined to raise some lesser male's kids.

But the killing can be quite indiscriminate. So when, say, the Gerbil King becomes a father, something has to stop him from killing his own offspring right along with his rival's, lest he abruptly eliminate himself from the Darwinian sweepstakes. And, sure enough, males of infanticide-prone species are brought into a "paternal state" just before the birth of their offspring. The hormonal profile of that state is very similar to that seen in the Canadian volunteers: lower testosterone levels and increased estradiol and prolactin levels.

I don't want to leave the reader with the impression that a man's pregnancy behavior can be explained simply by charting his hormone levels. Berg and Wynne-Edwards speculated about this in the conclusion of their Canadian study. "We do not anticipate a strict hormone-behavior relationship in men," they wrote in 1999. "Nevertheless, these changes, which involve hormones known or implicated in mammalian maternal behavior, may subtly alter hormone receptor expression, sensitivity to infant stimuli, or reactions to social stimuli in ways that enhance the psychosocial experience of becoming a father." In other words, hormones are simply one fascinating part of a much more complicated picture. More research is needed on a wider variety of men in different pregnancy situations. What happens to a soldier's hormones when he's shipped overseas early in his mate's pregnancy and returns after the birth? How about merchant seamen? Polar explorers? Pediatricians?

So that's the "why" of the matter. Altered hormones help turn a freewheeling Tarzan into a daddy. An expectant father is made more baby-friendly by his endocrine system, just as an expectant mother's behavior is altered to make her more responsive to her offspring. By the end of the pregnancy, if all goes well, a man and woman are transformed by hormones and shared life experience into something new and altogether different: parents. Driving the whole process is the fetus, pulling a myriad of chemical strings to bind both his mother and father to him long before he lets out his first cry.

The exact "how" of a man's hormone fluctuations remains a mystery, though scientists are steadily narrowing the possibilities. It's easy to see how a fetus can directly affect its mother's body, but how does it reach across open air to influence its father? Pheromones, those chemical messages that animals send to each other through the air, or via bodily secretions, would seem to be ideal candidates. It makes intuitive sense: a chemical scent travels from a woman to her mate, triggering changes in the workings of his endocrine system. The more exposure he has to his mate and her pheromones, the more his hormones change.

But the portion of the human brain devoted to picking up on scents—the olfactory center—has atrophied pitifully over evolutionary time. A dog's sense of smell is many thousandfold more acute than ours; it would seem unlikely that pheromones alone could account for the changes in a man's hormone profile during pregnancy. But lately it looks more and more as though that's the case—pheromones, or other substances very much like them, appear to act as chemical messengers between a man and a woman, just as they do in other mammals.

Dr. Charles Wysocki and his research team at the Monell Chemical Senses Center in Philadelphia have been investigating the role of scent in human mate selection for several years now. Here's the shorthand version of their findings: *We sniff, therefore we mate.* When pads steeped in male armpit sweat were placed beneath the noses of women volunteers, the women soon showed a spike in their blood levels of luteinizing hormone, the "fertility" hormone that controls the length of the menstrual cycle, the timing of ovulation, and the preparation of the uterus to receive an implanted egg. The women also reported feeling more relaxed and less anxious when smelling the pads, an effect that disappeared shortly after the pads were removed. Researchers at the University of California, Berkeley, have since isolated at least one of the chemicals in male sweat that triggers female hormone changes—androstadienone, a testosterone derivative—and demonstrated that as little as twenty sniffs of the stuff is enough to get a woman's hormonal attention. At first glance these findings sound like the ultimate adolescent guy-dream: walk around a bar with your arms in the air and the women come running.

But in 2002 a team of University of Chicago underarm investigators confirmed what every love-crazy young man eventually learns: women are a lot pickier in choosing a mate than that, and with good biological reason. Women, it seems, prefer the "odor print" of men with whom they share some genetic markers (the equivalent of third or fourth cousins) over either more closely related males or those with whom they share no markers at all. Put in evolutionary perspective, this means our female ancestors probably preferred to couple with distantly related men from their own group or tribe, rather than with their fathers or brothers or with complete genetic strangers. Such not-completely-random mating made for a healthy mixing of genes in each new generation.

So a man's smell, particularly the aroma emanating from under his arms, is a powerful attractant to potential mates. We now have evidence that a woman's hormones can be manipulated almost by remote control—remember that the subjects in Wysocki's experiments never met the men who donated their sweaty armpit pads to science. But does scent continue to work after the wooing and mating are over? Does the smell of a pregnant woman somehow trigger the "feminization" of a man's hormone profile, luring him into hanging around and becoming a protective daddy?

Alas, as of this writing we still don't know. Most human pheromone research to date has been devoted to chemical attraction and mate selection—and most of the studies involve women sniffing men, not vice versa. No one has yet stuck a pad soaked in "eau de pregnant woman" under the nose of a man and measured what happens to *his* hormone levels. Until that occurs, the best guess is that some form of chemical attraction—perhaps a variation on the one that draws a man to a woman in the first place, combined with some fetal influence—likely binds him to her, and to their child, long after the candy and flowers are gone.

Pity then the expectant father as labor approaches. He's an endocrine mess, with female hormones on the rise, manly hormones waning, and a wife who spends more time talking to her belly than to him. His body is acting up, too. Maybe he gets some heartburn, or gains some weight, or develops his own weird food cravings. He might even feel a little movement (gulp!) in his belly. No wonder he thinks he's going a little crazy.

Too bad he's not living in New Guinea back in premissionary times, when they understood the trials of a man in labor. There they'd have tied him up with leather strips, locked him in a dark hut, and shoved food under the door until his wife gave birth and his mind came back. Then they'd give him a bath and send him home. No big deal. Just another guy having a baby, that's all.

The French have a name for all this, one that English-speaking researchers have adopted: *couvade,* from the French verb *couver:* "to brood" or "to hatch." Couvade includes both the strange feelings that can plague a man during his mate's pregnancy, and the ways in which a society deals with him. The external, physical signs of a man's internal turmoil are collectively known as "couvade syndrome." A society's traditions surrounding a man's passage to fatherhood are known as "cultural couvade." We'll start with cultural couvade, the more colorful—and, unfortunately, slowly disappearing—of the two, and with the man who first wrote it all down.

Warren Royal Dawson was born in west London in 1888 and lived most of his life in the shadow of the British Museum. He was an insurance underwriter by trade and an Egyptologist by avocation. Though never schooled as an archeologist—his formal education ended at age fifteen, with his father's death—he became a self-taught worldwide authority on mummies, mummification, ancient tattoos, the magical and medicinal use of leeches, and couvade.

Dawson's interest in couvade sprang from his love of ancient Egypt. He spent years studying couvade practices from around the world in a passionate but failed attempt to prove that human civilization had first blossomed in the land of the Pharaohs. The book that resulted from his research, *The Custom of Couvade* (1929), drew on the reports of more than two hundred adventurers, from ancient times to the end World War I. (Dawson, a classic "armchair anthropologist," rarely left London himself.)

The Custom of Couvade is a fascinating read. From cultures as diverse as the Ainu of northern Japan, the Bushongo of East Africa, and the peasant farmers of Yorkshire, a pattern emerges: every culture that Dawson studied had prescribed roles for a father to play as the birth of his child approached. "These [couvade] customs," he wrote, "require that the father of a child, at or before its birth and for sometimes after the event, should take to his bed, submit himself to diet and behave generally as though he, and not his wife, were undergoing the rigours of the confinement."

Couvade rituals were strikingly consistent across great stretches of time and geography. Here's Marco Polo, traveling in thirteenth-century Turkistan: "And when one of their wives has been delivered of a child, the infant is washed and swathed, and the woman gets up and goes about her household duties, whilst the husband takes to bed with the child by his side, and so keeps his bed for forty days; and all the kith and kin come to visit him and keep up a great festivity."

Compare that with British explorer John Cain, who wrote six centuries later and a thousand miles away of the "peculiar habit" he observed among the Erekula people of southern India. There, the father-to-be put on his wife's clothing at the onset of labor and climbed into bed in a dark room, covered only by a long cloth: "When the child is born, it is washed and placed on the cot beside the father, [medicines] are then given, not to the mother, but the father . . . the man is treated as the Hindus treat their women on such occasions. He is not allowed to leave his bed, but has everything needful brought to him."

In some cultures the practices were merely symbolic—men of the ancient Tibareni tribe in Asia Minor simply "[took] to their beds with their heads tied up while the women pampered them with tasty food"—while in others they involved starvation or severe pain. The late-seventeenth-century Caribs of the West Indies certainly take the cake in terms of making a man think twice about fatherhood. After being forced to live on only cassava root and beerlike *ouycou* for forty days after the birth, the new father's friends "hack the skin of the poor wretch with agouti teeth and draw blood from all parts of his body" and then rub the wounds "with a peppery infusion . . . the poor fellow suffers no less than if he were burnt alive." Once they've finished marinating him, his friends put him back to bed and then "go and make good cheer at his expense."

Another consistent pattern to these rituals: the wife was excluded, or nearly so, from the festivities, and was sent back to the fields or kitchen shortly after giving birth. The "perfect form" of this symbolic role reversal struck Dawson. Whatever form couvade might take—and however unfair to the mothers, since no one ever thought to ask them what they made of all this—the underlying principle was clear. A man's transition to fatherhood was something to be celebrated, often with great extravagance.

Ironically, cultural couvade was fading away even as Dawson labored to connect all his far-flung dots to Egypt. Dawson's late-nineteenth and early-twentieth-century sources, mainly British military officers and explorers, viewed couvade through the cultural prism of late Victorian and Edwardian era morality. A civilized Englishman could hardly see the behavior of Bombay's Deshasht Brahmans, who insisted that a new father jump fully clothed into the family well before being allowed to touch his new baby, as anything but a godless superstition. To Dawson's correspondents, couvade behaviors simply reinforced the "primitiveness" of Her Majesty's colonial subjects.

The advance of Western civilization, with its tendency to consider third world customs as quaint, at best—and at worst, deserving of annihilation—doomed the practice to near extinction, except in the more remote, missionary-proof parts of the planet. Even as he worked on *The Custom of Couvade,* Dawson saw the coming of the inevitable. He fully expected that couvade practices would soon disappear from the earth.

But ritual couvade was more than just an aboriginal oddity. It was a society's way of recognizing impending fatherhood as one of life's great passages, almost on a par with childbirth itself. Banning couvade traditions didn't take away the reality of the often difficult transition to fatherhood. Couvade didn't disappear as modern Western culture swept much of the globe. It just went underground, only to resurface in the most unlikely of places—the doctor's office.

In 1982, New York medical researchers Mack Lipkin and Gerri Lamb turned their attention to a largely neglected area of human childbirth: *couvade syndrome,* or a father's physical experience of his mate's pregnancy. A man's discomfort during pregnancy had been the butt of jokes since Shakespeare wrote of Benedick's pregnancy-induced toothache in *Much Ado About Nothing,* and no doubt long before that. But Lipkin and Lamb's research was among the first to establish that there really was something going on inside fathers-to-be, and that it was more common than anyone realized.

Lipkin and Lamb reviewed the urgent care clinic visits of 267 expectant men in a New York HMO over a fourteen-month period. They rated the visits for the presence of traditional couvade symptoms, a rather broad category that includes bowel complaints, concerns about appetite or weight, and a number of odd ailments such as leg cramps, faintness, and fatigue that, like toothache, had no other obvious physical cause. Then they compared the number of urgent care visits each man made to the clinic in the six months before the estimated date of conception, in the nine months of his mate's pregnancy, and in the six months after the birth of his baby. Their findings: nearly 25 percent of the men had sought treatment for couvade symptoms during their wives' pregnancies. (The authors called this a "conservative" estimate; the month-long wait for appointments no doubt discouraged some men from seeking help, and non-traditional couvade complaints like genital burning, "dizziness when laughing," and one man's sense that "something" was trying to push out of his lower chest were not included.)

The couvade-afflicted men had twice as many visits and complained of four times the number of symptoms as they did in the periods before the pregnancy and after it ended. They received twice as many prescriptions, too. The medications most commonly prescribed were decongestants, antiflatulents, and Valium, leading to the inescapable conclusion that pregnancy leads to stuffier, gassier, more anxious men.

Interestingly, the condition of expectant fatherhood was rarely noted in the medical chart, and none of the doctors involved made the connection between a man's complaints and his wife's pregnancy.

The lack of medical attention to couvade syndrome was nothing new. Prior to the 1960s, American men who complained of physical or emotional symptoms during a mate's pregnancy were dismissed as neurotic weaklings. The prevailing view was that the vast majority of men sailed through a wife's pregnancy unscathed, barely noticing it at all except for those late-night trips to the store for orange Popsicles and Grape-Nuts. The assumption of a carefree male pregnancy experience was so pervasive that nobody, particularly doctors, gave it much thought.

But as Lipkin and Lamb showed to such startling effect, a great many men were experiencing uncomfortable pregnancies. Subsequent studies of Western males (and in non-Western societies, such as Thailand) have shown that, depending on how hard you look for it, the majority of men show some degree of couvade symptoms, and they do so in predictable ways. The complaints—mainly of the type that Lipkin and Lamb chose for their study—tend to cluster in a U-shaped curve, worst at the beginning and end of pregnancy, with a relatively calm second trimester. Though a man's specific complaints don't necessarily correspond with his mate's, the timing is perfect: as any pregnant woman can tell you, the first and third trimesters are the most uncomfortable.

Speculation on the basis of couvade syndrome has long been something of a cottage industry in psychiatric circles. Nineteenth-century observers attributed ritual couvade to everything from magical thinking to satanism. Couvade syndrome was blamed on a weak constitution, a fear of women, even "severe henpecking."

More modern theories hypothesize that an afflicted father is identifying with his expectant mate, or that couvade symptoms are an expression of ambivalence about fatherhood, or a rivalry with the fetus, or envy of the pregnant spouse. Psychiatrist Hilary Klein writes that a couvade-afflicted father is manifesting evidence of deeper intrapsychic phenomena, and with that I can heartily agree. Most expectant fathers can tell you that something weird is going on. And given that the archetype for Western males has long been that of the strong, silent, rugged individualist—not the kind of guy who would willingly join a fathers' support group—the ailments can fester.

But it's likely that couvade is less about ambivalence, henpecking, or the devil than it is about the hormonal changes roiling inside an expectant father. A growing body of evidence supports this and points to prolactin as the likely "couvade hormone." Couvade symptoms have long been known to be more common in cultures in which a man spends a lot of time with his pregnant mate. Hormone levels have now been shown to correlate between partners. When her prolactin level rises, his does too, and men with higher prolactin levels tend to have more couvade symptoms.

The decreases in testosterone and increases in estrogens and prolactin a man experiences during his mate's pregnancy are the only known times in his life that his relatively straightforward hormones are naturally tampered with. Some men no doubt feel this hormonal swing more strongly than others, and to many it can be a troubling experience. Toss in an expectant father's worries about his readiness for parenthood or the financial obligations of family life, and it's not surprising that he gets a stomachache.

So there you have it. A man in the act of racing his laboring wife to the hospital is not the same man who got her pregnant in the first place. His altered hormonal state has made him more baby-friendly—and perhaps more important, less baby-hostile. He has been chemically modified, as it were, to be more attentive to his child, to take a greater role in caring and providing—the constellation of behaviors we think of as "fatherly." The transformation isn't uniform; many men don't seem to respond at all, while others become so babycentric as to border on the pathological.

But a man usually changes for the better, from both a family and a societal standpoint. And, as preliminary studies of fathers in second and third pregnancies show, his hormone profile never quite returns to what it was before that first pregnancy. The change is permanent; he'll never be the same old guy again.

As for me, what kind of man had I become in those months leading to my first nonprofessional trip to the delivery room? I'd like to say that a dramatic change swept over me, but I don't recall feeling a lot different than I did before the pregnancy. I didn't suffer from lassitude, leg cramps, or movement in my belly. I did have a gold crown put on a cracked molar, but this had less to do with Shakespeare's pregnancy toothache, I think, than with my childhood reluctance to floss.

I may have been primed, hormonewise, given the daily exposure to pregnant women in my line of work. Too, I already liked babies, which is kind of a job requirement for a pediatrician. And I'd been in daily contact with a pregnant mate, so those pheromones or voodoo stares or whatever Elisabeth was wafting in my direction to trigger my dad hormones had had plenty of time to work.

But I wasn't couvade-free. I gained weight right along with Elisabeth, and I had trouble sleeping, particularly toward the end. I worried a lot about whether I was up to the challenges of fatherhood. I remember lying awake one warm spring evening, looking out our bedroom window at the full moon and realizing with a sudden chill that by the time another lunar cycle rolled around, I'd be a father. Ready or not.

Two years later, just a few weeks before the birth of my second child, I nearly chopped off a couple of fingers in a rather ghastly table saw accident. Couvade, or just plain clumsiness? Who knows? Whatever the reason, I think that the Land Dyaks of Borneo, who insisted on keeping sharp tools away from expectant fathers, were onto something.

My actual labor room performance will be dissected in the next chapter. Suffice it to say that I got Elisabeth to the right hospital at the right time—way ahead of time, as it turned out—and I did not chain myself to her bed or demand morphine for my own labor pains. I didn't panic, faint, hyperventilate, or split open my head in full view of the nurses. I avoided all of the pitfalls I'd witnessed in my years of watching daddies, but I was not without sin. In the midst of those most dramatic moments of any man's life, as my daughter inched her way out of her mother and into my life, I fell asleep.

Chapter 7

The Gang's All Here:
A History of Birth Attendance

It's six in the morning and I'm camped in Labor Room 3, where a budding emergency awaits: a woman, a fetus, and an obstetrician in the middle of a worrisome birth. I'm focused on a quick equipment check—in a minute or two I'll be handed a baby who might be very sick—so the tap on my shoulder barely registers.

The tapping resumes, this time more insistent. I turn to find an intense, bespectacled young man staring back at me. He is wearing a khaki vest with a dozen pockets stitched to the front, each of them containing a lens, a meter, or some other bit of camera equipment. I recognize him as Eric, the man at whom the laboring woman has just finished yelling.

"Do you mind?" he says, his tone of voice suggesting that I already know the purpose of his question, which in fact I don't. He sighs, rolls his eyes, and points to the window behind me, where the rising sun is just burning its way through the morning fog. "Move," he says, waving me toward the baby bed in the corner with fluttering *artiste* hand gestures. "You're standing in my light."

Eric was hired to videotape the woman's labor and delivery—all twelve hours of it—and just as things were getting cinematically interesting, just as he had trained his twin cameras and bank of lights on the fetus's emerging head, his client, the woman having the baby, changed the plan.

"Shut off the lights, Eric." She had said this in a calm, direct voice, which Eric, apparently unaccustomed to working with a woman in transition—that painful part of childbirth when the baby's head first appears, the part during which Tonya had threatened to cut me to pieces years before—unwisely ignored. "No can do, Terri," he said in an unctuous, directorial voice. "You know we need light."

Terri's second request, following on the heels of her next contraction, could not be so easily refused. *"Shut off the damned lights, Eric!"* she shouted. "They're blinding me!" Startled by his patron's unexpected ferocity, Eric obeyed, which led him now to his improvised backup lighting plan: shooing me away from the window and the rising sun.

I feel a bit sorry for Eric and his failing masterpiece, so I shift as far as I can, which isn't far at all. He and I are up against the far wall of a 15-by-20-foot delivery room that contains, besides Eric and his cameras and me and my baby table, a laboring woman in a large bed, a father-to-be, an obstetrician, three nurses, two prospective grandmothers, and a couple of other friends or relatives, one of whom, from her chanting and amulet-strung clothing, appears to be a shaman. Shoehorned in like that, somebody was bound to block his light.

Things happen quickly. The baby's head and shoulders suddenly appear, and then with Terri's final push he lands in the obstetrician's hands. There's meconium—baby poop—in the amniotic fluid, a sign of fetal distress, so the obstetrician quickly clamps and cuts the cord, then hands the baby over to me. I push my way through the bevy of spectators back to the baby table and get to work.

Now, it is not an easy thing to attend to a distressed newborn while simultaneously deflecting the attention of a determined documentary filmmaker. Eric appears at my side with his handheld camera, the red "on" light flashing maybe six inches away from my head. "Can you tell us what's happening?" he asks, as though he's a television anchorman and I'm a reporter in the field, interviewing witnesses at the scene of a house fire. "No," I say, and Eric responds with a muttered oath, something about my being uncooperative, and then an expletive that I assume can still be heard on Terri's birth video, barring Eric's editing skills.

Fortunately, everything goes smoothly. I suction the meconium away from the baby's windpipe; better able to breathe now, he perks up and cries out. The nurse dries him off, wraps him in a warm blanket, and then, after a minute or so of watching to make sure he's okay, she places the baby in his mother's waiting arms. I answer Terri's questions and reassure her that despite all the hubbub of the previous few minutes, her baby is just fine. Then I weave my way past Eric, the grandmothers, the friends, the shaman, a couple of older men who've just arrived—presumably the new grandfathers—and a young man making a feeble attempt to pop the cork on a bottle of champagne.

"Thanks!" the obstetrician shouts to me from her stool in the middle of the throng, her waving hand just barely visible in the laughing and crying crowd gathered around Terri's bed. "You're welcome," I call back. "Good luck in there."

Childbirth hasn't always been like that, and I don't just mean the cameras, the stage lighting, and the champagne. There once was a time, back before obstetricians, pediatricians, nurses, and shamans, when nobody attended to a female in labor—not her family, not her friends, and certainly not the guy she called her mate. It's been a long, strange, uniquely human journey from going it alone to birthing for an audience.

Back in the opening chapter I talked about the human female pelvis and its evolution in response to our shift to upright walking and our need for ever bigger brains. Our shoulders got broader as we gave up the knuckle-dragging locomotion favored by our ape cousins; the pelvis responded by widening to make room. When the fetal brain and head enlarged, the pelvis got rounder and twisted itself into an imperfect cylinder—more or less a toilet paper roll with the upper third slightly pinched from side to side.

All this pelvic remodeling caused a major change in birthing mechanics: the human fetus emerged from the birth canal facing its mother's backbone, rather than the face-frontward "sunny-side up" position common to every other large primate species.

That flipped-over exit from the womb had much greater implications for the human race than simply making birth more difficult. It also made it nearly impossible for a mother to do it alone, an anatomical oddity that led, a million years or so later, to Eric and me and that early morning elbow-to-elbow crowd.

Recall the example of the gorilla mother: she has her baby alone at night, in about half an hour. She doesn't require any assistance, in part because her small fetus passes easily through her large birth canal. And because the fetus is facing her as it emerges, she can easily reach down and clear mucus and blood from her baby's mouth to help it commence breathing, or unwind a tight umbilical cord from around its neck if need be.

Compare that with a human birth. It takes thirty times longer than a gorilla's, for one thing—much more time for something to go wrong. A human mother's arms are relatively shorter than a gorilla's, and her bulging belly is more prominent, too, making it more difficult for her to reach her fetus as it emerges. Adding to her troubles, the fetus comes out facing away from her; she can neither see nor easily touch its face. If she pulls the fetus's head back to try to clear the nose and mouth, she could seriously injure its neck. Finally, the fit between head and pelvis is so tight that it can be hard for an obstetrician to release a tightly wound umbilical cord from the fetus's neck, let alone a mother who can barely reach her baby's head.

Our ancestors reached a fork in the reproductive road a few million years ago. Solo birthing had become an evolutionary dead end. The pelvis had grown about as big and wide as it could, and it was far too late to put the big-headed genie back in the bottle. We couldn't simply regress, become less intelligent, and climb back into the trees—that niche was already filled by dozens of other primate species, and they weren't likely to take kindly to an invasion of bubble-headed competitors. If nothing changed in the birthing process, big-headed, broad-shouldered, wrong-way-birthing humanity was, literally and figuratively, stuck.

But prehuman ingenuity prevailed. Somewhere along the way, in whatever passed for language at that point in our history, a mother called out for help. At first that help may have come simply in the form of someone watching over her, driving away any hungry predators that happened by during her labor. Sooner or later one of those bystanders, maybe an empathic female with a fresh memory of how complicated and sometimes frightening birth could be, decided to help out directly. She may have done the job of clearing the fetus's nose and mouth as it emerged, or freed the umbilical cord, or maybe she just held the laboring female's hand, reassuring her that things were going well.

Whatever form that first level of help took, it increased the chances of survival for both mother and baby. The tendency to ask for and receive help became self-reinforcing, too: the daughters of a female with the sense to seek help and protection during labor would likely inherit her tendency to do the same. Likewise, the children of those who thought to offer help would be more genetically apt to do the same when they reached adulthood. As heads got bigger, those mothers who sought birth assistance had an increasing evolutionary advantage over those who did not. Having skilled birth helpers handy allowed the fetal head and brain to grow even larger. Birth assistance led directly to increased intelligence.

Beyond a certain point in human evolution, birth helpers became mandatory; solo childbirth simply got too dangerous. Anthropologist Wenda Trevathan coined the term "obligate midwifery" to describe this point of no return, which is the peculiarly human situation that exists today. No other large primate species has birth helpers. Beyond being watched from a distance or offered a bit of protection, a laboring chimp or gorilla female is on her own.

Obligate midwifery is hardwired into the modern human brain. While women do occasionally give birth alone, they rarely choose to, and their chances of surviving are much greater if skilled helpers are on hand. (An unattended breech birth, for example, is nearly always fatal to mother and child.) The biological need for birth attendants, and a woman's desire to seek their help during labor, transformed human birth into a social activity.

"Midwife" is a Middle English term, nearly a thousand years old. It's a combination of the words "mid" (with) and "wyf" (woman): a midwife was literally a person who stayed with a woman during her labor. Midwives have existed in virtually every culture and time, known by strikingly similar names. To ancient Jews the midwife was a "wise woman," the same name she goes by in modern France (*sage-femme*). In ancient Rome she was *cum-mater,* a term that survives in present-day Spanish and Portuguese as *comadre:* literally, "with mother."

Little is known of the role of birth attendants in early civilizations, though we can assume any society that worshipped as many childbirth divinities as did the ancient Egyptians—including the frog goddess Heqet, the hippopotamus goddess Tauert, and Bes, a dwarfish, lion-faced, bowlegged deity who moonlighted as the god of entertainment and a protector from snakes—likely had a sophisticated midwifery system.

The Egyptian midwife is found only in depictions of royal or divine deliveries, since less exalted births were considered impure and thus unworthy of description. The best mythological account of a midwife's work comes from the nearly four-thousand-year-old Westcar Papyrus, in which Isis and a quartet of assisting gods help Ruddjedet, a priest's wife impregnated by the god Ra, give birth to triplets. More or less shaming the three into emerging ("You should not be strong in her belly," she tells the first one), Isis "slides" the newborn godlets one by one from the womb.

In inscriptions found in temple birth halls the midwife is called "the sweet one" or, in her divine form, Nekhbet of el-Kab—"she with gripping thumbs." Divine though she may have been, her duties were much like those of midwives everywhere. Working with assistants who supported the mother's back and arms, she delivered the baby, cut the umbilical cord, washed and laid the newborn on a special bed, and then went back to attending the mother.

We know much more about the midwife's world in the first and second century A.D. Greco-Roman world, thanks in large part to Pliny the Elder (A.D. 23–79) and Soranus of Ephesus (A.D. 98–138), who wrote of childbirth and its traditions from radically different points of view.

Pliny was a Roman military commander, naturalist, and incredibly prolific writer. He was the author of more than a hundred books—including ones on grammar and childhood education, a twenty-volume history of Rome's wars with Germany, and even a how-to book on the use of the javelin as a cavalry weapon—but his greatest work was his *Historia Naturalis* (*Natural History*), still considered one of the most influential books ever written in Latin.

Pliny wrote about nearly everything in *Historia Naturalis,* from a survey of the world and its peoples "who now exist or formerly existed" to the question of the ethnicity of Rome's first barbers. (Sicilians, he figured.) Human biology was a particular interest. Mixed in among discussions of malaria, the fireproof nature of teeth, and the "remarkable circumstances" of menstruating women—how their very gaze withers crops and "takes away the polish of ivory," among other dubious monthly superpowers—is an extensive discussion of folk medicine as it related to childbirth in the Roman Empire.

Read with a modern eye, much of what Pliny described is mystifying. How did the idea come about, for example, that placing a hyena's right foot on a laboring woman's abdomen ensured an easy delivery? Or that doing so with its left foot caused death? Or that the smoke of burnt hyena loin fat—there seems to have been a lot of hyena-based medicine in those days—strengthened uterine contractions?

Other remedies sound downright repulsive. Sprinkling powdered sow dung in a drink helped relieve labor pain. So did drinking a concoction made from goose semen mixed with "the liquids that flow from a weasel's uterus through its genitals," which raises a practical question Pliny fails to answer: How did they collect this stuff?

Pliny goes on to describe an extensive array of herbs and plants used in labor, as well as amulets and other items, including a number of objects placed on a woman's thighs to ease delivery: a snake's shed skin, a dog's afterbirth that had not touched the ground, and "a stick with which a frog had been shaken from a snake," an object that sounds about as easy to hunt down in the heat of labor as the broomstick of the Wicked Witch of the West.

Pliny didn't make light of the staggeringly strange variety of treatments he found. From the tone of his writing he seems to think that employing them was sound maternity practice, and since most people lived in small villages and rural areas where folk medicine was the norm, it's safe to assume that the majority of women in the Roman Empire of Pliny's era relied on them.

How well did these folk remedies work? Pliny remains silent in that regard, but the fact of their persistence over generations indicates that the empire's citizens had a high degree of faith in their effectiveness. Perhaps they provided a placebo effect. If a woman truly believed that drinking sow dung would lessen her pains, it may well have done so. Recall the experience of acupuncture in modern-day Sweden—though the majority of midwives who performed acupuncture did it completely wrong, most of their patients still reported that it substantially reduced their pains. Substitute sow dung or the chanting of the shamanlike woman next to Terri's bed for acupuncture needles, and the story is remarkably similar.

Whatever else can be said of the hyena-foot-and-goose-semen school of maternity care, it was personal and probably reassuring to the mother. The labor-intensive nature of the remedies no doubt required the constant company of her female companions and the midwife, and, as we'll see, it was likely the continuous labor support, more so than the remedies themselves, that provided her with the most benefit.

Soranus, a physician who practiced in Alexandria and Rome in the second century A.D., a half century after Pliny's death, was more scientific in his approach to childbirth and dismissive of what he called "vulgar superstition," "omens," and the "customary rites" of the kind found in *Historia Naturalis*. Soranus wrote what amounts to a job description for the midwife, or *maia,* in his famed treatise, *Gynecology.* "A suitable person," he wrote, "will be literate, with her wits about her, possessed of good memory, loving work, respectable." She must also be physically strong, robust in character, sympathetic, well versed in the theory and practice of childbirth, sober, "unperturbed, unafraid in danger," possessed of a "manly patience," and "endowed with long, slim fingers and short nails at her fingertips."

Soranus also spelled out the on-the-job equipment the *maia* would need: warm water, olive oil, pain-relieving ointments and poultices, soft sea sponges, pieces of wool to cover the woman during labor and cloth to swaddle her baby afterward, smelling salts, a pillow to lay the baby on, and, most important, a birthing stool.

Soranus' birthing stool looked like an ordinary wooden chair, but with a crescent-shaped seat, open in front, for the laboring woman to sit on as birth approached. The stool had a gently tilted wooden back "so that both the loins and the hips may meet with resistance to any gradual slipping," and siderails "shaped like the letter pi [Π] . . . on which to press the hands in straining." For modesty's sake, the area below the seat was enclosed with boards or draped in fabric, except immediately in front, where the midwife worked.

With only minor modifications, Soranus' advice to midwives in *Gynecology* remained the standard of labor and delivery care for more than a thousand years. Women were attended by midwives of varying skills and training, practicing a mix of science and folk medicine that persisted well into the modern era when, starting about the time of the invention of forceps in the early 1600s, doctors slowly began to take over the business of birthing babies, pushing midwives to the periphery.

There were notable exceptions. Louise Bourgeois (1563–1636), midwife to the French court for twenty-six years, successfully battled the powerful obstetricians of her time who sought to discredit her. Her English contemporary, Jane Sharp, published *A Midwife's Book* in 1671 and was insistent in her demands for professional respect. Elizabeth Nihell, an outspoken opponent of doctors and their forceps, was famous for her battles with William Smellie and William Hunter, the most prominent British obstetricians of the eighteenth century.

But as respected as they may have been, midwives were often viewed with intense suspicion as well. This was particularly true in the American colonies. Margaret Jones, a midwife and healer, owns the dubious distinction of being the first New England woman executed for witchcraft, in 1638—fifty-four years before the Salem witch trials. That same year Jane Hawkins, another midwife, was accused of witchcraft and exiled from Boston to Rhode Island. A streak of infighting among rival Puritan factions had a lot to do with the charges against the two women, but the fact remains that midwives, with their mysterious potions and "women's work," were easy targets: twenty-two of the seventy-nine New Englanders eventually tried for witchcraft made their living birthing babies.

Midwifery survived the accusations of witchcraft. Midwives continued to provide the bulk of American labor and delivery care, mainly in homes, until the early twentieth century, when a new challenge to the profession—hospital-based birth—proved nearly insurmountable. It's difficult to overstate the impact of the move from home to hospital on American midwifery. Of the four-million-plus babies born in the United States every year, fewer than one in ten is delivered by a midwife, compared with nearly seven out of ten worldwide. And of all births attended by midwives in the United States, 96 percent take place in hospitals.

So far, this has been the story of the people who actually deliver babies: midwives and doctors—even me, in that action-packed summer of '77. But running parallel to the need for a person skilled in handling the complications of birth is the story of the other people who gathered around the mother-to-be: the friends and family who fetched the clean sheets, olive oil, or sow dung. Technically, anyone could fill that role, but in nearly every culture it was the woman's closest female friends and relatives who stood at the ready with soothing words, cool forehead compresses, and a firm grip when birthing time came.

Childbirth was a public act until well into the nineteenth century, for rich and poor women alike. Not the birth itself—that was accomplished under a mound of modesty-preserving blankets that often required the midwife to work by feel rather than sight. The birthing room, though, was open to the comings and goings of any number of people: friends, relatives, and neighbors bringing food, offering prayers and good wishes, or working to stuff cracks and seal windows lest a chill or an evil spirit enter the room to harm mother and baby. As delivery neared, the crowd usually winnowed to the midwife and a chosen circle of female family members and friends. The end result of all that traffic: from the onset of labor to her recovery, a woman was very rarely left alone.

Ironically, the birth of a prince or princess in Renaissance and Enlightenment Europe was often less personal and private than that of a peasant child. To confirm the birth of a legitimate heir (and prevent the possibility of a royal switcheroo—the furtive exchange of a live baby for a stillborn heir, for example), representatives of the court routinely gathered around the regal labor bed. Civil officials and even members of the general public were sometimes invited to observe the proceedings, too, though "common" witnesses usually had to watch from afar, sometimes from behind curtains or partitions.

The practice reached a pinnacle of sorts during the reign of France's Louis XVI. In her *The Private Life of Marie Antoinette*, Madame Jeanne-Louise-Henriette Campan, the queen's lady-in-waiting, described the chaotic scene that surrounded the birth of Princess Marie-Thérèse in 1778. When the royal physician, a Dr. Vermond, loudly announced that Marie Antoinette's labor had begun, all hell broke loose: "The floods of the curious that rushed into the room," Madame Campan wrote, "were so numerous and so tumultuous that this movement nearly killed the queen." Anticipating the crush, Louis had ordered the tapestries in the room secured with ropes the night before; if not for that precaution, Madame Campan reported, "they would surely have fallen on her." But even that safeguard wasn't enough.

The room soon filled to capacity and beyond. Spectators climbed onto the furniture, loudly jostling one another for a better look, a scene Madame Campan described as so boisterous that "one might have thought oneself on a public square." The queen, overwhelmed and overheated in the stifling room, soon passed out. Dr. Vermond cried out for fresh air and warm water, and commenced bleeding the queen's foot in an attempt to revive her. Leaping into action, the king himself broke open the chamber windows "with a force that could only have come from his tender feelings for the queen, these windows being very high and glued with bands of paper over their entire length." Once he'd smashed the windows, Louis went after the ill-behaved horde, ordering his manservants to forcibly eject "the indiscreet curious who did not stir themselves."

The crowd was quickly reduced to a dozen or so VIPs: the king and the doctor, of course, and "the princes of the family . . . the chancellor and the ministers [who] certainly sufficed to witness the legitimacy of a hereditary prince." Madame Campan and an unknown number of servants remained as well. With the room thus quieted and frigid December air blowing in through the broken windows, the queen came to.

Marie-Thérèse was born safely, but Marie Antoinette nearly died from postpartum hemorrhage, possibly aggravated by the rattled Dr. Vermond's handling of the delivery. She recovered, of course—her date with the guillotine was still fifteen years off—but she was not about to go through a birth circus like that again. As soon as the queen "returned from the gates of death," as Madame Campan put it, she decreed an end to the come-one, come-all tradition of royal birth. A much smaller crowd of officials gathered in 1781 to witness the birth of her son, Louis-Joseph.

As the nineteenth century dawned, the rituals and techniques of childbirth (royal births excepted) were much the same as in Soranus' time. Most births still occurred at home, attended by a midwife and the mother's chosen circle of female attendants. Doctors were called infrequently, mainly when things turned dire and forceps or craniotomy were required to end a troublesome labor. By the end of the century, though, things had changed dramatically—especially in the United States. As millions of women left rural towns and villages to seek factory work in large cities, slum conditions and overcrowded lying-in hospitals broke down the traditional social network of women helping women in labor.

That network had been quite extensive and, thanks to the nineteenth-century passion for letter writing and diary keeping, was well documented. The historian Judith Walzer Leavitt mines this material brilliantly in her book *Brought to Bed: Childbearing in America, 1750–1950,* in which she draws on personal journals and letters sent from woman to woman to show just how much things changed in the social upheavals of the time.

It's abundantly clear from the writings that when labor started, a woman wanted her female family members around her, in particular her own mother. Nettie Fowler McCormick, a young Wisconsin woman contemplating her first labor in 1890, illustrates that desire: "Dearest mother mine," she wrote in one of an impassioned series of letters she exchanged with her mother, "all would be complete if you were here."

Giving birth with relatives at hand became more difficult as families spread out across the country, but Leavitt shows how determined women were to keep that connection alive. Dorothy Lawson McCall, for example, traveled four times by train and wagon from her home in Oregon to give birth at her parents' house in Massachusetts. Another woman wrote of her grandmother traveling fifty miles on horseback to be with her own mother as her first labor approached, then riding back with babe in arms a few weeks later. Tales of pregnant women traveling long distances to join their mothers and sisters (and vice versa) were common.

Women unable to attend to their laboring daughters or sisters often felt a great deal of distress. In 1863 Mary Louise Fowler wrote to her pregnant sister in Europe: "I think of you in anticipation of your coming *trial*," her letter reads. "Will you, can you have among strangers, in a foreign land, that tender care which we all require at such a time[?] . . . it would relieve me of great anxiety if you were in *our* best little bed-room where I could nurse you as only a *mother* or a *sister* can." Albina Wight, on missing her sister's 1870 confinement in rural Wisconsin, confided to her diary, "Poor poor girl how I pitty [*sic*] her. She says the two wimen [*sic*] that were there were as kind and good as Sisters could be. I am glad of that. . . . Oh how I do wish I could be with her."

If family members were unavailable when labor began, women sought the companionship of any woman available, and they almost always got it: neighbors, servants, slaves, even complete strangers pitched in to help. Cultural differences usually disappeared in the birthing room—childbirth was a strong common denominator for women everywhere—but not always entirely. When Susan Allison delivered her baby prematurely in 1869, shortly before her planned trip to her mother's home, she relied on the help of a Native American woman: "Suzanne was very good to me in her way," as she later described her. "She thought I ought to be as strong as an Indian woman but I was not."

The scene inside the typical nineteenth-century American birthing room Leavitt describes was overwhelmingly female. Fathers were allowed a quick hello visit now and then, but those who lingered were soon turned out. In an 1836 account, an eager Minnesota father-to-be who tries to enter the birthing chamber is quickly dispatched by a Mrs. Warren, who "interposed, and the happy father was compelled, with reluctant steps, to quit the spot."

Most men respected the exclusion, understanding it was best to have experienced women attending their wives in the birthing room. As one father who clearly sympathized with his wife's ordeal explained it, "His life had not been in jeopardy. Except in sympathy his nerves had not been wracked, his muscles strained, his joints wrenched, his fibers torn, his blood spilled." Or, as a female physician put it in 1860, "Only a woman can know what a woman has suffered or is suffering."

The attitude of many women toward even the most well-intentioned men was neatly summed up by a fictional turn-of-the-century South Carolina woman contemplating her first birth in Grace Lumpkin's 1932 novel, *To Make My Bread*: "As she gulped down the warm coffee she wished in herself there was a woman who would know what to do without telling. And she wished the men were where they belonged when a woman was in travail—somewhere out on the mountains, or at a neighbor's."

Nearly all of this—the tradition of woman-to-woman birth assistance honed over thousands of years of human births—disappeared in the United States in the relative blink of an eye. When doctor-assisted hospital birth beckoned in the early twentieth century, with its promise of increased survival and decreased pain, women abandoned the ways of their mothers and grandmothers. By mid-century the transition was complete. Home birth was an unlamented thing of the distant, dusty past, a relic of pioneer times.

But that shift away from home and family had hidden costs. The traditional circle of female attendants didn't mesh well with hospital routine. Doctors increasingly saw family members, with their incessant questions, as meddlesome obstacles to efficient, "ideal" childbirth. By the 1940s, nonmedical birth attendants had largely disappeared; childbirth became a matter of a doctor, a nurse, and an often unconscious laboring woman.

My mother's birth experiences are a poignant example of the cold, impersonal nature of mid-twentieth-century hospital birth. She had seven babies in thirteen years, and each time she labored almost entirely alone. Her first delivery was particularly stark. Her labor began nearly two months prematurely, in the middle of January 1948. My father raced her to the hospital and was immediately dispatched to the fathers' waiting room. My mother was wheeled to a sparsely furnished room—a bed, a nightstand, and a straight-backed chair—where she spent her thirteen-hour labor in almost total isolation.

She remembers a couple of brief check-in visits from nurses, and a quick hello from a distant female cousin of my father's who worked at the hospital, but otherwise, as she recalls today, "I just laid there. Nobody told me anything." When delivery time came she was wheeled to a larger room and knocked out with sedatives. She woke up some time later, back in the room with the empty chair, frightened, nauseous, and alone.

My brother, James Bernard Sloan, died two days later from complications of his premature birth. My mother never saw him when he was alive because the doctors thought it would have been too frightening for her to see him struggle to breathe; and not after he died, either, because, they judged, that simply would have been too traumatic.

My mother's isolation extended well past James's death. She was kept in the hospital for nearly two weeks, customary at the time for an immediately postpartum woman. Visitors were allowed, but they were expressly forbidden by hospital staff to make any mention of James. Conversation was awkward in the extreme. "They could talk about the weather, the news, anything they wanted to," she remembers, "except for the fact that I'd just had a baby and that he died." She wasn't allowed to go out, not even to attend the funeral. All she has of James today is a fuzzy three-inch photograph taken of him at his wake, lying in a tiny white casket on a table in the living room of my grandparents' house.

It's not surprising that all this lonely laboring would spark a backlash against the increasingly mechanistic Western way of birth. What was surprising, at least to the mainstream obstetrics world of the mid-twentieth century, was that the strongest challenge would come from a man within its own ranks: an eccentric, yoga-practicing obstetrician by the name of Grantly Dick Read—the father of the natural childbirth movement.

Read, the son of a farmer, was born in Norfolk, England, in 1889. He set out to become a missionary as a young man, but his experiences as a medical officer in the trenches of World War I left him exhausted, shell-shocked, and decidedly skeptical of traditional religion. After he recovered, he turned his missionary zeal to a career in obstetrics.

From the beginning, Read took a radically different view of birth than his more intervention-prone colleagues. He stood virtually alone in his belief that normal childbirth "was never intended by the natural law to be painful," and that modern women—not to mention their doctors—had strayed far from nature's ideal. Read wrote admiringly of the birthing practices of women of "the more primitive type." At the start of labor, he wrote, the "primitive" simply sets aside her hoe or grinding stone and "isolates herself . . . in a thicket." Then, much like the female gorilla, she gives birth quickly and quietly.

Birth was fast and easy for the primitive woman, Read wrote, because she had "no knowledge of the tragedies of sepsis, infection and hemorrhage," and, better still, "no midwives [to spoil] the natural process." Should she die in childbirth, her tribe did not mourn her because they instinctively knew that "if [she] were not competent to produce children for the spirits of their fathers and for the tribe, [she] had no place in the tribe."

Read believed that modern women had lost the knack for easy, painless births (and grief-free deaths) through no fault of their own. He blamed the effects of modern culture that "protected [girls] from the hard facts of life" and never allowed young women to exercise their "natural instincts." Childbirth, Read noted, was often the "first primitive, fundamental physical act" a modern, acculturated woman was called upon to perform.

Not surprisingly, given such poor preparation for childbirth, Read's "modern" woman was terrified of labor. And it was the pain produced by that fear, compounded by the loneliness of hospital birth, that led to obstructed labors and the tendency of impatient obstetricians to intervene with drugs and forceps. Eliminating loneliness and the "fear-tension-pain" syndrome, Read fervently believed, would allow women to achieve a quick, primitive, painless birth.

Where and how Read came up with his primitive birth ideal is unclear. He was inspired in part by his war experiences, in which he claimed to have watched a smiling Flemish peasant woman pause to "drop a quick one" in a field and then return to her planting with barely a pause, her newborn baby in tow. But his obstetric experience—a decade in a private practice in a London suburb and later an urban practice in white South Africa—wouldn't seem to have provided him with access to many "primitive" births.

Read's research, such as it was, was definitely long on speculation and short on science. He rarely quoted scientific studies in his work, preferring to depend on his own observation and judgment. His technique of "natural childbirth"—Read was the first to popularize the term—relied on prenatal instruction, specific exercises for pregnant women, and yoga-based relaxation techniques he had picked up from an Indian junior officer during the war. It also required a doctor to remain with his patient, attending to her throughout the course of her labor, a decidedly uncommon practice in the mid-twentieth century. If followed to the letter, Read insisted, his technique nearly always resulted in childbirth "as God intended": joyous and absolutely pain-free, without need of any obstetric meddling.

Read's nearly science-free research and missionary zeal led to predictable clashes with mainstream obstetricians, but his natural childbirth techniques resonated with women, many of whom were deeply dissatisfied with the solo, knocked-out, forceps-guided delivery that was becoming the norm in hospital maternity wards. When his first book, *Natural Childbirth,* appeared in 1933, Read had already attracted a small but devoted group of supporters. By the time its sequel, *Revelation of Childbirth,* was published in 1943, Read's fans had grown in number and boisterousness. At a conference on labor pain management sponsored by *Wife and Citizen: A Journal Advocating the Economic and Social Emancipation of*

All Women, a group of Read's female supporters heckled the panel, most of whom supported the kind of isolated, medicated childbirth that Read abhorred.

Ironically, Read's unshakable faith in his beliefs and near-messianic enthusiasm for promoting them made him a growing target for his critics. Physicians grew tired of Read's sarcastic dismissal of any questions or criticism, and of his habit of appealing directly to the public, which many considered unethical. Given Read's tendency to freely contradict himself and his unwillingness to show any hard data to back up his claims of a nearly 95 percent success rate, it's not surprising that the public face of natural childbirth would eventually come in for a professional bruising.

That roughing up came in a 1950 article in *The Journal of the American Medical Association,* when two American obstetricians systematically dismantled every aspect of Read's "fear-tension-pain" theory, in particular his claim that childbirth is naturally a painless event. Read's response was angry but undaunted. His attackers either hadn't read his work, he wrote in reply, or they simply weren't smart enough to understand it. But a further blow came in 1953, when Dr. Frederick Goodrich, a supporter of Read's at Yale University, was forced to admit that only 2 percent of the women attempting natural childbirth in New Haven reported no pain at all, and slightly more than half of them took "mild" sedatives or stronger medications during labor.

The Read-versus-mainstream-obstetrics battle took on a new twist in 1956 with the publication of *Painless Childbirth,* a book written by Fernand Lamaze, an obstetrician at the Metal Workers' Union Hospital in Paris. Lamaze had traveled to Leningrad in 1951, drawn by Russian claims of a Pavlovian technique that resulted in painless childbirth in 90 percent of labors. Lamaze gave full credit to Russian obstetricians for devising the technique, in the process dismissing Read's work as emotional and unscientific by comparison.

Read took Lamaze's challenge as an affront to both his work and his country. He pointedly reminded the public that Lamaze was a known Communist sympathizer whose writing heaped praise on Stalinist Russia. Wrapping himself in the British flag at the height of the Cold War, he renamed his technique the "English" method, and even went so far as to Britishize himself by hyphenating his name. Plain old Grantly Dick Read became the much more stiff-upper-lip-sounding Grantly Dick-Read.

Despite Read's appeals to patriotism, Lamaze and his technique grew in popularity, especially in the United States, where Elizabeth Bing and Marjorie Karmel would soon found the organization Lamaze International. Then, just as it appeared that Lamaze's fame would eclipse his own, Read acquired an unlikely new ally: the pope. Speaking to a conference of several hundred gynecologists at the Vatican, Pope Pius XII endorsed Read's natural childbirth techniques as ethically and theologically sound. He briefly credited the Russians for their innovations in the field, then praised Read for "perfecting [the] theory and technique." Lamaze went unmentioned, his work reduced to a vague papal reference to "a Communist hospital in France."

It's not completely clear why Pius jumped into the Read-Lamaze fight. On the surface he was simply responding to a question from a gynecologist at the conference. But from his long, formal reply (the text was published the next day in *The New York Times*), it's clear Pius had been mulling over the issue for some time. He may have looked at natural childbirth from a practical point of view. After all, any technique that made childbearing more attractive had the potential to produce waves of new Catholics. More likely, his support of Read was rooted in Cold War politics.

Pius was a staunch anti-Communist. It must have pained him to praise a Russian innovation, however backhandedly, but he had to admit that the Leningrad researchers were onto something. Read was a bit of a problem for the pope, too, having once labeled Christianity's emphasis on the fall of Eve and God's painful-labor curse as a major cause of childbirth pain and fear. But Read's flag-waving patriotism probably made him more palatable to Pius than the Communist Lamaze.

Read's case was helped further by an unexpected tragedy. Caught in the mire of internal French Communist politics, Lamaze was fired from the Metal Workers' Union Hospital in October 1956. Exhausted after months of fighting to keep his position, he died of a heart attack the next day.

With his papal endorsement in hand and his chief rival now dead, 1957 became the year of Grantly Dick-Read. He released a recording of a natural birth, eleven hours of labor condensed to forty minutes of the mother's breathing and calm reassurances from Read, capped by the newborn's first lusty cries. It sold remarkably well. Later that year Read performed history's first televised birth and embarked on a successful American lecture tour. He created a stir wherever he went: one British newspaper compared him to Elvis Presley in terms of his ability to whip up mass hysteria.

When Read died in 1959, he was popularly eulogized as a brilliant, enthusiastic advocate for women. Physicians judged his career a bit more harshly. Dr. Frank Slaughter, an American surgeon and novelist, described Read and his followers as "a sort of cult, with considerable mumbo-jumbo and much popular discussion." Read's methods, Slaughter wrote, "spelled quackery to a suspicious medical profession."

As peculiar as some of his theorizing looks in hindsight, Read's work was important because it once again made the laboring woman the focus of childbirth. Where conventional obstetrics practice in the early twentieth century had increasingly turned its attention to the workings of the uterus, with or without a woman's conscious participation, Read recognized the soullessness of such an approach, and the impact that loneliness had on childbirth and much of a woman's life afterward.

Read also saw the value of continuous labor support in the delivery room, a time-honored concept that had been lost in the transition to hospital birth. Read couldn't see entrusting such an important task to female family members or friends, though. It was the physician's job, he declared, to provide that support by his continuous, reassuring presence throughout labor—an idea that earned him no end of scorn from many of his obstetrics peers.

Read did encourage one particular family member to be present in the delivery room: the husband. Granted, he had to earn his way in—Read banned men who hadn't taken his childbirth classes and insisted that nervous types be "kept downstairs" for their wives' sakes. Read's idea of the husband's role was limited, too. During the first stage of labor, he was to remind his wife of the lessons they had learned in class, helping her breathe correctly and "relax when relaxation was indicated." But when the pushing started, he was exiled to a stool in the farthest corner of the room to watch in silence, gowned and masked, as Read worked his magic. One peep out of him and "downstairs" with the nervous nellies he went.

In welcoming qualified husbands to the hospital delivery room, Read set in motion a trend that would revolutionize Western childbirth and the role of expectant fathers everywhere: witness the dawn of the father as labor coach.

At four in the morning on June 13, 1990, Elisabeth phoned me at the hospital to tell me her labor had started. I was in the call room, my head just hitting the pillow after a sleepless night of sick babies. Her bag of waters had broken in the bathroom a couple of hours earlier, she said. She was starting to have contractions.

This struck me as wrong. She wasn't due for ten more days. "Are you sure?" I asked, in the first of many clueless moments that day. "The bathroom floor is flooded," she patiently replied. "I'm very sure." The reality finally pierced my fuzzy-headed call night fog: I was about to become a father.

I took a deep breath. I was ready for this, I reminded myself. I was a certified labor coach, after all—I knew all about breathing and the stages of labor, about how to keep a woman comfortable and not take any cussing or punches to the head personally if the going got tough. God knows I'd seen enough babies born to understand the process. I was one fully prepared dad-in-the-making.

My task was straightforward. I'd go fetch Elisabeth and bring her back to the hospital, where we'd walk the floors awhile, count to ten a few times and—voilà!—we'd have a baby. Excited, confident, and hopelessly naïve, I called in the backup pediatrician, ran to the parking lot, jumped in my car, and headed for home.

We lived right on the northern California coast in those days. Our house sat on a bluff in an area dotted with dairy ranches, two hundred feet above sea level, staring straight out at the ocean. From our window we had a lovely if sometimes unsettling view of the San Andreas Fault as it dives into the ocean; the epicenter of the 1906 San Francisco earthquake lay just a few of miles offshore.

Twenty miles of serpentine country road lay between my laboring wife and me that morning, a bumpy two-lane strip of asphalt lined with pastures, oak trees, and acres of Ansel Adams photo ops. I usually made it home in about forty minutes, but traffic was notoriously unpredictable. Around every curve was a potential slowdown. Some days I'd sail through unmolested, while others were a stop-and-go gauntlet of wheezy school buses, antique farm machinery, and loose livestock. A particularly dreaded obstruction was the farmer who often picked commute time to move his glacially slow tractor from one field to the next, responding to the angry line of honking cars that trailed his five-mile-an-hour journey with a stiffly raised middle finger.

But I was cool as I pointed my car westward toward the sea. My brother and his wife were staying with us at the time, and John Henry was a doctor, so he'd know what to do if anything went wrong before I got there. I steered past the first potential roadblock—a dozen dairy cows, udders in full swing on the way to the milking barn, lined up on their own side of the fence. Things were going smoothly. Besides, what could go wrong in a mere forty minutes?

But forty minutes is a long time in the life of an immediate father-to-be, especially if he's alone in his car with no way to call his wife in those pre-cell-phone days. What had Elisabeth meant when she said that she'd be fine "until I got there"? Was she planning on *not* being fine after that? Had she been hiding something from me, just being brave so I wouldn't panic?

And wait a minute . . . John Henry was a physical medicine and rehabilitation specialist, the kind of doctor who fixes broken necks and old people's strokes, not an obstetrician. What did he know about delivering babies? Visions of my little brother filled my head: the one with all the stitches, the kid who'd tumbled down more stairwells than I could count, the boy who knocked out his front teeth—*twice*. This was the guy who might end up delivering my baby? My cool began to melt.

More worries: What if Elisabeth gave birth at home? I'd left my equipment back in the call room, and we certainly didn't keep an oxygen tank under the kitchen sink. What if there were complications? An ambulance would probably take an hour to get there. *My wife! My baby! Yikes!!* And just like that I was transformed from a calm, collected baby doctor into a sweaty, wild-eyed Every Dad. Damn the livestock—they crossed the road at their peril. And just let that crabby old farmer try and pull out in front of me. I'd bite his finger off.

A blur of scenery, a swerve around a hay wagon, and then a world record: home in just under thirty minutes. The overheated Honda fishtailed into the driveway, spraying gravel onto our brand-new landscaping. I sprinted to the front door like a hyperactive caveman, fully intending to sweep Elisabeth off her feet and carry her out to the still running car, then retrace my path to the hospital and race her up to labor and delivery just before our baby popped out.

Elisabeth greeted me at the door, a cup of tea in hand. She was dressed in her nicest maternity outfit, a suitcase at her feet. "You might as well take a shower," she said, sticking a pin in my adrenaline-charged balloon. "I don't think this is going to happen real soon." I surveyed the scene, speechless. *How could she know?* I eyed her with a mixture of anxiety and awe. She seemed pretty sure about the timing, and she was the one having the baby. I went back to the car and shut it off.

So I shaved and showered and had a cup of coffee. My brother and his wife gathered around to wish us good luck. I loaded the suitcase and a brand-new infant car seat into the Honda, and then, under her own power, Elisabeth climbed in. I drove her back to the hospital, just as I'd originally planned, but under strict orders to stick to the speed limit this time.

An hour later—no tractor encounters, but the school buses were out in force—we reached the hospital. I rolled up the curved driveway to the patient drop-off area, where a row of gleaming wheelchairs sat to the side of the entryway like so many cabbies awaiting a fare. Before I could move to fetch one, Elisabeth grabbed me by the arm. "I do *not* need a wheelchair," she said, and so, holding on to one another like a slow-moving couple in a three-legged race, we hobbled down the hall and took the elevator to the third floor.

The labor and delivery unit looked pretty much the same as it had the last time I'd been there—four hours earlier, attending the delivery of a baby with some minor problems that had quickly resolved. We walked to the nurse's station, pausing on the way for a strong contraction.

Some of the nurses at the station had been on duty when I left, but things were different now. They weren't looking at me, the pediatrician, pointing me to the room where the sick baby was. They were looking at Elisabeth. One of the nurses smiled, took her by the arm, and led us into a labor room. She asked Elisabeth the kind of questions women have no doubt asked one another since humans first walked the planet: How are you feeling? When did your contractions start? Any fevers or bleeding?

I trailed behind with the suitcase, relieved that my first fatherly hurdle—getting mom to the hospital on time—had passed without a hitch. Had I been my own father in 1953, taking my mother to the hospital to have me, that would have been it. I'd have gone home or shuffled off to the waiting room to watch the other dads smoke. But I'm not my father, and this wasn't his generation. My very long day of labor had just begun.

• • •

A father was a relative delivery room rarity when I started my career in the mid-'70s; by 1990, the year my daughter Claire was born, he was a fixture. Not only was his attendance mandatory, for the first time in human history he was expected to run the nonmedical end of things, too. He was the go-to labor support guy, for everything from breathing exercises to ice chips to foot massages. Ready or not, *like* it or not, the mantle of labor coach (and was that manly sports-metaphor title intentional?) had been laid on his shoulders.

Pity the father who tried to opt out. He was seen as a lesser father, an unenlightened man who chose to ignore the overwhelming weight of evidence that being present at the birth, actually seeing his newborn arrive in the world, was critical to forming a lifelong bond with his child.

The importance of paternal birth attendance and father-infant bonding moved center stage during the 1960s and '70s. Young Americans were in full rebellion against much that their parents stood for, and the detached fathering style of the 1950s and earlier was a prime target. In less than a generation the cultural pendulum swung from the image of father-as-distant-breadwinner to one of a man so immersed in his children's lives that he could never really be *too* involved. That intense involvement extended to the delivery room. A number of studies in the 1970s and early '80s seemed to confirm the critical importance of a father's birth participation. Miss those crucial first minutes of your son's life, and you blew it— might as well pack the kid off to boarding school while he's still in diapers.

One problem with the dire predictions of unbonded fatherhood, though: they weren't true. Much of what passed for evidence linking paternal birth attendance to father-infant bonding in those early studies was really a classic case of research bias. Scientists "found" what they set out to find—that birth was a critical, not-to-be-missed moment for father and child—and the public passionately embraced their findings. The pressure on fathers to attend soon became so strong that researchers found it difficult to find "non-attenders" for their studies.

Dr. Rob Palkovitz, a developmental psychologist at the University of Delaware, was the first to critically review the existing research on paternal birth attendance and bonding. His landmark 1985 study challenged the received wisdom of the time, pointing out the flaws in many of the studies that had been used to "prove" the need for a father's labor room presence.

Much of that research drew sweeping conclusions from very small numbers of men, for example—as few as fifteen in some studies—as well as after-the-fact surveys and brief labor room observations. The measures of bonding were a bit suspect, too: a "bonded" father was defined as one who, presumably due to his having been there at birth, changed more diapers at six weeks of age. Or did more housework. Or carried his baby more often.

But, as Palkovitz noted, a father's presence or absence in the delivery room was the only variable the researchers examined. No attempt was made to look at what a particular man brought to labor with him: his preexisting level of "helpfulness," his previous experience with babies, the strength of his marriage, or even his desire to be a father in the first place. It was like linking a father's birth attendance to his future willingness to help with his child's math homework, as though no other factors—whether he's any good at math himself, say—might come into play.

Pro-attendance researchers were highly selective in what they took away from previous studies, too. A 1974 study by Dr. Martin Greenberg, based on a survey of just thirty men, was the first to document the impact of the birth experience on fathers. "Attenders" seemed more comfortable with their babies a couple of days after birth than "non-attenders," he found, and were more confident that they could identify their babies on sight.

Greenberg's small, largely subjective study became a touchstone for the pro-attendance researchers who followed him. Here was conclusive evidence of the importance of birth attendance, they said, and based on his findings they developed the "be-there-or-else" theories that soon made a father's attendance virtually mandatory. Yet none of the researchers mentioned Greenberg's actual conclusion: that there really wasn't any significant difference between the fathers who were present at birth and those who weren't in terms of attachment to their babies.

Palkovitz went on to cite studies that contradicted the idea that a father who missed his child's birth had caused irreparable damage to their relationship. One stood out: in 1983, Dr. Betsy Lozoff surveyed 120 cultures and found that only one in four of them permitted the father to be present at birth, mostly just as an observer, and yet there was "no increase . . . in paternal involvement when fathers were allowed at childbirth." Lozoff speculated that if a father's attendance at birth really was crucial to a child's well-being, humans would have figured it out long ago and made it a universal practice.

His own research led Palkovitz to conclude that the benefits of birth attendance are probably indirect. A father's involvement in pregnancy, labor, and delivery help strengthen his relationship with his partner (if she wants that kind of attention, Palkovitz noted) and contribute to his feeling that he's part of an evolving family. But despite what fathers were being told at the time, there was—and still is—no strong evidence that birth attendance by itself directly promotes father-infant bonding. To assign too much importance to that one factor among so many in the complicated process of becoming a father, Palkovitz wrote, "is a disservice." Birth attendance, he concluded, is "neither necessary nor sufficient for the establishment of positive father-infant relationships."

Given all that pressure on a 1970s-and-beyond father to be there at birth, it's not surprising that he wound up as labor coach. He was the person most attuned to his partner's needs, the thinking went, from all those months of painting the nursery and picking baby names, so who better to guide a woman through her labor?

Most men agreed. They enjoyed the intense emotional experience of birth, and the tasks themselves—breathing exercises, back rubs, and such—weren't all that difficult. And anyway, a man had his own support system in the labor room. There were always nurses around to take over for a while if he needed a break, right?

A funny thing happened to hospitalized childbirth along the way. First, the female family members and friends disappeared, chased out by doctors and nurses in the heyday of Twilight Sleep. Then, under pressure from natural childbirth advocates, hospitals relented and allowed a single family member back into the delivery room—the father/coach, who depended a great deal on the nurses for advice and assistance. Then, slowly, the nurses themselves began to disappear.

The vanishing delivery room nurse was a trend that had started decades earlier, as her role shifted from providing nurturing care at the bedside to performing medical tasks. By the 1980s she became even more scarce, thanks to the introduction of electronic fetal monitoring (EFM). Before EFM, a nurse checked on a laboring mother frequently, sometimes every five to fifteen minutes, using a stethoscope on the mother's belly to manually count the fetus's heart rate. That close contact allowed her to keep an eye on the father, too, reassuring him that the labor was going according to plan and preparing him for what was to come. The laboring couple was rarely alone for long.

But EFM changed all that. With a mother connected to an electric monitor, nurses could keep track of several women at once, often from a central nurses' station. Visits to the room became fewer and further between; "face time" with the couple decreased. As labor progressed and the mother grew more focused on the workings of her body, the father was increasingly left to stew in his own fears and anxieties. It gradually became apparent that just maybe, given the fact that he was dealing with some significant issues of his own, the father-to-be wasn't always the best person for the job of supporting his partner.

A spate of research in the late '80s and early '90s explored the inner world of the expectant father and discovered there's a lot going on in there. Labor was stressful for all fathers, researchers found, and many spent more time hiding their feelings or worrying about being useful than doing any actual coaching. Fathers were generally positive about being there to see their babies born, and many turned out to be excellent coaches, but most had a lot of insecurity, anxiety, and worry for themselves, their partners, and their babies mixed in. Men in the studies consistently reported fears of seeming "unmanly"—of vomiting or fainting, for example. They worried about their relationships, about being replaced in the mother's affections by the baby. And there was the big-ticket worry: What if their partner or child died?

Maybe we're expecting too much of men, the researchers concluded. After all, a man doesn't have an entire patch of his brain devoted to the rhythms and hormones of childbirth the way a woman does. Maybe all those unexpressed worries about life, death, and the responsibilities of fatherhood, coupled with the experience of seeing a loved one in intense pain, perhaps for the first time, get in the way of providing the kind of support a laboring woman really needs. Maybe it's enough that he's just *there,* without burdening him with the coaching job, too.

Back to 1990. Safe in the labor and delivery unit, Elisabeth changed into a hospital gown and climbed into bed. The nurse squirted jelly on her abdomen and placed an electronic stethoscope over where she figured our baby's heart would be. *Whoomph! Whoomph! Whoomph!* Sounded like the fetus had a battering ram in there; the nurse turned down the volume. "Healthy heart," she said and moved on to taking Elisabeth's pulse, temperature, and blood pressure. The two women talked briefly about what to expect next, and then the nurse went over a few of the hospital basics with us: the alarm button's here, the TV remote's there, we're right outside, just call if you need anything. Then she left us alone with the door almost closed, the sounds of a busy labor unit seeping through the crack.

I had been in Labor Room 5 many times. I knew everything in it, from the monitor attached to Elisabeth's abdomen to the swatch of a 1920s baby blanket in the plastic display box on the wall, right at a laboring woman's eye level. But the room looked different now, a matter of changed perspective. I had stood by the small table in the corner, the one with all the equipment and the direct view of the fetal monitor and the emerging baby, what—a hundred times? Now I was sitting in the comfy chair next to the bed where the expectant fathers always sat. I thought about all those men—how scruffy and bleary-eyed they looked by the time I was called in at labor's end. How had I looked to them, I wondered, with my scrubs, stethoscope, and mumbling explanations?

We were all alone now, and though Elisabeth diplomatically says I hid it well, I was no different from the men in those research studies—I was scared. I could rationally tell myself that she and our baby-to-be were safe, that it was only a matter of a few hours until I'd be calling the relatives with a name, a weight, and the news that mother and baby were just fine. But I'd seen too many births go awry in my career; what if this was the one case in however many that didn't end happily? What if Elisabeth or the baby was injured, or even died? And what about me—even if everything turned out okay, was I ready to be a father? My one overriding anxiety: *Will we ever be the same again?*

"Hey." Elisabeth's voice snapped me out of my reverie. "Aren't you supposed to be helping me with my breathing?" I held Elisabeth's hand and counted with her.

A couple of hours later I was calmer. We talked between contractions, mostly about names. A girl would be Anna or Claire, we finally decided. A boy . . . well, we still weren't sure. Girl names were so pretty, so melodious. All the boy names we could think of sounded like variations on "Thud" or "Bam-Bam."

Elisabeth's womb fell into a rhythm: a contraction every three minutes or so. With each one I kicked into the labor coach role I'd learned in our childbirth preparation class, helping Elisabeth focus on breathing until the contraction passed. I reached into my grab-bag of comfort measures—neck rubs, cups of water, cold compresses for her forehead—and prepared for the few hours I thought remained.

Three hours and several dozen rounds of coached breathing passed. The nurse midwife, a calm, slender, comforting woman named Gina, examined Elisabeth around three o'clock and announced that she was dilated to four centimeters. "Great progress!" she told us, but I could do the math. At a centimeter an hour we were looking at another six hours to delivery. Turned out that my math was a little off—twenty-four hours off, to be exact.

Adrenaline is a fickle thing. It's your body's way of getting you to do things you couldn't normally do, like fighting off a wild animal or charging into a burning building to save a child. But after the adrenaline rush departs, *bang!* You fall asleep. As day dragged into evening and I passed my thirty-sixth sleepless hour, I couldn't keep it up anymore.

We had just returned from walking another of our seemingly infinite loops around the labor and delivery hallways. Elisabeth eased herself back into bed and I straightened the blankets over her. She was sweating and red-faced; this was labor in every sense of the word. I fetched her some water, sat down in my comfy chair, and without so much as a blink, fell sound asleep. Three minutes later I was awake again, called by Elisabeth. I stood and helped her through another contraction.

My legs were going wobbly now. I pulled my chair as close to the bed as I could, so that I could hold Elisabeth's hand and breathe with her without actually getting up. But even that didn't help—I ended up with my head on Elisabeth's shoulder, passed out between contractions. Somewhere in the middle of the night, after a series of three-minute catnaps, she told me to just go to sleep. I retreated to my chair with a blanket and did as I was told.

The rest of the night was a foggy blur. Nurses, obstetricians, and anesthesiologists came and went. Elisabeth was exhausted. In order to get some rest and hopefully avoid a cesarean, she reluctantly agreed to an epidural. For a few blissful hours we both slept while her uterus continued to do its job on a kind of biological autopilot.

I awoke for good at five-thirty. The sun hadn't yet cleared the office building across the street, but the sky was cloudless and bright. Gina, our midwife from the day before, had returned, a little surprised to see us still there. She did an examination: eight centimeters. This time Elisabeth didn't moan. Her energy was back; she was ready to get this done.

Right around the time we were struggling through Elisabeth's labor, the hospital-birthing world came to realize that an expectant father wasn't necessarily a woman's best labor supporter. But if dads weren't the best coaches, then who? Looking back through human history, the answer seemed obvious: female relatives and friends had done the job for millennia, so why not now? The door to the labor room opened a bit wider; absent for decades, the circle of female relatives and friends slowly returned to the bedside.

There were still problems, though. These women were different from the circle that had gathered around their great-great-grandmothers. For one thing, courtesy of smaller family sizes and a mobile society, there were fewer of them and they often lived too far away to rush to a daughter's or sister's side when labor began. Many of them lacked personal experience with natural vaginal birth, too—remember that one-fourth of births at the time were cesareans, and the experience of vaginal birth was often altered by epidural analgesia. Many women simply didn't—and still don't, as cesarean and epidural rates continue to climb—have the older, birth-experienced relative or friend who was critical to pre-twentieth-century labor support. Who, then, could a woman turn to as her due date grew near? Enter the *doula*.

"Doula" is a Greek word meaning "woman's servant." First used in the United States in 1976 to refer to a woman who helped other women with breast-feeding problems, the name soon became synonymous with a trained female birth companion. A doula (pronounced DOO-lah), especially one who has been certified by an organization like the Seattle-based Doulas of North America, provides nonmedical physical and emotional support to a woman during her labor and sometimes well beyond. She offers information about pregnancy, birth, and hospital or birthing center routines, provides continuous support and comfort during labor, and acts as something of an interpreter between mother and medical staff when needed. Her job, in sum, is to support a woman's prenatal desires for the birth of her child while helping her adjust to the realities of the actual labor.

The doula movement was given a huge boost in the 1980s and '90s when research by Drs. Marshall Klaus and John Kennell showed the striking benefits of continuous labor support, particularly as provided by a trained doula. The two physicians found that an experienced labor companion was more than simply a comfort to a woman—her presence also dramatically improved the outcome of her labor.

Klaus and Kennell's original study was done in 1980 in a busy urban hospital in Guatemala, where, by hospital policy, women routinely labored alone. The first experiment was simple. Women early in their first labor were randomly placed in one of two groups: half of them labored alone, following usual hospital routine, while the other half were kept company from admission to birth by an unfamiliar, untrained woman who did nothing more than hold the woman's hand and chat with her. The positive effect of such basic human interaction was startling: the average length of labor was cut by more than half, from 19.3 hours for women who labored alone to 8.7 hours in the accompanied group.

In 1986, Klaus and Kennell followed up with a larger study in the same hospital. In addition to confirming that accompanied women had shorter labors, the study found that continuous labor support drastically reduced cesarean rates: 7 percent of the supported women ended up in the operating room, compared with 17 percent of those who labored alone. Still, American hospitals didn't flock to change their policies—this was a hospital in Guatemala, after all, with many other differences that might have affected the outcomes. American doctors wanted to see American results.

So Klaus and Kennell proved their case on American soil. In 1996 they published the results of a study done at Jefferson Davis Hospital in Houston, an urban hospital whose crowded labor and delivery unit served mainly low-income women. This time they divided the women into three groups: those who followed usual hospital policy and labored alone, those who labored with a trained doula, and those who labored with an observer in the room—a woman who never spoke, didn't touch the laboring woman, and remained as inconspicuous as possible.

The Houston results were nearly identical to those from Guatemala: the doula-assisted women had shorter labors (7.4 hours versus 9.4 hours) and fewer epidurals (7.8 percent versus 22.6 percent) and cesarean births (8 percent versus 18 percent) than those who labored alone. Particularly striking were the results from the "observed" group—those who had the silent woman simply sitting in the room. Their labor lengths and epidural and cesarean rates were midway between the doula-assisted group and the laboring-alone group. In other words, the mere presence of a person in the room was enough to improve labor outcomes, though whether this was due to a direct effect on the mother herself or on the staff who took care of her wasn't clear. Perhaps the presence of the silent woman reminded the staff of the study and discouraged them from jumping too quickly to epidurals and cesareans.

Still, the case for continuous labor support had been made. Studies from Belgium, Finland, France, Greece, Canada, and South Africa soon confirmed Klaus and Kennell's findings: continuous labor support reduced cesareans, epidurals, forceps use, and labor length. Remarkably, the effects could still be seen several weeks after birth. Women in the South African study who had been attended by a trained doula had higher self-esteem, less anxiety, and lower depression scores than those who had labored alone, and they were more likely to still be breast-feeding their babies six weeks later.

It's important here to emphasize the word *continuous*. From Grantly Dick-Read onward, research has shown that, in terms of improved labor outcomes, *intermittent* labor support is barely better than laboring alone. The fear and anxiety that often accompany labor increase a mother's production of catecholamines, those fight-or-flight hormones I discussed in "Pain and Politics," which can slow labor and intensify pain. It takes a constant, reassuring presence to keep the catecholamines at a healthy level, and it turns out that a supporter who comes and goes isn't really much help.

The person providing that continuous support doesn't necessarily need to be a doula, of course. The support provided by an experienced female relative or friend will likely yield the same benefits as that provided by an unrelated, sometimes unfamiliar doula, but as we've seen, that kind of start-to-finish, high quality birth support from family or friends is getting harder to find.

It appears that dad, though, really isn't the best person for the job. Figures don't lie: labor outcomes in the studies—cesarean rates, epidural use, and such—were significantly better when couples were supported by a doula than when they labored by themselves, even when the expectant father had completed a childbirth preparation course. Much of the difference had to do with the doula's having been through childbirth herself, and her focus on the mother's needs. With no emotional issues of her own to deal with, she did more touching and holding, had more verbal interactions, and remained physically close to the mother for longer periods than did the father.

That's not to say the father doesn't belong in the labor room, of course, or that he can't be a wonderful birth attendant. His presence is important to his partner, their relationship, and their baby—it's a life-changing experience a man shouldn't miss. But he doesn't need to be a coach. With a doula or a female relative or friend doing what women have done since time immemorial, he's free to be what a father in a labor room should be: a comforting presence in what for him is a very strange land.

The final hour that Elisabeth pushed was one of the most wonderful, surreal hours I've ever spent. A tiny tuft of red-blond hair played a game of hide-and-seek with us, peeking out when Elisabeth pushed, retreating when she rested. Each time a little more hair remained visible between contractions. Gina, the midwife, joked about braiding it. I didn't know yet whether I had a son or a daughter, but this much was clear: he or she was a hairy-headed little thing.

Gina and the nurse had taken over coaching now—two women helping another to have a baby, the way it was always done before hospital routine got in the way. I became an observer, a hand holder, and a fetcher of things. Nobody sent me to boil water or gather firewood, but if they had, I'd have jumped on it.

Finally, at 3:36 in the afternoon of June 14, nearly thirty-six hours after Elisabeth first called me, our baby arrived—first her head, then her shoulders, then the rest of her, guided by the midwife's sure grip. Gina cradled our daughter in her lap, cut the cord, and laid her on Elisabeth's chest. We decided right then she was a Claire, with her spiky strawberry-blond hair. An Anna would have been darker.

This was the point in a birth when I usually left. Everyone was fine, no need for a pediatrician here. I have a habit of looking back one last time as I leave a delivery room, and the scene is almost always the same: mother and baby in the bed, father standing to one side, his head turned to look at his newborn's face, reaching out to touch a finger. But this time I didn't leave. This time that guy was me.

•　•　•

If I could have a redo of Claire's birth, knowing what I know now, I'd do a lot of things differently. For starters, seeing that "due dates" are at best educated semi-guesses, I'd trade away all my June call nights well in advance. Next, Elisabeth and I would seek out a birth-experienced woman to support the two of us—mainly her, of course—so that I could be free just to hold Elisabeth's hand, mop her brow, and silently worry all my expectant-father worries.

We didn't lack for candidates back then. Elisabeth's mother and sister, both birth-experienced intensive care nursery nurses, would probably have jumped at the chance to help, but we just didn't think to ask. There may well have been doulas in our area, too, but I didn't know of any. Besides, we thought, why would we need anyone else? This was right in the middle of the father-knows-best period of birth attendance, and every pregnant woman we knew planned on laboring with her husband or male partner as coach, the two of them a self-contained birthing unit. Even our prepared childbirth teacher, a self-described "anti-establishment birth educator," didn't bring up the idea of the traditional experienced woman as a companion.

Still, if I had been aware of the research already out there in 1990, and especially if I could have foreseen the studies that have come to light since then, I would have realized that a father-to-be can understand only so much about having a baby. Though prepared childbirth classes are helpful, there really is no substitute for having someone with personal childbirthing experience there from start to finish. Most likely we'd have had our baby the old-fashioned way, with Elisabeth's mother or sister present.

So, then, the redo: Freed of my call night grogginess, I'm there when Elisabeth's water breaks. Skipping the crazed ride home, I see right away that she instinctively understands what's happening, that birth is still a long way off. While Elisabeth showers and packs her things, I call her mother or sister or whoever the woman is we've chosen to help us through labor and delivery. She meets us at the hospital, and there, through all the grueling hours of labor, I watch as she and Elisabeth do the intimate, elaborate birthing dance that women have done with one another since nearly forever.

Maybe then I could have relaxed and enjoyed Claire's birth even more than I did. And maybe then I could have avoided the vague, gut-level sense that I failed as a labor coach, a feeling that took me a long while to shake.

The smallest group of birth attendants I've ever seen was at the very first birth I witnessed—just me and Tonya, nearly alone to the end. The crowd at Terri's birth, the one that Eric tried so valiantly to film, was the biggest: twelve people in the room when I arrived and sixteen when I left, including the brand-new baby.

However many people gather around a woman at birth, whether they're friends or relatives or hospital staff, this much is true: in the end there's always one more. And it's the newest one, that squalling seven or eight-pound bundle of a family's hopes and dreams, that soon steals all the attention.

PART IV
Looking at Babies

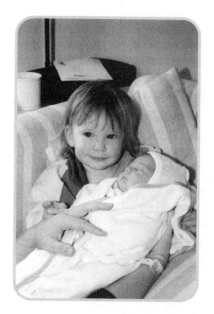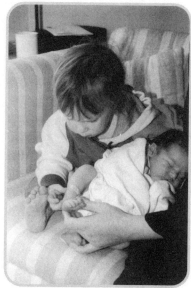

Claire examines her brother, January 3, 1992

Chapter 8
Inside Looking Out:
The Five Senses at Birth

Victor was four years old, a compact, dark-haired bundle of boy energy contained for the moment inside an open-in-the-back clinic gown. Seated on the exam table in my office, he eyed me warily, on the lookout for anything with a needle attached to it. Victor was seeing me for his kindergarten checkup. He knew that sooner or later, someone, somewhere, was going to give him a shot.

I rolled up my sleeves to show Victor I wasn't hiding any syringes. "Shots come later, in another room," I said. "In here, I'll just be looking at you." He relaxed a bit, though his fingers still gripped the toy doctor's bag in his lap. As I started my exam, he held it out to me. "You can use my stuff if you want to," Victor said, his voice so quiet I had to lean forward to hear him.

I took the bag and opened it. Inside were a half-eaten granola bar, a Power Ranger (the red one), and several garishly colored plastic replicas of the tools of my trade: a stethoscope, an otoscope, a reflex hammer, and a blood pressure cuff. I took them out one by one, oohing and aahing as I laid them on the table next to the real things. At the bottom of the bag, under the granola bar, I found a small, expensive-looking flashlight, the kind you see in those high-end gadget stores that sell reclining massage chairs and electronic watch-winders.

"What do you use this for?" I asked, figuring it was an unofficial Power Ranger weapon of some kind. Victor's eyes widened. His mouth opened, then closed. He cast a sidelong glance at his mother, who was seated in the wooden chair next to the table. "Show him what it's for, sweetie," she said. "It's okay. He's a doctor."

Victor hopped off the table, flashlight in hand. He switched it on and waited as his mother pulled up her blouse, exposing her ample third trimester belly. Then he pressed the flashlight gently into her navel. "It's okay, brother," he said, laying his head on his mother's abdomen while he patted her tightly stretched skin. "It's okay."

"He's worried it's too dark in there," Victor's mother said. She smiled and stroked her son's cheek. "He doesn't want his brother to be scared of the dark, so every now and then he shines in some light." Victor looked up at his mother, then at me. "It *is* dark in there," he said, a trace of irritation in his voice.

I boosted Victor back onto the exam table and helped him reload his bag. "I know what you mean about it being dark in there," I said. And I did—I knew exactly what he meant.

My aunt Joan is the first pregnant woman I can ever remember noticing. We were at a family gathering at a lake house in Wisconsin, the early-sixties kind of reunion where the dads gathered around the barbecue while the moms took turns fishing each other's kids out of the lake. I was probably six or seven, old enough to have seen a few pregnant women by then—my mother was already two babies past me, after all, and her sisters were in the midst of a remarkable flurry of cousin making. But somehow, until that afternoon, I hadn't really noticed any of them *looking* pregnant.

Aunt Joan was standing on the little patch of beach in front of the house. I hadn't seen her in a few months, and the change in her appearance was startling. "Why is Aunt Joan so fat?" I asked my mother, who was reading a magazine in a shady hammock nearby. "I don't know," she said absently, without looking up. "Why don't you ask her?" So I did. I crossed the beach to my aunt and asked her, point-blank: *Why are you so fat?* Aunt Joan blinked at me through her thick glasses, then she laughed. "Oh, honey," she said, tousling my hair, "I'm going to have a baby!"

Which of course made no sense whatsoever. I was still in my babies-come-from-the-hospital phase of childbirth understanding.

She might as well have told me she was fat because she was going to have her hair done or her house painted. What did having a baby have to do with it? I nodded in feigned comprehension, walked back to my mother, and told her what Aunt Joan had said.

Maybe it was the look on my face, or maybe Mom thought I needed a bit more childbirth education than the nuns at Sacred Heart were ever going to give me. Whatever the case, she sat up in the hammock, closed her magazine, and pulled me near. "The baby's in her tummy," she whispered, like we were spies exchanging nuclear secrets. "That's why she's fat."

Wow. You could have knocked me over with a puff of swampy, mosquito-laden midsummer Wisconsin air. *The baby's in her tummy.* I watched, stunned, as my aunt waded in and out of the lake shallows. *That's why she's fat.* And the first thing that occurred to me, once I could think again, was this: *It must be really dark in there.*

Except it probably wasn't. I didn't know then that the world inside the womb isn't always pitch-black, that as Aunt Joan stood in the warm sun in her summer-weight cotton blouse, some light was actually passing through the skin and muscles of her abdomen, all the way into her womb. Nor could I have known that when I stood close to my aunt and blurted my question, my third trimester cousin-to-be—Jimmy, it must have been—might well have seen the shadow of my head pass over him, like a mini solar eclipse. Or that if I posed my *Why so fat?* question loudly enough, he might even have heard me.

I thought about telling Victor what it's really like in the womb for an almost-born baby, about what his brother could already see and hear, smell and taste, but I stopped. At four, it was enough that he felt good about protecting his brother from the darkness, a feeling that would only grow stronger when he finally laid eyes on him a few days later.

"It's nice that you're taking care of your brother," I told Victor a few minutes later, as we finished up and he buttoned his shirt. "I'm sure he appreciates the light."

• • •

The late term fetus does spend most of its time in the dark. Maternal clothing, skin, fat, muscle, and the wall of the uterus itself add up to a relatively lightproof barrier. But every so often the inside of the womb isn't pitch-black. It's red.

The ability of light to reach the fetal eye from the outside world varies with the color of the light. Virtually all lower-wavelength light—violet, blue, and green—is filtered out before reaching the inside of the uterus. Given the right conditions, though, about 10 percent of red light makes it through. That's just enough to give the interior of the womb a dim, glowing, Martian-sunrise look when a lightly dressed mother stands in direct sunlight, as my aunt did on that Wisconsin beach a half century ago.

Surprisingly little research has been done on fetal vision, at least in comparison to what's been done on hearing, the research champion of the fetal senses. This is partially due to the different rates at which vision and hearing develop. Sound penetrates the womb much more easily than light, and aural input is important to the development of fetal hearing. Given the paucity of visual stimulation in there, though, it's not surprising that eyesight at birth is comparatively underdeveloped. Vision, in fact, is the last of the senses to fully mature.

The human eye on the day of birth is definitely a work in progress. It's big, more than two-thirds the size of an adult's, but performancewise it lags far behind those of its sister senses: hearing, smell, taste, and touch. A newborn's vision is a blind-as-a-bat, Mr. Magoo–like 20/400. Coincidentally, that's about how well I see, too. I got my first pair of glasses at age nine—probably should have had them years earlier—and was astounded to discover that there really is a man in the moon. In practical, grownup terms, 20/400 vision means I have to stand twenty feet from an object to see it as clearly as an adult with 20/20 vision can from four hundred feet.

I would have more sympathy for the newborn and her poor eyesight if it weren't for the fact that 20/400 vision fits her needs just fine. Unlike my younger, squinting, spectacle-less self, a newborn doesn't really care what's going on four hundred, twenty, or even five feet away. Everything he needs in life after birth is no farther away than the length of his mother's arms.

Most fetal vision experiments have been straightforward stimulus and response studies: do something and see if they jump. Scientists learned early on that bright light causes a "rise and shine" reaction in the fetus. First comes a rise in the pulse rate, then increased body movement as the fetus more or less climbs out of bed.

The response to bright light is so predictable that not long ago a team of obstetrics researchers at the University of New Mexico proposed it as a test of fetal well-being. When they beamed a halogen light directly against the abdominal walls of fifty-three healthy women with uncomplicated pregnancies, they found the usual fetal response in all but one: increased heart rate and body movement. The only fetus who didn't respond as expected turned out to have a placental abnormality and ended up with an emergency cesarean delivery. (And here's how well maternal tissues work as a light filter: the very bright halogen beam used in the experiment was nearly as intense as sunlight; by the time it reached the fetus it was estimated to be only about as bright as a 25-watt bulb.)

Mothers have no doubt known about the fetal response to light far longer than researchers, though. Tales of fetuses set in sudden motion by sunshine, floodlights, and other very bright lights are fairly common. I remember a woman once telling me her fetus moved and kicked whenever she and her husband watched a movie on the wide-screen TV in their darkened living room. Perhaps she was right, but there's more to a movie than light. Was it really the movie's brightness that woke up her fetus, or might it have been the dialogue, music, and crashing sound effects—in short, the noise—that came with it?

• • •

The human fetus went deaf in 1885 and stayed that way for three-quarters of a century. That was the year German scientist Erklärung von W. Preyer declared, after some informal experiments, that the fetus can't hear a thing. Preyer's word on the subject was good enough for the Western scientific community, most of which was too busy battling tuberculosis and cholera to worry about whether or not a fetus could hear. Very little research on the subject was done in the decades that followed.

The news that the fetus was deaf may have made sense to Preyer's colleagues, but it must have come as a surprise to the women in their lives, many of whom no doubt had experienced a sudden fetal jerk or kick in response to a loud noise—a slamming door, for example, or the clang of a falling kitchen pot. That experience was nothing new; in Luke's gospel the Virgin Mary tells her cousin Elizabeth that the fetal Jesus "leaped in my womb for joy" at the sound of her family's loud, friendly greeting. Still, a woman's subjective impression was no match for the iron will—and male viewpoint—of nineteenth-century science.

Common sense and scientific thought eventually meshed. Preyer's countryman Dr. Adolf Pieper was among the first to challenge the deaf-fetus theory. In 1925 he came up with a rather straightforward experiment to test fetal hearing. Pieper sat himself between a pregnant woman and an automobile, with one hand resting on the woman's belly. On command, an assistant blared the car's horn from a distance of three feet. Pieper then made a check mark in his notebook each time he felt the fetus kick, which by his reckoning happened once in every four honks. (The make and model of Dr. Pieper's car are long forgotten, but given the year of the experiment I have to assume the test stimulus was a loud "aah-*oooh*-gah.")

Science slogged onward. Using buzzers, bells, and snapping rattraps as noisemakers to stimulate the fetus, and stethoscopes, stopwatches, and hands on the belly to measure its response, by the 1930s researchers had built a small but impressive body of evidence that the fetus could hear at least very loud noises. Still, the scientific and medical powers-that-were responded with a collective yawn. The findings of Pieper and others were ignored or dismissed; perhaps Pieper was actually measuring the mother's movements, they suggested, rather than those of the fetus. In 1937, Preyer's 1885 findings were republished, verbatim, in *The American Journal of the Medical Sciences*. The fetus stayed officially deaf until the middle of the twentieth century, right around the time I became one.

Undaunted, a new generation of researchers in the late '40s and '50s improved their experimental technique by bombarding the fetus with more precisely measured noise. Taking advantage of advances in the field of electronics, they broadcast sound through loudspeakers at various distances from the uterus, even directly against the mother's abdominal wall. They soon confirmed Pieper's findings. The fetus seemed to react to loud noise, all right—usually with the sudden, startled movements and jump in heart rate we associate with fear—but no matter how refined the noisemaking became, test results were often hard to interpret. Fetal researchers were held back by a simple obstetrical fact: they couldn't directly observe their subjects.

What scientists longed for was a way to peer into the womb and watch the fetus in action, to see its responses to noise firsthand. The inventions of obstetric ultrasound and electronic fetal monitoring in the 1960s were the breakthroughs they needed: they now possessed objective, noninvasive ways to spy on the fetus.

Armed with refined noisemakers to stimulate the fetus, and electronic monitoring and ultrasound to watch its reaction, fetal hearing research entered a remarkably productive "golden age." By the mid-1990s, studies had proven that there's a lot more going on in the womb than Preyer and Pieper could have imagined. In the span of one decade the fetus was discovered to have quite a list of hearing-related talents—feats made all the more remarkable when you consider that the sound quality in the womb is roughly equal to that of a cheap boom box played underwater.

During the most recent century and a half of its existence, the third trimester uterus has been viewed as: a) a soundproof booth; b) a place so noisy that by all rights you should hear it from across the room; and c) a quiet, heavenish place filled with background "white noise," punctuated only by the soothing sounds of a mother's heartbeat and her reassuring voice. In reality, it's a world filled with a wide variety of noise, both internal and external—everything from lullabies and traffic noise to a mother's gurgling stomach—all of it important for the development of hearing and, ultimately, a child's ability to communicate with the world around it.

But when sound from the outside world penetrates a mother's abdominal wall, not all of it gets to the fetus, and what does is greatly modified. To begin with, in order to be heard at all, a sound has to be louder than the "noise floor" in the uterus itself. Noise floors—a fancy name for background noise—aren't unique to the womb, of course. Here's a real-time writer's-life noise floor example: I'm sitting in a coffee shop as I type these words, and I'd love to know why the couple at a nearby table is having such a heated conversation, but I can't quite hear them. There's too much noise from the coffee roasting machine, the murky reggae thudding from the speakers overhead, and the rowdy table of preschool kids getting tanked on hot chocolate while their mothers chat away. That's my "noise floor" for the moment. Unless the couple gets into a shouting match that's louder than all of that, I'll never know why the man looks as if he's afraid his girlfriend's about to smack him.

The noise floor in the pregnant uterus consists mainly of biological noises produced by mother and fetus. The mother contributes the sound of her breathing, her speech, heartbeat, placental blood flow, body movement, and gastrointestinal noise. (A sobering thought: more commonly heard by the fetus than its mother's sweet voice is the sound of her intestinal gas.) The fetus contributes the noise of its own heartbeat, movements, and pulsating umbilical cord. Just as in my coffee shop example, any sound that makes it to the fetus from the outside world will have to be louder than all those noises put together. So how loud does that have to be? How noisy *is* it in the womb?

The first studies of the uterine noise floor were done forty years ago, when intrepid researchers inserted small microphones into the still open wombs of some remarkably complaisant women who'd just given birth. Results varied quite a bit. Some studies found the womb a quiet place, with only 30–50 decibels (dB) of noise—a loudness somewhere between a quiet whisper and a normal conversation. Others described it as "very noisy," as loud as 96dB—the equivalent of a subway train heard at two hundred feet, which, assuming there was no actual train running by the labor room at the time, raises a legitimate question: How could the researchers have heard themselves think over all that noise coming out of the womb?

It turned out that the "loud womb" studies were wrong. Much of the noise they picked up was from the room itself: machinery, voices, and other stray hospital sounds that don't reflect the actual noise level inside the womb in the days and weeks leading up to birth. More recent studies on pregnant ewes—sheep are remarkably similar to humans in terms of uterine noise floor and fetal hearing—show that the noise level in the womb is similar to that in the surrounding room and varies according to the frequency, or pitch, of that noise.

There's a lot of bass in there. Sounds with a frequency of less than 100 hertz (Hz)—that's about two octaves below middle C, for any musicians out there—pass into the womb easily, while higher-pitched sounds are muffled or missing altogether. The difference is due to the sound-absorbing characteristics of the abdominal and uterine tissue that sits between the fetus and the outside world. Low-frequency sounds pass though skin, fat, muscle, and body fluids almost unchanged. Higher frequencies are largely absorbed by these tissues; the higher the pitch, the less of it passes into the womb. So by the time sound passes through maternal tissues and amniotic fluid, it's already been filtered in a bass-heavy, treble-light way. And that's just fine with the fetus, since it doesn't hear high-pitched sounds well until after birth anyway.

A fetus's ear doesn't work like an adult's, either, unless that adult happens to be underwater. For one thing, eardrums don't have much to do with hearing in the womb—they're for detecting sounds that travel by air, which the fetus obviously won't encounter until after birth. Like the fetal lungs and liver, the eardrums in utero are basically along for the ride, just growing and developing in those final weeks before they're put to lifelong work.

Think about how things sound when you're underwater, the closest you'll ever again get to being in the womb. There's a peculiar hard-to-locate quality compared to sounds that travel through air. It's difficult to tell where a sound is coming from. That's because underwater sound is sensed by bone conduction: sound waves travel through water and vibrate the bones of the skull, which in turn conduct sound directly to the hearing centers in the inner ears. It's the same thing that happens when a doctor touches a vibrating tuning fork to the center of your forehead. If your hearing is normal, the vibrations will travel through your skull and reach both your inner ears at the same time, giving the noise a coming-from-nowhere-in-particular quality.

That's how fetal hearing works. Sound waves passing through maternal tissue and amniotic fluid are transmitted to the inner ear by bone conduction, bypassing the eardrums altogether. The sounds that reach the inner ear are mainly low in frequency, matching what the fetus is best able to hear. That combination of low-frequency sound transmission and low-frequency-dominated hearing combine to shape the late term fetus's understanding of the world around itself, both within the womb and beyond. And as it turns out, even with almost no high-pitched sound coming through, the fetus understands quite a bit.

· · ·

Once scientists finally understood that the fetus could hear, they asked the next logical question: Was it listening, too? And if so, was the fetus capable of learning from what it heard? The answer to both, they quickly discovered, was yes.

In 1948, D. K. Spelt of Pennsylvania's Muhlenberg College set out to prove that the fetus could learn by classical conditioning—that is, with practice, the fetus could learn that a seemingly minor stimulus meant that a second, more significant one was on the way.

Spelt's experimental setup looked like something straight out of a Cold War–era science fiction movie. On one side of a screen lay the pregnant subject, with three pairs of movement-detecting electrodes taped to her abdomen and a fourth attached to her chest, to record her breathing. Hovering over her belly in a wooden frame was a small metal rod, something she likely didn't recognize for what it was: the vibrating "striker" from an ordinary electric doorbell.

On the other side of the screen the wires connected to pens that left continuous ink trails on a "long-paper kymograph," a bed-long contraption that looked a lot like an earthquake-measuring seismograph. Sitting on the floor by the head of the bed was Spelt's homemade noisemaker: a long oak clapper attached to a large square pine box by means of a steel spring. When Spelt pulled a cord, the spring released and the clapper "struck the face of the box sharply." Voilà: the noise stimulus.

The setup must have puzzled Spelt's subjects, but they knew better than to ask about it. In those pre-informed-consent days, the women had no idea what the wires, noise, or vibrating rod were for. They weren't even told they were part of an experiment, only that the doctors wanted some "special information" about their babies. The reward for going along quietly was significant: free labor and delivery care. Thirteen women quickly signed up.

Here's how the experiment worked. Spelt would touch the vibrating striker to the woman's abdomen, sometimes following that with a loud oak-on-pine "thwack" from the noisemaker, sometimes not. The buzzing from the striker by itself didn't cause any fetal reaction, but the sudden loud noise caused it to jump, its movements captured by the pens on the kymograph. Then Spelt began to follow each buzz with a thwack.

After about twenty attempts, the fetus started to catch on: when it felt the buzz, a thwack was on its way. Soon the buzzing alone, which hadn't caused a reaction at the start of the experiment, was enough to get the fetus moving.

Though there were some problems with the study—the subjects had an inconvenient habit of going into labor before finishing the multisession experiment, for one thing—after several hundred buzz-and-thwack cycles, Spelt had shown fairly convincingly that the fetus can learn to anticipate a loud noise.

Researchers later found that the fetus can do much more than simply predict a thwack: it can learn to ignore it, too. "Habituation" is familiar to just about everyone on earth. It's the ability to tune out irritating background noises: a loudly ticking clock, say, or a droning after-dinner speaker. When a fetus hears a novel sound, its heart rate increases: excitement! After a while, when the repeated sound becomes old hat, the heart rate drifts back to normal: boredom. Add a new sound and the heart rate goes up again—until the novelty wears off, that is. Like everybody else, a fetus can learn to ignore a repetitive noise.

There's one sound a late term fetus can listen to all day, though: mama's voice. In the late 1970s researchers confirmed what women had long suspected: the fetus prefers to hear its mother's voice over any other sound. When a pregnant woman speaks, her fetus often slows down its movement and heart rate, a condition recognized in newborn infants as the quiet, alert state. In other words, when mom speaks, her fetus pays attention.

Even a recording of mother's voice played back from outside the womb is more appealing to a fetus than a stranger's spoken voice, but given a choice between a maternal recording and the real thing, the mother's live voice wins nearly every time. But is it what she's saying that captures her fetus's attention, or how she says it?

Like all other sounds that enter the uterus, a mother's voice is filtered so that the low-pitched tones are most prominent. When the fetus listens to its mother it hears mainly vowels—longer, low-frequency tones—and almost no consonants, which tend to be the kind of brief, high-frequency sounds maternal tissues filter out. Think of the adult voices in those *Peanuts* TV specials, with their nonsensical *wah-wah* trombone quality. That's pretty much what a fetus hears of its mother's voice.

As a result, the fetus pays more attention to the rhythm, pitch, and rise-and-fall patterns of its mother's speech (together known as prosody) than what she's actually saying. This accounts for the fact that a fetus pays more attention to its mother when she speaks in her native tongue, even if she's fluently bilingual. The rhythms of her preferred language are more familiar, more interesting, more like, well, *mama*.

The same is true of music: the fetus likes to listen. A large number of studies have demonstrated fetal interest in music, and at first the interest seemed to be particularly strong for classical music. But just as Brahms-loving researchers were asserting their bragging rights over their Beach Boys–obsessed colleagues, someone figured out that the supposed fetal yen for classical music actually related more to the tastes of the people doing the research—it's what they played in their experiments—than to any innate fetal love of Mozart. In reality, almost any musical style will do, a fact dramatically underlined by a study that got fetuses hooked on the theme song from a popular British soap opera.

Highbrow/lowbrow debates aside, what fetuses like most about music is the rhythm, since, as with language, most of the higher frequencies are never heard. The overtones of both Brahms's Lullaby and "Good Vibrations" are lost en route to the womb. The fetus goes through its last trimester floating in a musical world that sounds like what you hear when one of those bass-blasting hot rods pulls up next to you at a stoplight.

But bass-heavy hearing didn't stop the fetus from racking up an impressive list of experimental achievements during the golden age of fetal hearing research. By 2000 the fetus had shown that it could distinguish different voices and different pitches; recognize a story read by its mother (and ignore it if she read it in a different language, or if someone else read it); respond to sounds as diverse as *Peter and the Wolf* and jet noise from a nearby airport; and even show a preference for familiar musical pieces and stories over newer ones, a preference that persists after birth. The ability of the fetus to learn about the environment outside the womb is almost eerie; after reading a dozen or so of these studies, I half expected to find one with scientists tapping Morse code on a mother's belly and the fetus tapping right back at them.

In short, fetuses actively learn from the internal and external environment around them, picking up the fundamentals of speech, language, and musical rhythms over the course of the last few weeks of pregnancy. The awareness of in utero learning has led many researchers and parents to explore the idea of actually teaching the fetus—playing Mozart concertos through "belly-phones" to promote musical talent, for example, or stimulating math skills by playing increasingly complex electronic "heartbeat" patterns—but it's here that the issue of fetal learning veers into uncharted, unproven territory.

A quick Internet search turns up a number of sites promoting "teach the fetus" materials, most of which tout the early developmental benefits of their products. But the "results," such as they are, are often no more than testimonies from satisfied customers, most of whom have sunk a lot of cash into the advertised program and would hate to think they've wasted their money. There's no real evidence that such programs work—or indeed, that they're not actually harmful.

Human hearing evolved in the relatively protected environment of the womb. Until the last two hundred years or so, that environment was largely free from the kind of industrial and mechanical noise that is now known to contribute to hearing loss in modern children and adults. We've seen that the womb isn't soundproof—the noise level is similar to that of the room a woman finds herself in at any given moment. If a pregnant woman works in a loud factory, she may in fact be putting her child's hearing at risk—you can't stick protective earplugs in a fetus's ears.

Adding even more noise to that environment, even if it's "good" noise like classical music or recorded maternal heartbeats, without any evidence that it helps a child develop "better" than he or she would if simply left alone, is another example—like elective primary cesareans—of putting our kids through a large, uncontrolled experiment we may come to regret.

Shortly after Aunt Joan patted my head and sent me back to my mother's hammock, I went swimming under the dock. I couldn't have known it at the time—I'd just learned about wombs, after all—but I was doing a passable job of imitating my cousin Jimmy's third trimester sensory world. The water was warm and dark under the dock, a bit like the womb was for him. My vision was limited, too, though by foggy goggles rather than the wall of the uterus. And when I dived down in search of snails, clams, and a vaguely seahorse-looking kind of pipefish, the low-pitched throb of passing motorboats vibrated in my head—and probably Jimmy's, too—bone-conducted all the way.

There were a couple of big differences, though. I couldn't smell a thing, courtesy of my too-tight, nostril-smashing nose clips, and when I opened my mouth I tasted an organic, fishy, petroleum-seasoned mix of lake water and dilute outboard motor fuel. Jimmy had the better deal. He was smelling and tasting the pretzels Aunt Joan munched as she waded in the water, just as he had smelled and tasted everything else she ate in her third trimester.

Historically speaking, testing a fetus's sense of taste and smell hasn't been nearly as much fun for scientists as testing its hearing. There's no equivalent of Adolf Pieper's honking car or D. K. Spelt's wooden thwacker in taste and smell research. You can think up all kinds of ways to transmit noise to the fetus, be they vibrating rods, tape-recorded nursery rhymes, or blaring Bach sonatas, but the abdominal and uterine tissues are impervious to tastes and smells. Rub all the peanut butter and jelly you want on a mother's belly—none of it will ever reach the fetus. That's why the stack of fetal nose-and-tongue research papers on my desk is a lot smaller than the one for ears.

Let's start with smell. The idea that a fetus could detect odors was long dismissed in scientific circles, mainly by the same people who assumed that the fetus was deaf, too. There were three main objections offered as proof: First, the nasal passages of newborns (and so, presumably, fetuses) are usually filled with mucus, amniotic fluid, and other secretions at birth. How could a fetus smell with all that gunk stuck up its nose? Odor detection is an airborne phenomenon in the out-of-the-womb world, too—how could the fetus detect odors when there's no air in there? Lastly, what would the fetus smell, anyway? Amniotic fluid was thought to have the same, uniform odor throughout pregnancy. Even if the fetus could smell it, wouldn't it eventually tune it out, just as adults do with the smell of their own breath or body odor?

Those questions had to be answered indirectly, since direct testing of the fetus—injecting smelly chemicals into the amniotic fluid and seeing if the fetus reacts, for example—was an ethical nonstarter. But determined smell researchers, working from animal studies and detailed examinations of both term and premature human newborns, enjoyed their own "golden age" of discoveries. By the end of the 1990s, they had established a clear picture of the human fetus's olfactory capabilities.

By means of detailed ultrasound studies, they examined the fetal nasal cavity. Rather than being a stagnant, mucus-plugged backwater awaiting liberation at the hands of a delivery room nurse with a suction catheter, the third trimester nose was found to be wide open and free-flowing. Every swallow, hiccup, or breathing movement circulates a bit of amniotic fluid; as a result, the fluid in the nasal cavity is constantly turned over.

They discovered, too, that the nasal chemosensory system—the nerves that detect odors—is well developed and functional by the beginning of the third trimester. There are actually four interconnected sets of nerves that make up our sense of smell, but only two of them are major players in detecting odors.

The first is the *trigeminal system,* which is more or less an early warning system for the nose; it's responsible for that tickling, burning, stinging, or itching sensation you get with a cold or allergies, or when smelling salts get waved under your nose. The second is the *olfactory system,* which does the heavy lifting of sorting out the odors of everything from fancy perfume to spoiled milk. The two other systems, the *terminal system* and the *vomeronasal organ,* play roles that are probably minor and certainly not well understood.

Those four systems don't operate in isolation; they work together in helping an out-in-the-world human detect, memorize, and recall smells. The fact that they are already up and running in premature babies means that the olfactory system must work well in the late term fetus, too. So, if the third trimester fetus's nose works just as well as an adult's, what is it actually smelling in there?

Those of us who attend a lot of births know that the odor of amniotic fluid isn't uniform; for one thing, it's often altered by a recent maternal meal. A mother who has a nice Italian dinner in the hours before giving birth may well have garlic-scented amniotic fluid when her membranes rupture. I well remember the strong odor of asparagus on a baby whose mother had been munching stalks of that vegetable—a craving of hers—just before going into labor.

That the smell comes from the amniotic fluid itself and not somewhere else—the mother's breath or intestinal gas, or the abandoned take-out box sitting in the far corner of the labor room, for example—was proven in a study in which third trimester women not yet in labor swallowed garlic powder capsules before having a medically necessary amniocentesis. An hour later, when the amniotic fluid was withdrawn from the womb for testing, it smelled strongly of garlic.

We notice strong-smelling foods in amniotic fluid at birth, but that's just the tip of the in utero food pyramid. We can't detect the subtler ones—foods with milder odors that are overpowered by the other smells that come with childbirth. But a fetus bathes in those smells throughout pregnancy, especially in the last trimester, when the placenta allows more maternal food molecules to pass into the amniotic fluid, bringing a complex potpourri of odors directly to the fetus.

The fetus not only smells the foods in its mother's diet, it remembers them after birth, and it tends to like what it remembers. In one study, newborn babies whose mothers regularly ingested anise during pregnancy repeatedly showed interest in that licorice-like aroma by turning their heads toward the source of the smell. In another, third trimester women were given a daily drink of carrot juice; months later, when it came time to start solid foods, their babies showed a preference for carrots.

That memory can last for a long time, even several decades, if my own experience is any guide. I learned in my family research for the "Daddies" chapter that one of my mother's main cravings when she was pregnant with me was Grape-Nuts cereal. My father told me he'd keep two or three boxes on hand in the kitchen, afraid of running out in the middle of the night in those pre-convenience-store times. Sure enough, just like those anise- and carrot-loving babies, I was hooked on Grape-Nuts from early childhood until just a couple of years ago, when its pebbly crunchiness started to make my aging teeth ache.

The smell of amniotic fluid probably plays a role in the development of cultural food preferences, too. A child who is exposed to a heavy rotation of curry in the womb, for example, will likely develop a yearning for curry dishes later on. It's also why a fetus and infant never exposed to curry—one hooked on Grape-Nuts, say—might not learn to enjoy Indian food until well into adulthood.

The fetus *tastes* the same things it smells in the amniotic fluid, of course, but taste seems less important than smell in imprinting cultural food preferences. The tongue of the late term fetus and newborn can detect sweet, bitter, and sour (the ability to detect saltiness doesn't come until weeks later), skills that seem much more hardwired and less flexible, less emotional than the sense of smell.

That makes intuitive sense: notice how even favorite foods taste bland when you have a stuffed-up nose, or how the smell of freshly baked chocolate chip cookies lures you straight to the kitchen, salivating, long before you spot them on the countertop. The two senses work together; taste does the basics of measuring sweetness and such, but the emotional connection to food resides in the sense of smell.

So, then, is there a purpose to the fetus's apprentice-gourmet habit of savoring every bit of maternal food? And what's the point of all that intrauterine listening and learning? Would it really matter if Erklärung von W. Preyer had been right—that the fetus is more or less walled off inside the womb, oblivious to external sensory input?

It's good to remember, once again, that nature does nothing without a reason. The answers to these questions can be found in those first few minutes of life outside the womb, that welcome-to-the-real-world moment when the fetus suddenly discovers that there's no longer such a thing as a free lunch.

Asked to imagine what it's like to be a newborn in the first hour outside the womb, most people conjure something along the lines of what I call the Big Surprise: *Colors! Lights! Noise! People!* Kind of like being tossed—naked, soaking wet, and screaming—onto Main Street Disneyland at noon in high tourist season.

The Big Surprise may be a fair description of birth from an adult perspective, but it's nothing at all like that for the baby. The experience of being bodily evicted from the womb, the only home it has ever known, is no doubt a sizable shock to a newborn's system. But it's a shock adults can't really fathom, even though we've all been through it, because the world a newborn enters isn't simply a bigger, bolder version of the one he just left. A baby is born into a world he never knew existed, a world filled with unimaginable sights, sounds, tastes, and smells. It's not naked-in-Disneyland; it's naked-in-an-alternate-universe.

Consider that the voices the baby heard in utero, those muffled noises that arrived from nowhere in particular, now come blaring out of giant, blurry *somethings* moving around in an incomprehensibly vast space. The baby soon finds himself zooming through that space, passed from one loud, bizarre creature to the next. Strange objects move in and out of sight, new sounds bombard his ears, and everywhere he turns, his new world is filled with dazzling, nearly blinding lights and colors.

And the smells! These aren't the familiar, comforting aromas of amniotic fluid and mother's diet anymore. These are strange odors, perhaps even a bit repulsive, smells he will someday recognize as his mother's sweat, his father's cologne, and the rubbery scent of a doctor's gloves. But for now, they're all mixed together into a sensory shock the likes of which we can't begin to imagine.

It's enough to make a baby cry, and so he does—but only for a short while, just long enough to drive the fluid from his lungs and reassure everyone around him that he's up and running. Then he settles into an almost eerie period of quiet alertness, his eyes searching for something his prenatal sensory life has primed him to expect: a certain voice, a face, a nipple, a lifetime connection.

One of the most amazing moments in a newborn's first day is one that too often isn't allowed to happen. In our mania for weighing and measuring, for passing babies from relative to relative and photographically documenting their every blink and startle, a magical moment that connects us with other mammals and our primate ancestors is frequently missed. Because when placed on his mother's abdomen and left undisturbed by visitors and medical staff in the first minutes of extrauterine life, a freshly born baby will make a remarkable journey.

At first the baby lies quietly. His eyes wide and hardly blinking, he scans his mother's face—in particular her eyes and mouth—and listens intently to her voice. After a few minutes of mama-gazing, he begins to make mouthing movements, smacks his lips, and starts to drool. Then, slowly, he begins a laborious crawl to his mother's breast.

That crawl looks a bit like a horizontal, slow-motion version of a rock climber scaling a particularly tricky cliff wall. The baby searches for toeholds in his mother's abdominal skin; finding them, he pushes himself forward one small step at a time. Every so often he adjusts his side-to-side position with a kind of two-handed push-up. Along the way he stops frequently to rest, sucking and smelling his fingers while he gathers energy for the next big push. This is hard work, particularly considering all the energy he's just used up being born, but inevitably, after a breather, it's back to the climb.

It can take a half hour or more, but eventually he succeeds in scaling Mount Mama. Cradling his mother's breast between his arms, he moves his head back and forth, licking and smelling her nipple. At last he latches on and begins to suck, all the while watching his mother's face. Mission accomplished: in less than an hour he has figured out where the food is, how to make it appear, and who he can count on to make more of it. He uses all his senses in that journey; a newborn sees, hears, smells, feels, and tastes his way to his mother's breast, guided by the sensory learnings of the womb.

Newborn vision is perfectly designed for this search. As we've seen, babies are born very nearsighted. They see objects most clearly from eight or ten inches away, which makes sense, since that's exactly the distance from a nursing baby's eyes to his mother's face. From a newborn's perspective, anything farther than that isn't worth looking at anyway.

From the moment of birth, or at least as soon as the crying is done, a baby visually homes in on his mother. He knows what he's looking for. He's born with an innate visual interest in certain things: curved patterns, roundness, light-and-dark contrast, and things that move about. If that sounds suspiciously like a face, with its darting eyes and expressive mouth, you're right—babies are born with the ability to recognize the elements of the human face. This was demonstrated in an elegant series of experiments in which newborns were shown a cartoon drawing of a normal face and another in which the facial features were scrambled—nose on top, both ears on the same side, and such. The infants consistently sought out the "real" face and ignored the surrealistic one.

There is a debate among developmental psychologists as to whether the newborn brain has an innate, hardwired ability to recognize the human face per se, or whether the baby simply seeks out facelike features. Experiments with black squares placed in different arrangements on white, lightbulb-shaped figures seem to show that the newborn actually seeks patterns—two "eye" squares in the "forehead" part of the lightbulb shape, with a "nose" and "mouth" lower down—not actual human features. This face-versus-pattern developmental debate strikes me as a bit strained. The pattern newborns preferred in the study looks a lot like a face, even to my adult eyes. Anyway, how many black-square-covered lightbulbs is a newborn likely to come across? Nature makes the human face powerfully attractive to the newborn, with good reason.

That face recognition skill, whatever its source, is present in both full term babies and those born a few weeks prematurely. This means that a late term fetus could probably recognize the elements of a face, too, though no one has yet figured out how to project a scrambled-face slide shows into the womb.

The idea that their fetuses already know the basics of what a human face looks like never ceases to amaze the parents-to-be who come to my prenatal classes. But newborns do more than simply see faces—they memorize them, too. A baby can often distinguish his mother's face from another woman's as early as four hours after birth. Babies quickly become sensitive to changes in that special face, too. In a somewhat mean-sounding study, mothers of few-days-old babies were given masks to wear during nursing. Their babies were clearly rattled by the change. They scanned the masks frequently during the "masked lady" feedings, searching, it seemed, for that familiar face. They took less milk during the masked feedings, too, and were more restless when put down afterward to nap. Fortunately, when Mom's reassuring face returned, they settled back into their happy-baby nursing patterns.

Hearing is important to a newborn's first journey as well. A mother's voice, so pervasive and nondirectional in the womb, now comes to the baby from her mouth, a sound that reverberates in her chest. Following that familiar voice, so reassuring among all the strange noises that echo around the room after birth, helps direct the baby to the breast.

The sight of a mother's face and the sound of her voice may set a baby's first journey in motion, but the newborn's sense of smell is actually the key to finding his mother's nipple. Without it he might sail right past her breasts, inching forward until he bumped into her chin. This is more than speculation—in a study in which one of a mother's nipples was washed immediately after birth, the baby nearly always ignored the clean nipple and headed for the unwashed one instead.

What draws the newborn to his mother's nipple is, remarkably, the smell of amniotic fluid. Anyone who has attended a birth knows that amniotic fluid has a distinct aroma, one that isn't entirely pleasant. Researchers have variously described its smell in terms more commonly associated with the bouquet of a really bad wine: rancid, urinaceous, musty, spicy, oily, or milky, even "goaty" and "fecal." Adults, or at least the ones who performed the studies, tend to find the aroma of amniotic fluid "displeasing."

Rancid or not, newborns are crazy about that smell—it reminds them of their dear departed intrauterine home. That's what the baby is doing when he pauses to sniff and licks his hands en route to his mother's breast: he's comforting himself with the familiar smell and taste of amniotic fluid. He notices, too, that something nearby has that same wonderful aroma. Inspired, he continues his search, at last finding the source: his mother's nipple. This, to me, is one of the most amazing elements of the newborn's first-hour journey: a mother's nipple secretes a chemical that smells exactly like amniotic fluid.

There was a time in our evolutionary history when the crawl from a mother's belly to her breast was much more than simply an emotion-filled moment for parents to watch and treasure. The skill to climb quickly to the nipple was once a matter of newborn survival, and it still is in many mammalian species.

Look no further than modern mammals who give birth in litters, like dogs, pigs, and even rats. Newborns of those species scramble like mad to the mother's nipples at feeding time. The quickest and strongest get the most nourishment; the slower, weaker "runts" often die. It's the smell of the mother's nipples, with their reassuring aroma of the womb, that draws the babies to their food.

Even those mammals who give birth to a single infant, where competition isn't an issue, depend on smell to connect mother and baby. Not long ago I was fortunate enough to observe a minutes-old elephant seal pup and its mother at Point Reyes National Seashore, about an hour from my home in northern California. I watched through binoculars as the pup and its mother sniffed one another's faces, memorizing the unique scent that would bind them through their month together on the beach. After twenty minutes of nuzzling, the mother rolled onto her side, exposing her nipples low on her abdomen. Moving in the opposite direction from that of a human baby's crawl, the pup sniffed its mother's neck, then her chest and abdomen, and very slowly worked its way down to where the food was.

The human baby, then, is lured toward his mother's breast by a combination of sight (mama's smiling face), hearing (her familiar, calming voice), and smell (her amniotic fluid-scented nipple). The newborn quickly associates that face, that voice, and that nipple with food, warmth, and comfort. The lifelong bond between mother and child begins—or rather it continues, as it's already been nine months in the making.

• • •

I haven't forgotten about the fifth sense. I've saved the discussion of touch until now because its benefits aren't obvious until after birth, when the flashier senses have done their thing and the baby is happily nestled against his mother's breast.

Though we don't often think of it that way, the skin is the body's largest sense organ. A newborn has a very well developed ability to sense heat, cold, pressure, moisture, and pain. We often think of those sensory abilities in negative or protective terms. That's understandable—much of the skin's sensory ability is designed to warn the baby and his parents that something is amiss. A baby who's too cold or too hot, uncomfortable from a wet diaper, or in pain from an older sibling's "affectionate" earlobe pinch, will signal his parents with a loud and clear *Fix it!* cry.

But the skin, particularly on the lips and hands, is covered with nerve endings that sense the pleasurable aspects of touch as well. All babies comfort themselves by sucking on things—their hands, mother's nipple, a pacifier—and all of them like to be picked up and held. The close parental contact a baby craves does more than simply calm him. Human touch is actually key to a baby's overall health.

The physical benefits of touch have been proven in research done with premature babies in intensive care nurseries. Infants who underwent brief periods of gentle massage three times a day gained weight much faster than babies who did not, and were more alert and active with their caregivers. They also went home nearly a week earlier than did the babies who were not massaged.

In fact, a lack of human contact can be disastrous. A baby who is fed enough calories to grow on, but otherwise receives little or no contact with his caregivers, often "fails to thrive"—the medical term for a child who refuses to gain weight and whose physical and emotional development are often severely stunted. The hands-off style of care that was once the norm in orphanages and foundling homes led to many cases of failure to thrive. Sadly, failure to thrive hasn't disappeared. It's still seen in babies who are victims of neglect and abuse.

The benefits of touch can easily be overlooked by parents, since most need no encouragement to touch and cuddle their babies. Vision, hearing, taste, and smell may be flashier—*Look! He's following my face!*—but touch is the sensory glue that holds it all together. Without parents' instinctive urge to touch and hold their baby, all that seeing, listening, sniffing, and tasting would be for naught.

In our direct ancestral line, the ability to quickly identify mama by sight, smell, voice, and touch was often a lifesaver in a different way. Consider ancient hominid birth, back in the time before birth attendants provided some measure of protection. A female with a just born baby was a prime target for predators. If attacked, her fight-or-flight hormones kicked in, sending her scampering up a tree or into the underbrush to escape, a task for which she needed all four limbs. In that flurry of clashing bodies, the newborn needed to know whose fur to cling to, which body represented danger and which one safety. The sensory learning that took place in the womb—the ability to instantaneously identify mother—was critical to survival.

Humans don't give birth in litters, of course, even if the mother of triplets I once took care of strongly disagreed with me on that point. And lion, tiger, or bear attacks in the course of a modern hospital birth are exceedingly rare. The drive to find mama's breast immediately after birth isn't as critical to physical survival as it once was, not with legions of doctors, midwives, nurses, and breastfeeding specialists standing by and, when the need arises, the willingness of people to adopt and raise other women's children as their own.

Everyone alive on earth, including me and my cousin Jimmy, and Victor and his baby brother, has been through some variety of that in utero sensory learning experience. It is a testament to the adaptability of the human newborn that an entire generation of American babies—those of us born in that mid-twentieth century era of "scientific" birth, who were separated from our knocked-out mothers for the first few hours of life and denied the chance to breast-feed—never completed that womb-to-world sensory connection, yet we survived and still ended up loving our mothers.

Fortunately, the pendulum is swinging back. Most hospitals today practice a less interventional style of obstetrics for uncomplicated births. Weighing and measuring and such are put off until that initial bonding period passes. Even in the deliveries I'm called to attend, in which it's often necessary to separate a sick baby from its mother until all is well, we work hard to reunite mother and baby as quickly as possible.

The intrauterine environment is so rich in sound, smell, taste, and, to a lesser degree, visual stimulation that we instinctively expect a brand-new baby to know what to do next. Once he is born, a baby's drive to find his mother's breast is so strong that lack of interest in doing so is a worrisome sign.

When that happens, when the sensory connection from the womb to a mother's breast somehow fails, the pediatrician or neonatologist steps in to figure out what's gone wrong and correct it. Because sometimes that most natural connection on earth—the one that starts in the womb, changes radically at birth, and then continues through the rest of life—needs a little human encouragement to get started.

Chapter 9

"The Newborn Worth Rearing":
Infant Resuscitation, from Aristotle to Apgar

I cried right away when I was born. I know this for a fact because my nurse, Miss Glover—her first name is lost to history—put a neat check in the box marked "Cry: Immediate" on the second line of my Newborn Infant's Record at Mercy Hospital in Dubuque, Iowa. The date, March 18, 1953, is written across the top of the form in the kind of flowery longhand script that no one learns anymore.

Miss Glover was in a position to know. She was there when Dr. Richard Storck knocked my mother out with a Twilight Sleep–like combination of drugs, clamped a pair of forceps on my head, and pulled me into the world. Once my immediate squawking had been duly recorded, Miss Glover weighed and measured me (7 pounds, 14 ounces; 21 inches), gave me a shot of vitamin K in the thigh, doused my eyes with silver nitrate drops, set my bowels in motion with five drops of castor oil, and then settled me into a bassinet.

Whatever else Miss Glover may have done to me, she didn't think it important enough to write down. She tossed off my "Physical Examination at Birth" in three words: my eyes and skin were each "OK," my cord "clamped." The spaces on the Newborn Infant's Record next to "Head," "Heart," and "Extremities" went unfilled. I'm sure I had those body parts at birth—I have them now—but Miss Glover was no doubt a very busy woman, working the night shift at Mercy as the baby boom neared its peak.

Dr. Storck apparently lost interest in me, too. He left the space labeled "Doctor's Comments" blank, and never even got around to signing off on me. He probably figured that a crying baby was a healthy baby, so why bother? He, too, had his hands full dealing with that endless wave of births.

One more thing is missing from my newborn record, as I read it from my twenty-first-century pediatrician's perspective: there are no Apgar scores. With the exception of Miss Glover's lone check mark, there's no assessment of how well I made the transition from fetus to newborn, no comment about what, if anything, Dr. Storck and Miss Glover had to do to get me wailing. A baby boy born in 1953 either cried or he didn't, and that was that, at least as far as his paperwork went.

Fifty-odd years later, most expectant parents have heard of Apgar scores, but many don't really understand their significance. "Apgars" measure how well a baby makes the womb-to-world transition in those first five minutes of life—no more and no less. A score of zero points (bad), one point (so-so), or two points (good) is given to a baby in each of five categories: *heart rate, breathing effort, skin color, muscle tone,* and *reflex irritability*—the latter being a baby's reaction to having his nostrils tickled with a catheter. At the low end of the Apgar scale is a baby in serious trouble: limp and blue, pulseless and breathless. At the other end is the baby every parent hopes to have: pink and wiggling, strong of heart and lungs, ready to take on the world.

Apgar scores are assigned today at one minute and five minutes of age for all babies, and at ongoing five-minute intervals in the case of a very sick baby. A score of seven or more at any time is a sign of a healthy transition. "Perfect tens" are uncommon. It's the skin color category that trips babies up—very few newborns are pink all the way to the tips of their fingers and toes, which is the requirement for two color points. Since a newborn's immature circulation can keep the hands and feet of a normal baby blue for several hours, an Apgar score of nine is as good as most babies will get.

And that's all they really need. Except in the case of very low scores, which may point to a child at risk of serious complications,

Apgars don't mean a whole lot. They certainly don't predict a child's future. A newborn with a score of seven or less at five minutes may end up winning a MacArthur "genius" grant; a baby with a ten may still end up being lousy at math.

This point is sometimes lost on parents, particularly the go-getters with rule-the-world plans for their children. Once, after calling out a five-minute Apgar of nine on a perfectly healthy new-born, I felt a tap on my shoulder. It was the baby's father, a tanned, beefy, intense fellow in reflector sunglasses and a corporate golf shirt. "He's not a nine," he said in a deep, cigarette-sanded voice. "He's a ten." I laughed, going along with what I assumed was a proud father's joke. *Yes, of course,* I agreed, nodding amiably. *Every baby's a ten.* But he wasn't joking. "You're going to change that, right?" he said, folding his arms across his chest.

This was an odd moment for me. Two decades into my career, I'd never been challenged by a parent about something as routine as Apgar scores—it was like arguing over the baby's birth weight. I told the man that no, I wasn't going to change the score, but before I could explain why—his son's hands and feet were still blue, even as we spoke—he cut me off with a curt wave of his hand. "We'll see about that," he said, and turned his back to me.

The man—I came to think of him as Apgar Guy—then set out on a determined two-day campaign to have his son upgraded to a ten. After I left the labor room he harangued the obstetrician for a scoring change, but she was happy to point out that once the cord was cut, babies were my jurisdiction. He then cornered a couple of nurses, but they, too, demurred. All avenues of appeal led back to me.

Apgar Guy zeroed in on me later that afternoon. I saw him com-ing from the far end of the postpartum unit, bulling his way through the maze of patients and staff until at last he stood directly in front of me. He whipped off his sunglasses and fixed me with an icy-blue stare. "Take a look at this," he said, stuffing a small paper bag into my hand. "You'll see my point." I opened the bag to find a single sheet of paper—an Apgar scoring chart on which he had circled "pink hands and feet"—and a videotape marked "My Son's Birth." Then he clapped me, hard, on the shoulder. "We'll talk tomorrow," he said, and marched back to his wife's room.

I didn't watch the tape. During discharge rounds the next morning, I handed it back to him. "Sorry," I said. "His hands and feet were blue. That's a nine." Apgar Guy's face reddened; a large vein bulged in the middle of his forehead. Just as he opened his mouth, his wife, apparently accustomed to refereeing her husband's confrontations, spoke up. "Honey, give it a rest," she said wearily. "It's not like he hurt the baby." The rest of the visit went quickly. I examined Apgar Junior and fielded his mother's questions while his father smoldered in a chair in the corner of the room.

I saw Apgar Guy one last time, as he boarded the elevator that afternoon with his wife and son, headed for home. He glared at me from behind his wife's wheelchair, held up ten fingers, and nodded his head. "Pink hands and feet," he called out. "You know I'm right."

I felt a little bad as the elevator doors closed. It wouldn't have killed me to give his baby a ten, I thought. After all, there's a little bit of Apgar Guy in every parent, even me. I remember trying to coax my daughter Claire's hands and feet into turning pink by the five-minute mark, as though it really mattered, as though that would protect her from everything I knew could go wrong with a newborn. Being rational about your own baby isn't part of most new parents' emotional toolboxes.

Wishing didn't make it so. Claire's hands and feet stayed blue, and she ended up with a nine. Not wanting to be some other doctor's Apgar Guy, I accepted the verdict and left the on-call pediatrician alone.

Sometimes lost in the debate over nines and tens is the fact that before there were Apgar scores, there was an actual Apgar. Dr. Virginia Apgar was born in 1909 in Westfield, New Jersey. She decided to become a doctor early in life, a career choice that may have been inspired by the fate of her brother, who died in childhood from tuberculosis. Apgar earned a degree in zoology at Mount Holyoke College, where, in addition to helping pay her tuition by catching stray cats for the physiology lab, she established herself as a gifted violinist and cellist. Four years after leaving Mount Holyoke she graduated with high honors from Columbia University's College of Physicians and Surgeons, one of only four women in the class of 1933.

Apgar did a three-year surgical internship and residency at Columbia, and by all accounts performed brilliantly. But the chief of staff, who had seen other female graduates fail to make a living in the nearly all-male world of general surgery, discouraged her from continuing her surgical career. He suggested she try her hand at surgical anesthesia instead, at the time a task handled almost entirely by nurses. Apgar resisted at first, but after two frustrating years spent trying to establish a surgical practice, she returned to Columbia, where she built the anesthesiology department into a nationally recognized program.

Apgar made her greatest contributions in the area of obstetric anesthesia. Her career coincided with a time of much experimentation in obstetric pain medications and delivery systems, often with little attention paid to the effects those treatments had on the fetus and baby.

It was a well-known fact that babies born by cesarean delivery, usually performed under general anesthesia, were groggier than their vaginally born counterparts. They fed poorly and often showed signs of asphyxia—a sometimes life-threatening lack of oxygen during the birth process. Yet no one had developed a systematic way of evaluating the condition of a newborn at birth. Without that key assessment, Apgar wondered, how could obstetricians and anesthesiologists really evaluate the effectiveness and safety of their treatments?

The Apgar score was born at a Columbia breakfast meeting in 1949, when a medical student asked Apgar to describe how she assessed a newborn's health at birth. "That's easy," Apgar replied. She jotted down on a napkin the five signs of good health she looked for in the delivery room and then, in a "Eureka!" moment, decided to test a scoring system for newborns based on those signs. She tried out her system on more than two thousand babies, publishing her findings in 1953—two months after I was born—in a paper entitled "A Proposal for a New Method of Evaluation of the Newborn Infant."

Note that Virginia Apgar didn't call her scoring system "Apgars"—that was an honor bestowed on her years later. And she never warmed to the somewhat forced acronym APGAR—Activity (muscle tone), Pulse (heart rate), Grimace (reflex irritability), Appearance (skin color), and Respiration (breathing effort)—that has led many a parent and medical student to think of her as a jumble of letters rather than a pioneering woman physician.

Apgar's research confirmed her clinical observations: cesarean-born babies exposed to prolonged periods of general anesthesia had significantly lower scores than vaginally born babies—fives compared with nines. She also found that spinal anesthesia, the precursor to today's epidurals, caused only a modest decrease in the score. She recommended further research in spinal anesthesia, predicting that with the right combination of newer anesthetic agents, "elective cesarean section might be made as successful as . . . an uncomplicated vaginal delivery," which is exactly the situation we find ourselves in today, for better or worse.

In the beginning, then, Apgar scores weren't so much about documenting the nines and tens of normal newborns as they were about measuring the harm caused to babies by anesthetic medications. And in that way Apgar's work was simply a continuation of that done by centuries of doctors and midwives who sought ways to help a baby in danger. It was also an answer to the birthing room question asked by generations of worried parents: Is my baby okay?

The evaluation of the newborn in the first minutes of life is a process as old as human history. In ancient times, when neonatal mortality was an everyday fact of life, the purpose of evaluating a newborn wasn't to decide whether an Ivy League college was in his future, but to decide whether a baby was even worth the effort of raising. The evaluation could be harsh, even cruel, depending on the culture into which the child was born. Aristotle (384–322 B.C.) approvingly recorded this test of newborn fitness: "To accustom children to the cold from the earliest years is also an excellent practice, which greatly conduces to health, and hardens them for military service. Hence many barbarians have a custom of plunging their children at birth into a cold stream." Those babies who couldn't handle the "hardening" were left outdoors to die.

Soranus of Ephesus, the prominent second-century A.D. Greek physician (and the first Western physician to write about child health), strongly disagreed with such practices. In a medical treatise entitled *How to Recognize the Newborn That Is Worth Rearing*, Soranus opened a window on how doctors and midwives of the time approached the assessment of newborns.

Soranus starts with the basics. Good maternal health was essential: "The infant which is suited by nature for rearing will be distinguished by the fact that its mother has spent the period of pregnancy in good health, for conditions which require medical care . . . also harm the fetus and enfeeble the foundations of its life." Next, prematurity was a bad sign: "[It should be] born at the due time, best at the end of nine months, and if it so happens, later."

At birth the baby was subjected to a quick check for congenital deformities and a "worth rearing" assessment that sounds almost Apgarish: "When put on the earth [the baby] immediately cries with proper vigor; for one that lives for some length of time without crying, or cries but weakly, is suspected of behaving so on account of some unfavorable condition . . . and by conditions contrary to those mentioned, the infant not worth rearing is recognized."

Once a baby had made the grade, though, Soranus saw no need for harsh fitness tests. He disapproved of Aristotle's enthusiasm for "hardening" the newborn: "The majority of the barbarians, as the Germans and Scythians, and even some of the Hellenes, put the newborn into cold water in order to make it firm and to let die, as not worth rearing, one that cannot bear the chilling but becomes livid or convulsed[.] We reject all these." Soranus goes on to make the obvious point: just because a child dies from exposure to cold water doesn't mean he wouldn't have lived a healthy life "if unharmed."

Next up on Soranus' neonatal checklist: baby salting. The point of the salting—he specified "fine and powdery" salt, with care taken to avoid the eyes—was to cleanse the baby and "have an astringent action," and to harden the skin against rashes. This may seem like an odd practice at first glance, but salt is a fine if sometimes harsh antiseptic, and when I think of the castor oil and the silver nitrate eye drops I received at birth, it doesn't sound so strange after all.

Salting was apparently an exact science, though key bits of information, such as how much salt to use, were left out of the recipe. Too much of it and the skin became "pungent," even "corroded"; too little salt resulted in skin "not rendered sufficiently firm." If the child was deemed "too delicate" for direct salting, he or she was basted head to toe with a mixture of salt, honey, and the juice of barley, mallow, or fenugreek. The mixture was then washed off, reapplied, and washed off again, this time with warmer water. Once the second coating was removed, the baby was lightly salted and then returned, well marinated, to his mother.

Missing from Soranus' elaborate plans for evaluating, cleansing, and salting a newborn baby is this: What do you do with a baby who looks as if he *might* be worth rearing, but is born pale or limp or not breathing very well? What do you do with the baby who needs a little help getting started?

I learned about mouth-to-mouth resuscitation when I was ten or eleven years old. It was in a water safety class at our local municipal pool, the kind for slightly chubby kids who had passed beyond the fall-in-and-drown level but were never going to be actual swim team material. The instructor, a mean, skinny lifeguard who clearly wished he were anyplace but where he was, taught us that mouth-to-mouth resuscitation was the modern technique for rescuing a nearly dead swimmer. He emphasized the word *modern* as he lectured us, as if this were space travel he was talking about, or heart transplants.

He scoffed at older resuscitation practices—pumping the victim's arms and legs, for example, or rolling him over a barrel to drain the water from his lungs. *Might as well just throw him back in and let him die,* he said with a sneer—something I feared he'd have been happy to do with our entire class, given half a chance.

The lifeguard "volunteered" the best-looking older girl in the class to be his mouth-to-mouth demonstration dummy. He laid her down on the pool deck, tilted her head back, pinched her nose to demonstrate proper positioning, and then, to the terrified girl's immense relief, stopped just short of making actual mouth-to-mouth contact. Then he stood, pulled out a balloon he'd been hiding somewhere in his skimpy Speedo, and blew it up. *In goes the good air,* the lifeguard said, and then he let the balloon-lung loudly, flatulently deflate. *Out goes the bad.* What could be simpler? What could be more modern?

Mouth-to-mouth resuscitation made perfect sense to the budding scientist in me. If a half-dead swimmer were too weak to breathe, why, you simply blew air into him until he came around and started breathing for himself! It made so much sense that I wondered: What took people so long to figure it out?

I later learned that the lifeguard was misinformed, or maybe just showing off to the girls in the class. Mouth-to-mouth resuscitation isn't a modern thing at all—it's at least as old as the Old Testament. Open the Bible to II Kings 4:34–35 and there it is: the prophet Elisha revives an apparently dead Shunammite boy by "put[ting] his mouth upon his mouth . . . and the flesh of the child waxed warm . . . and the child opened his eyes."

Death from respiratory failure at birth had long been recognized. The Chinese emperor Hwang-Ti (2698–2599 B.C.) described it in premature infants, and accounts of babies rescued with mouth-to-mouth breathing date from earliest recorded history. Hebrew midwives practiced the technique as early as 1300 B.C., and in the Babylonian Talmud, written between 200 B.C. and A.D. 400 permission is given to birth attendants to provide "all assistance possible" to a mother laboring on the Sabbath, when working was otherwise not allowed, such as "pull[ing] out the young by pressing the sides" and "breathing air into its nostrils, and leading it to its mother's breast, so that it may suck."

Other remarkably modern techniques surface in ancient writing, too. In addition to mouth-to-mouth breathing, the Talmud describes a newborn lamb revived by a man who inserted a reed into the lamb's windpipe and blew into it. Aristotle—he of the icy-stream-dunking school of newborn fitness testing—observed that midwives were known to squeeze the umbilical cord of "the child [who] appears to have been born dead," thus forcing blood from the cord into the baby's body. Aristotle couldn't have known how cord squeezing helped revive a baby—the extra cord blood raised the infant's blood pressure and sent oxygen to his ailing organs, just as a blood transfusion does today—but he was impressed. "The child that a moment before was bloodless," he wrote, "[comes] back to life again."

Methods of newborn resuscitation came and went over the centuries, often forgotten and then reinvented as politics and geography kept far-flung scholars from learning from one another. Maimonides (1135–1204), the renowned Jewish physician, scholar, and rabbi, described newborn respiratory arrest in his writings from Egypt, as well as a method of resuscitation. Three centuries later, the Italian physician Paulus Bagellardus published a book on childhood diseases that included a description of mouth-to-mouth resuscitation for the newborn. It isn't known whether Bagellardus ever saw Maimonides' work.

Progress in reviving near-dead babies and adults remained a hit-or-miss affair until the seventeenth and eighteenth centuries, when expanding university libraries and improved communication meant that a doctor researching the subject was more likely to have access to the work of other physicians and scientists, near and far.

One of the main obstacles to resuscitation research was the well-entrenched belief that divine intervention, and not that of a doctor or rescuer, was responsible when a seemingly dead individual was revived. Raising the dead simply wasn't within human capabilities. When William Tossach, a London surgeon, used mouth-to-mouth resuscitation in 1745 to revive a coal miner who had apparently died from smoke inhalation, the Royal Society dismissed his claim, noting that "life ends when breathing ceases." If the miner was breathing now, the Society reasoned, he must have been breathing then, too. Dr. Tossach was simply mistaken.

But interest in resuscitation soon made the Royal Society's definition of death obsolete. Founded in 1774, the Institution for Affording Immediate Relief to Persons Apparently Dead from Drowning (which briefly changed its unwieldy name to the spookier-sounding Society for People Apparently Drowned, and finally to the Royal Humane Society) was the first organization to promote resuscitation education and to issue certificates to those who completed their training program. The curriculum was a bit rough by modern standards, though. Mouth-to-mouth breathing and keeping the victim warm were emphasized, as they are today, but so was blowing tobacco smoke into the rectum with a bellows.

Advances in newborn resuscitation followed on the heels of progress made in adults, particularly in drowning victims, since the waterlogged lungs of a man pulled half dead from a lake or river resembled, at least superficially, the amniotic-fluid-filled lungs of an asphyxiated newborn. In 1749 William Smellie, the famed Scottish obstetrician, wrote of reviving a newborn after exhausting the "common efforts," which included rubbing the baby's head with liquor and putting mustard up its nostrils, by "blowing into the mouth through a . . . catheter." By 1752 Smellie had developed a straight endotracheal tube—a coiled wire wrapped in leather, inserted through the mouth into the windpipe—which he frequently used in resuscitating newborns.

Physician reports of apparently dead infants revived by mouth-to-mouth breathing became so frequent that in 1774 the Royal Humane Society declared it should be routinely attempted on all apparently stillborn infants. But the idea of direct mouth-to-mouth contact with an unwashed newborn was considered repulsive by many influential doctors. The Scottish obstetrician William Hunter described mouth-to-mouth as "the method practiced by the vulgar to restore newborn children" and developed a small bellows to do the job of inflating an infant's lungs. Cowed by Hunter's reputation, the Royal Humane Society rescinded its endorsement of mouth-to-mouth in 1776, less than two years after first promoting the practice.

Bellows-assisted resuscitation soon became the norm, and remained so for nearly fifty years. Then, in 1827, a French physician reported that bellows breathing—and by implication, mouth-to-mouth breathing—often ruptured delicate newborn lungs, possibly killing more babies than they saved. Bellows and mouth-to-mouth ventilation soon fell out of medical favor, replaced by a variety of truly novel resuscitation techniques. The Age of the Swinging Baby had begun.

If I had been born in 1873 instead of 1953, and if I had been lifeless-looking at birth, any one of a number of things might have been done to me. I might still have been resuscitated with mouth-to-mouth breathing, since midwives never really abandoned the practice. But I might also have had my chest vigorously squeezed (the Prochownich Method), perhaps while having my arms raised and lowered like a pump (the Sylvester Method), or I might have had my tongue rhythmically yanked (the Laborde Method). I might have been shaken or screamed at, dunked in hot and/or cold water, tickled, slapped, or pinched, had my rectum dilated with a corncob, a clay pipe, or a raven's beak (en route to having tobacco smoke blown in), or been shocked with electricity. Or, like many European babies of the day, I might have awakened to find myself high over the doctor's head, gazing down at him like a cherub on the ceiling of the Sistine Chapel.

The over-the-head technique, better known as the Schulze Method, shows how far infant resuscitation practice had drifted from its mouth-to-mouth heyday. In a two-panel illustration accompanying a lengthy 1871 monograph describing the method, a long-bearded doctor in a dark frock coat and shiny black shoes—presumably Dr. Bernhardt Schulze himself—is shown in the act of reviving a baby. In the first panel the doctor stands slightly bent at the waist, holding a limp, upright infant under its arms, facing away from him. The baby's toes almost touch the floor. In the second panel the doctor has swung the baby over his head and peers intently at its tiny, flipped-over bottom as though gazing through a telescope at the rings of Saturn. The detailed directions that accompany the engraving boil down to this: *swing up, swing down, repeat.*

The Schulze Method wasn't as crazy as it sounds. By swinging the baby up and down, Dr. Schulze performed an odd-looking but crudely effective form of artificial respiration. It's easy to see how it worked: you perform a "modified Schulze" on yourself every time you rise from a chair. When you stand up, air automatically rushes into your stretched-out lungs. Sit down again and your folding trunk compresses your lungs. Air flows back out.

At the peak of Schulze's swing, then, with the newborn head down and its trunk flexed at the hips, the baby "exhaled": amniotic fluid and oxygen-poor air poured out of its lungs. As Schulze reached the low point of the swing, the body straightened out, the lungs passively expanded, and oxygen-rich air flowed in: the baby "inhaled."

Schulze's method worked more often than not, or so he claimed. He spent a dozen years perfecting his technique before writing about it, and in his monograph he recommends it "warmly" to other physicians "because—if applied in time—it is rarely unsuccessful." The problem with the resuscitation practices of his time, as Schulze saw it, was that doctors wasted too much time fiddling with various folk remedies and homemade contraptions designed to force air into a newborn's lungs. Better to commence swinging as soon as a baby was in trouble.

The German medical establishment agreed. With only minor modifications—such as carefully drying the newborn "so that the swinging neonate did not become the flying neonate," as the Schulze biographer, Thomas Baskett, later put it—the Schulze Method became the standard method of neonatal resuscitation taught in German medical schools from the 1870s to the 1920s. Outside Germany, though, other scientists noted the head injuries and broken bones caused by inexpert use of the Schulze Method and sought safer ways to ventilate newborns in distress.

The Fell-O'Dwyer device, a gentler, foot-operated bellows originally designed to keep diphtheria sufferers from suffocating on their swollen tonsils, was adapted for newborn resuscitation in 1887. In 1889, Alexander Graham Bell, the father of the telephone, invented a negative pressure ventilator—the precursor of the "iron lung" that spurred frightened parents to vaccinate their children against polio in the 1950s—that breathed for the newborn by raising and lowering the ventilator's air pressure. Later a positive pressure ventilator appeared: a distressed baby was sealed inside a stainless-steel chamber at birth, pressurized oxygen was pumped inside and his progress was observed through a porthole. Everyone, of course, claimed that his own contraption worked best.

It's easy enough from my twenty-first-century perspective to trace the development of the instruments used in modern neonatal resuscitation—the endotracheal tube, laryngoscope, and oxygen delivery equipment that reside in every hospital labor room in the country—and to think of their appearance as preordained, a straight-line march of progress from the Old Testament to my next night on call. But when Virginia Apgar started chasing cats at Mount Holyoke in 1925, and even three decades later when she published her landmark neonatal scoring system, the treatment of the asphyxiated newborn was a very gray area, a messy mixture of old methods that refused to die and newer techniques that often didn't work.

A look at the medical texts of the time is instructive. Dr. L. Emmett Holt of Johns Hopkins University—one of the preeminent pediatricians of his time—spent several pages of his 1933 pediatrics textbook discussing the best way to revive a severely ill baby. Pinching and gentle spanking were okay, but "the more violent procedures such as swinging the child are to be condemned." Sicker babies were to be given accordion-like artificial respiration: the doctor held the baby's trunk in one hand and its thighs in the other as he vigorously flexed and extended the baby's trunk at the hips, a maneuver that sounds suspiciously like a horizontal version of the "condemned" Schulze Method.

Dr. Mary Crosse, who established the first ward for premature infants in Great Britain in the 1930s, recommended more gentle techniques: clearing the airway of mucus, raising the child's head, and administering oxygen through a soft rubber mask. She dismissed "manual methods . . . and older forms of artificial respiration [that] often do more harm than good," but kept a ready supply of injectable medications such as adrenaline and camphor-in-oil at hand to stimulate a failing heart.

In *The New-Born Infant* (1945), Yale obstetrician Emerson Law Stone recommended that all newborns initially be held upside down so that amniotic fluid could drain from the lungs, then be "stimulated to breathe" by anything from inhaled ammonia to the kind of bottom spanking that quickly became a cartoon cliché of childbirth. If that wasn't sufficiently stimulating, the baby was to be immersed up to the neck in a tub of warm water—Stone specified 110–115 degrees. While one resuscitator blew oxygen in the child's face, another held the baby around the chest and pressed with his thumbs, mimicking the chest wall movements of breathing. If that failed, a brief period of mouth-to-mouth breathing, with the baby still in the bathwater, ensued. Next came a dunking in an adjacent tub filled with ice water, then back into the warm water for more mouth-to-mouth and chest compressions. When all else failed, the doctor slid a small rubber catheter down the baby's throat and blew into it with "the pressure exerted [only] by the cheeks."

And that was that. According to Stone, "practically every case of asphyxia in the new-born is cured or succumbs . . . in the earliest minutes or hours of extrauterine life." Babies either lived or they died; "the need of continued intensive therapy over long periods of time is very rare indeed."

Little had changed by 1953. By the time I was born, a baby could be resuscitated upside down or right side up. He could be pinched and spanked and played like a squeeze box, or handled with kid gloves. He might receive oxygen through a mask connected to a canister, or have it blown directly into his lungs by a doctor with puffed-out cheeks. He could be dunked in hot water or cold water, or kept high and dry as smelling salts were whiffed under his nose. And every doctor could say with confidence that his or her own method worked best, because with no standardized, objective means of evaluating the baby, who could contradict them?

As wildly varied as the treatments for the obviously asphyxiated infant were during Apgar's early career, the initial assessment of mildly ill and even healthy newborns was equally murky, and highly subjective. L. Emmett Holt devoted only one sentence of his 1933 textbook—far less than Soranus had written eighteen centuries earlier—to the evaluation of the nonasphyxiated newborn: "It is good practice at this time [after the cord has been cut] to examine the infant thoroughly for injuries received during delivery and for congenital deformities and to observe the condition of the circulation and respiration." Holt included no guidelines, though, as to what distinguished normal from abnormal cardiorespiratory "conditions."

Like Holt, Dr. Wilfred Sheldon, in his *Diseases of Infancy and Childhood* (1936), spends considerable time on the treatment of the baby in shock, but only a single sentence on evaluating nonshocky, nondeformed newborns: "The standard of health has to be estimated by such special indications as the strength of the cry, the power of sucking, and the degree of drowsiness." How to estimate those "special indications" was left to the reader's imagination.

These guidelines weren't particularly helpful to the practicing obstetrician, pediatrician, or general practitioner attending a birth. A baby in shock was easy to spot—pale or blue, floppy, unresponsive—and so was a strapping, squalling, healthy one. What they needed was a quick assessment tool, a more objective, less seat-of-the-pants guide to evaluating babies that fell in between those two extremes.

Virginia Apgar turned her attention to that gray zone of neonatal assessment, commenting on the questionable science of newborn care in the opening paragraph of her 1953 paper: "Resuscitation of infants at birth has been the subject of many articles. Seldom have there been such imaginative ideas, such enthusiasms, and dislikes, and such unscientific observations and study about one clinical picture. There are outstanding exceptions to these statements, but the poor quality and lack of precise data of the majority of papers . . . are interesting."

Apgar changed the assessment of newborns, both sick and well, from the equivalent of a Cold War–era Olympic figure skating competition—where the same performance could receive widely different scores, depending on a judge's political allegiance—to a system that took much of the subjectivity and institutional bias out of the evaluation of the effects of medications and treatment. Her scoring system caught on quickly. By the end of the decade it became impossible for researchers simply to claim that an obstetric medication was harmless to a newborn, or that one resuscitation technique was better than another. Now they had to prove it. And that led, in a not quite straight line, to me standing over a sick newborn trying to figure out what to do next.

We don't lay babies on the earth these days to see whether they're worth rearing. We don't plunge them into icy streams to toughen them up, either. We don't slather them in honey, salt them like cocktail peanuts, or even give them castor oil, as Miss Glover did on behalf of my bowels. What we *do* do at every birth these days is follow a diagram—more accurately, a "treatment algorithm," a what-to-do-next flowchart posted on the walls of most delivery rooms, and in the brains of the people who attend deliveries.

The algorithm goes by the official, humdrum name of "Emergency Cardiovascular Care Guidelines for Neonatal Resuscitation," referred to in the business as the "NRP Guidelines," NRP being short for the Neonatal Resuscitation Program, a joint project of the American Academy of Pediatrics and the American Heart Association.

The NRP guidelines are directly descended from Virginia Apgar's cafeteria-napkin-inscribed scoring system, that first truly scientific attempt to bring order to the wild and woolly world of newborn resuscitation. The guidelines take available scientific evidence on the resuscitation of newborns and distill it into flowchart form for easy reference.

The algorithm itself is a cut-and-dried-looking arrangement of boxes and arrows. There are ten boxes in all—seven on the left side of the chart, three on the right. The seven left-hand boxes tell a pediatrician what to do next when things are going wrong; the three right-hand boxes indicate the level of care a child will need once things stabilize. The farther down the left side of the flowchart a baby gets, and the more boxes he hits, the more worrisome the situation.

Every newborn starts at the upper left-hand box with a basic, Soranus-like assessment: Is this a full term baby? Was there meconium (the greenish baby poop that's a sign of prenatal distress) in the amniotic fluid? Is the baby breathing or crying? Does he have good muscle tone? If the answers are yes, no, yes, and yes, congratulations! You're looking at a normal newborn. The baby goes right to mama's breast and over to the top right-hand box, "Routine Care." This is the kind of birth I never get called to, since there's no need to do anything else.

If, however, the baby fails the initial four-question assessment, or if he shows other signs of in utero distress, such as a low heart rate before birth, he gets a bit more scrutiny. The baby is placed under a warmer on a nearby resuscitation bed, dried off, suctioned of any mucus that might be blocking his airway, and then watched for thirty seconds or so. If he comes around quickly and his breathing, heart rate, and color are good, then the arrow directs him to the second right-hand box—"Observational Care," which is like routine care, but with a little more watching. Sometimes it takes a little extra oxygen blown in the face to help a baby come around, but, in general, a newborn who ends up with observational care will do just fine.

So far, so good. It's easy to follow an algorithm when all you have to do is fuss with a baby a bit and then watch as nature does its fetus-to-infant transition thing. But when a baby is born in serious trouble—limp, breathless, and nearly pulseless, usually from a prolonged period of oxygen deprivation in the womb—the first few boxes, with their polite questions and gentle suggestions, go right out the window. Things happen fast.

If the heart rate is less than 60 beats a minute (the normal newborn heart rate is over 100), chest compressions are started to get blood moving more quickly through the baby's body. This is the same basic CPR used on adults, but instead of the stiff-armed *wham-wham-wham* technique familiar to viewers of TV medical dramas, a doctor or nurse encircles the baby's chest with his or her hands and rhythmically compresses the breastbone with the thumbs. An endotracheal tube, which provides better oxygen delivery than the bag-and-mask method, is usually slid into the baby's windpipe at this point as well.

If the baby's color and heart rate improve, the chest compressions stop, the endotracheal tube is withdrawn, and "blow-by" oxygen resumes until the crisis has clearly passed. The NRP arrow then points the baby to the third right-hand box, marked "Post-Resuscitation Care," because any newborn who needs that much help to get started is at risk for a complicated neonatal course: low blood sugar, say, or the need for IV fluids, antibiotics, and more oxygen.

But if the baby doesn't respond to chest compressions and oxygen delivered through the endotracheal tube, we reach the seventh and final left-hand box: "Administer Epinephrine." Fortunately, this is rarely needed, because a baby who needs epinephrine is a baby in critical condition. More commonly known as adrenaline, epinephrine is used to jump-start a heart that refuses to rev up on its own. It can be squirted down the endotracheal tube directly into the lungs, or injected into the baby's bloodstream through a catheter quickly inserted into the umbilical vein, while chest compressions and endotracheal tube respiration continue. The need for epinephrine, especially if multiple doses are required, always signals a baby in serious trouble.

The fact that epinephrine is the only drug mentioned in the entire NRP algorithm illustrates how different newborn babies are from the rest of us. There is an adage that pediatricians often invoke when explaining treatment options to parents (and sometimes to our adult medicine colleagues): *Children aren't just small adults.* You can't simply perform a miniaturized version of an adult treatment on a child and expect it to work. In fact, that's a good way to harm a kid.

That adage is doubly true in the immediate treatment of sick newborns. Consider this: if a grown man is found unconscious on a sidewalk, the first maneuver attempted by arriving paramedics isn't going to be: *Let's rub his back and see if that brings him around!* The man will have his heart shocked with a cardiac defibrillator before he even reaches an emergency room bed, because the odds are he's having a heart attack. Yet you won't even find a neonatal cardiac defibrillator in a delivery room. In thirty years of resuscitating newborns, I've never had to use one.

That's because newborns don't have heart attacks. A baby born limp and lifeless-looking usually has a perfectly fine heart. The problem is respiratory—he's not breathing because the respiratory center in his brain is depressed from some kind of distress in the womb. The cause can be as straightforward as a long, difficult delivery—in which case the baby is simply exhausted and "beat up"—or narcotic pain medications his mother received, which can temporarily depress the respiratory center. Or it can be asphyxia, a serious lack of oxygen brought on by things like the placental abruption that set off Sean O'Connor's rocky start. But there isn't always a clear-cut reason why a baby refuses to take that first breath. Sometimes we just don't know what happened.

In most cases, the in utero distress occurs close to the time of birth and doesn't last very long—a cord tightly wound around the baby's neck, for example, that's relieved as soon as the obstetrician cuts the cord at delivery—and time, drying, and maybe a little oxygen is all that's needed. Once a baby starts breathing, either on his own or with the help of a bag and mask, the heart usually follows suit, speeding up to the normal range in short order. A newborn heart that doesn't promptly respond to oxygen therapy is one that has had a prolonged period of inadequate oxygen, long enough that its normal rhythms, which started very early in fetal development and are hardwired to last for decades, have been overwhelmed.

Epinephrine, chest compressions, and endotracheal tube respirations nearly always get the heart started again. But a baby who needs all that help has earned a bed in the intensive care nursery, because the same lack of oxygen that caused the heart to temporarily malfunction can affect other organs as well, particularly the kidneys, bowel, and brain. Recovery can be complicated and prolonged. Fortunately, very few babies end up in such a predicament. The vast majority end up leaving the algorithm after a box or two, moving on to breast-feeding and diapers and the rest of life.

The NRP chart hanging on the delivery room wall, with its neat boxes, bold arrows, and straightforward questions, looks simple enough—almost comically so to anyone who actually resuscitates babies. Consider that the entire algorithm, from weeding out normal newborns in the first box to squirting epinephrine down the endotracheal tube in the seventh, takes less than 90 seconds. It's far from a linear process, too, as illustrated by the five points along the way in which an asterisk gently suggests that maybe, just *maybe,* this would be a good time to skip all the rubbing and patting stuff and intubate the baby. Last, there are the space constraints. In a difficult resuscitation there can be several people at work—intubating, compressing, inserting catheters, and giving medications—on a patient who could fit in a large shoebox.

This all sounds so *modern*, as that skinny lifeguard would have put it. Modern, that is, until you realize that all the maneuvers on the NRP algorithm are old, many of them ancient. Remember that midwives were performing mouth-to-mouth breathing more than three thousand years ago, and that doctors were intubating babies with handmade endotracheal tubes in the eighteenth century. Umbilical catheters, chest compressions, epinephrine . . . they're all old hat. Even the laryngoscope, the fancy flashlight that allows me to see the opening of a baby's windpipe—in the old days they did it by feel—is older than I am.

The tools of the trade have improved greatly, of course— we traded leather endotracheal tubes for flexible plastic a long time ago—but there is truly nothing new under the sun, neonatal-resuscitation-wise. The NRP treatment algorithm is simply the culmination of a centuries-long pruning process. The weird and the strange resuscitation methods, like the ice baths and iron lungs and baby-swinging, have been cut away, leaving behind what seems to work best. Nothing is ever cast in stone, though. Every five years or so, since their first publication in 1987, the NRP guidelines are tweaked to reflect newer research findings. Ironically, the most recent edition in 2005 de-emphasizes the use of oxygen in mildly distressed babies. We now give nature a little more time to take its sometimes meandering course.

Notice that in this discussion of the NRP treatment algorithm I've never once mentioned Apgar scores. That's because they're not there—you won't find them in any of the NRP boxes. Virginia Apgar wouldn't have found that omission surprising.

Remember that her original scoring system was designed to evaluate the effects of various maternal treatments and medications on newborns, not to tell doctors how to treat babies. That's still true today. The Apgar score in a modern resuscitation simply measures how well what we've been doing is working.

An "Apgar timer" attached to the resuscitation bed buzzes at one and five minutes after birth, and then every five minutes until somebody shuts the thing off. At every buzz I take a mental snapshot of the five categories—the heart rate and color, the baby's muscle tone, breathing effort, and reflex irritability—assign a score, and then keep going. It's gratifying when a baby whose Apgar score was only one at a minute of age improves to a nine by five minutes—the rising numbers signal a successful resuscitation. But Apgars themselves are just signposts on the way to a child's recovery. That's exactly the way Virginia Apgar would have wanted it.

Which brings me back once more to 1953. What would my own Apgar scores have been if Virginia Apgar had published her paper a few months earlier, and if Dr. Storck and Miss Glover had seen fit to add such a newfangled tool to their busy hospital routine?

Working from the sketchy paperwork they left behind, I know I'd have gotten at least a two for respiratory effort, given my immediate cry. And from scoring a couple of thousand babies myself, I know that a loudly bawling baby has a normal pulse rate—it takes a strong heart to power all that noise—and good muscle tone, too. That's a six. And any baby worth his salt—the Soranus kind, come to think of it—would object to a catheter tickling his nose. Eight.

Alas, my color remains a mystery. It had to be good enough, since neither Miss Glover nor Dr. Storck gave me much of a second thought, but was I pink to the tips of my fingers and toes by the time I turned five minutes old? There's no way to know now, but given the signs—Apgar's paper was published the year I was born, after all, and her research was done at Columbia's Sloane Hospital—I can reach only one conclusion. There at the dawn of the modern era of neonatal resuscitation, I was a big, pink ten. Take that, Apgar Guy.

Chapter 10
Infant Origami: A Guided Tour of the Newborn Body

When all is said and done—when the pushing and pulling are finally over and the last of the relatives and friends have trickled away—what's left is a baby and his parents, alone together for the first time. It's then that the new-parent microscope makes its first appearance. Every square millimeter of the baby's body is scrutinized by an awed new mother and father. Every finger, toenail, hair, and pore is examined and, eventually, attributed to one side of the family or the other. In the course of that microscopic evaluation, anxiety often appears. *Should his ears look like that? Why do her feet curve so much? Isn't he breathing kind of fast?*

That anxiety is often rooted in family history: an uncle who was born deaf, a grandparent with clubbed feet, maybe a newborn cousin who died from pneumonia. At the bottom of all these concerns lies a single, fundamental question: *Is my baby normal?* It's my job as a pediatrician to answer that question.

I learned to examine newborns from a senior resident at a private hospital during my first medical school pediatrics rotation. Tom was a jolly, rotund fellow with smudged rimless glasses and an overall appearance he himself described as "one white beard shy of Santa Claus." He was also my first pediatric role model.

We met one morning in the hallway outside the newborn nursery. This was in the days before "rooming in," back when a newborn nursery was a hospital ward rather than a place where babies temporarily hang out while their mothers shower or catch a nap, as it is today. In the 1970s, babies were trucked out to their mothers for feedings and then brought back to the nursery for cleaning up and tucking in. If you wanted to see your baby in between times, you hiked down to the nursery and asked permission.

I remember the nurse in charge of the newborn nursery that morning. She was a no-nonsense type—they were all no-nonsense types to this easily petrified student—who kept the wheeled bassinets in rigidly straight rows, boys on the left side of the room and girls on the right. She surveyed her patients from a desk at the head of the aisle that separated the sexes, like a chaperone at a dance for tiny, diapered junior high students.

Tom unwrapped the first baby we came to: a girl, I knew, without waiting for the diaper to come off. She was on the "girl" side of the room, after all, and her blanket, cap, and name tag were a uniform pale pink. I looked across the aisle: a sea of baby blue. The nurse eyed us suspiciously. "Make sure you wrap her back up right," she growled. Tom smiled amiably. "Lady runs a tight ship," he whispered.

With the baby naked, sound asleep, and milk-drunk from a recent feeding, Tom stepped back from the bassinet and asked me what I saw. Well into my third year now, I dreaded questions like that—they were usually tricks, a sign of a resident about to pounce on a hapless student. An obscure medical condition no doubt lay before me, yet there was nothing obviously wrong with this child. What was it I was supposed to see?

"A baby?" I ventured, after what seemed like an eternity of pondering.

Silence.

"A girl baby?" Tom regarded me quizzically through his fingerprint-smeared lenses. I was running out of ideas.

"A healthy girl baby?" I closed my eyes, waiting for the usual deluge of resident sarcasm—*No, idiot, it's a two-headed kitten!*—but it didn't come.

"Bingo!" Tom said, punching my shoulder. "That's a healthy baby girl! Excellent diagnosis." Teaching and learning should be fun,

Tom told me much later, and he took no joy in tormenting students. A rare resident, in my experience.

"Now watch this." Tom slid his beefy hands under the baby and began, slowly and gently, to fold her: head onto chest, arms against ribs, legs tucked up on her abdomen—an exercise in infant origami. The baby was now in perfect fetal position, almost egg-shaped—uterus-shaped, really. Tom pointed out the still visible accommodations a fetus makes to the space constraints of the late term womb: her head slightly rounded on one side, where it had lain against the uterine wall; the indentations on either side of her rib cage, where her arms had nestled; the gentle curve of her legs and feet, gracefully molded by the womb.

It was important to see those fetal traces, Tom said. If I didn't know what was normal, I wouldn't know what was abnormal, when to *really* worry. He then took me on a guided tour of this naked baby girl, stopping to point out the differences between the newborn and adult body, and even that of a slightly older child. The whole lecture took about ten minutes, but it made an impression. Thirty years later, it's still the basis of my discussions with new parents.

On an average hospital morning, squeezed in between rounds in the intensive care nursery and the pediatric ward, I'll examine eight or ten healthy newborns. I see the "discharges" first—the eager-to-get-home families who peek out to the nurses' station from behind their bouquets and packed suitcases, wondering when in the world someone is going to come and set them free. Their babies have been examined at least once already, in the delivery room or out on the postpartum ward, and they've gotten answers to most of their questions. The bulk of the discharge visit is spent making sure follow-up appointments have been made and that somebody remembered to bring the still-wrapped-in-plastic car seat from home that morning.

Once the last of the discharged babies is headed home, I turn my attention to the admissions—the new babies, born during the night, when the on-call pediatrician would have examined them only if there had been an immediate health concern. These exams take longer than the discharges because there are usually a lot of questions, especially—and understandably—from first-time parents.

There is an art to examining a baby. The evaluation itself doesn't take much time; these are tiny bodies, after all, and I can do the basic heart-lung-neurological check in a minute or so. But that first exam is never just about the baby. A newborn is the physical product of two gene pools, but also the psychic product of the hopes and fears that a mother and father bring to the moment. Part of the art of examining a newborn baby is knowing when to speak, what to say, and, sometimes, when to shut up.

Tom had a few rules of thumb for talking to parents about their babies, but first and foremost was this: *Take a good look at both parents before opening your mouth.* I learned the wisdom of Tom's advice during my pediatrics internship a couple of years later, while trying to console a mother about an unusual birthmark on her son's face, a purplish blemish I'd never seen before. *Maybe it'll go away in time,* I stammered, not having any idea if that was at all likely. I babbled on, caught in an awkward rookie doctor trap: not knowing what I was looking at and lacking the self-confidence to simply admit it.

The mother listened patiently, unable to get an edgewise word into my nervous rapid-fire spiel. And then, just as I was swinging into my *he's-just-perfect-even-with-that-thing-on-his-face* grand finale, her husband walked into the room with a dozen roses, an armload of baby clothes, and the exact same birthmark smack in the middle of his forehead. My jabbering screeched to a halt. "We'll be fine," the mother said drily, stroking her baby's cheek. "I'm sure it won't matter to *his* wife, either."

Looking back, I can forgive my younger self for jumping the gun. To other parents, that unexpected blemish might have been worrisome, and my sincere if misguided attempt to help them cope with such an imperfection might have been welcomed. What I quickly learned, though, is that what looks like a problem to me isn't always a problem for them.

These days my technique is simple: I start at the top of a baby's body and work my way down. I hit the high points—count the fingers and toes, listen for heart murmurs, check the belly and hips and skin—and then let the discussion go where the parents lead.

The head is a logical place to start. This is partly because it's often the only thing peeking out of the baby blankets when I arrive, and also because a baby's head, bearing the brunt of a vaginal birth as it does, is usually the object of much parental concern. But once the lumps, bumps, and bruises are explained and those fears put to rest, the next stop on the tour of the newborn body is the face.

And what a face! With those searching eyes, Cupid's-bow lips, and button nose, a newborn baby's face is perfectly designed for two essential newborn tasks: finding food, and bonding with—if not outright hypnotizing—the food giver.

It was Konrad Lorenz (1903–89), the Nobel Prize–winning Austrian physician and zoologist better known for his work with newborn geese—he got them to "imprint" on him at birth, thus becoming more or less a surrogate Mother Goose—who first showed that infants of many mammalian species look different from adults in remarkably consistent ways. Consider puppies, kittens, bunnies, and human babies: all have larger heads relative to their bodies, more expansive foreheads, bigger eyes, and smaller, flatter noses than their parents do.

Lorenz went on to show that humans of all ages have a natural tendency to be attracted to baby-shaped faces. This is true even of babies themselves—put a couple of six-month-olds in a crowd of adults and they'll seek each other out, staring in happy fascination at the other little round-headed creature in the room. And if any other evidence of our love of round faces is needed, look no further than the phenomenal commercial success of dolls with babylike faces, from Raggedy Ann to Cabbage Patch Kids, and comic strip characters like Charlie Brown and Linus. We're suckers for chubby cheeks.

Humans may love puppies and kittens, but we are particularly susceptible to the allure of our own infants. A new mother and her baby, left undisturbed in the hour or so following birth, spend a long while gazing into each other's eyes. We tend to think of this moment from the newborn's standpoint—he's bonding with his mother, memorizing her face and smell, locking her image into his developing brain. True enough, but while he's doing all that he's also weaving a spell on his mother.

Biopsychologist Eckhard Hess, a contemporary of Lorenz's at the University of Chicago, pioneered the study of pupillometry—changes in pupil size—as a measure of emotional response. He found that a mother's pupils enlarge at the sight of her baby's face, a strong sign of a "favorable attitude." (Hess also found that men looking at what he described in his research paper as "pin-up" pictures—this was the 1950s—had a similar reaction, though not as strong.)

More recently, researchers at the University of Wisconsin have found that the part of the brain associated with processing pleasurable sensations—the orbitofrontal cortex, right behind the forehead—"lights up" on a brain scan when a woman is shown pictures of a baby; the response is strongest when the baby in the picture is her own. Fathers probably light up, too, what with their "feminized" hormone profiles at the time of birth—see chapter 6—but the Wisconsin team hasn't yet gotten around to sticking them in the scanner.

None of this research comes as a surprise to anyone who has ever watched a mother interact with her new baby. There is nothing so fascinating to her as the sight of her newborn's face, and most captivating of all, of course, are his eyes. He'll meet her gaze with those baby blues, stare for long stretches almost without blinking, even follow her face as she moves her head from side to side. Then, when he's had enough, he'll close them sleepily and drift off.

· · ·

Sooner or later in all that eye-gazing a parent notices their color, and the question arises: *What color will they be when he's grown?* The question is really a two-parter: Why do most newborns have blue eyes, and why do so many parents want them to stay that way?

Step number one in answering the eye color question: check the parents. If they both have blue eyes, the answer is yes, most likely their baby's eyes will stay blue. If the mother and father have different colored eyes, say dad with green and mom with blue, their baby could have blue eyes, but there's no way to know. And if both parents have dark brown eyes, the chances of having a blue-eyed baby are remote, but still not impossible. Add them all up and you get a resounding "maybe" in answer to the staying-blue question. Eye color, it turns out, is a bit of a gene pool crapshoot.

Science used to be so much simpler. Back in my high school biology class I learned that eye color was a simple matter of Mendelian genetics, so named for Gregor Mendel, the nineteenth-century Austrian monk who worked out the details of inheritance in his research on garden peas. Genes for brown eye color were dominant over blue; case closed. Brown-eyed parents might still have a blue-eyed baby, if they carried recessive genes from some blue-eyed ancestors, but blue-eyed parents could never have a brown-eyed child—or if they did, the mother had some serious explaining to do.

That never quite made sense to me. Anyone who has gazed longingly into the orbs of a loved one knows that eyes don't come in uniform shades of green, brown, and blue. There's amber and gray and violet, for instance, and that murky "hazel" category, which can range from light brown to yellowish green, depending on the lighting and who's doing the describing. And what about all the people with flecks of brown in their green eyes, or vice versa, or even eyes of two different colors?

Recent research paints a more complicated inheritance picture. It's now thought that there are two major eye color genes: one that controls for brown or blue and another for green or hazel.

These in turn are modified by several other genes. An almost infinite number of variations exist, which is one reason electronic iris recognition—the iris is the colored ring that surrounds the black-dot pupil—has been suggested as a foolproof successor to fingerprints for security checks.

Back to baby blues. Their characteristic blue-gray color comes from *eumelanin,* a blackish pigment produced by cells in the iris. Dark-skinned people have more iris eumelanin than fair-skinned people do, sometimes so much more that their newborns already have dark eyes.

After birth, genes determine how much *melanin,* the dark brown pigment that also colors the skin, will ultimately be deposited in the iris. A lot of melanin leads to brown eyes, a medium amount to green, gray, or hazel, and not much melanin gets you blue. The color change takes time and exposure to light, the same ingredients required for a deep suntan. Most babies reach their final eye color by a year of age, but for some it can take longer. In a small number of people, final eye color isn't reached until adulthood.

So eye color is more or less generic blue-gray for most babies at birth, and then changes over the first few months as a result of genetic influences and sunlight. But what about that other, unspoken part of the question of newborn eye color: Why do so many parents *want* their babies to have blue eyes?

That desire could be rooted in something as primal as our associations with blue: it's the color of a clear, sunny sky, or the sea on a beautiful day. It might also have something to do with sexual selection—bright coloration equals mating success in many species. Or it could have to do with a blue-eyed man wanting to be sure that the baby he's helping to raise is actually his.

Bruno Laeng and colleagues at Norway's University of Tromso found that blue-eyed men preferred blue-eyed women in tests of "attractiveness" performed with photographs in which eye color was digitally altered. They postulated that this evolved as a primitive sort of paternity test: a blue-eyed man, instinctively knowing that his children by a blue-eyed woman would almost always be blue-eyed as well, would immediately suspect something was amiss if his wife gave birth to a brown-eyed baby. Having a blue-eyed mate at least gave him some degree of assurance that his blue-eyed kids were probably his.

Well, not really. Having a blue-eyed baby in a part of the world where most of the men around you also have blue eyes—from the milkman to your semi-trustworthy next door neighbor—doesn't really provide a guy with much assurance. And anyway, as we'll soon see, newborn babies are pretty good at concealing who "daddy" really is, regardless of eye color.

He looks just like his daddy, doesn't he? If I had a nickel for every time I've been asked that question, I'd have a very large pile of nickels. Sometime in those first few minutes of life, especially if her partner is present, a new mother typically points out how much the baby looks like the putative father. When her family members arrive, they do the same thing. Friends soon join the chorus, and more often than not the hospital staff is drawn into the discussion, too.

The right answer to this question is always a resounding "Why, yes, he's the spitting image of his old man!" That's especially true for a busy pediatrician who doesn't have an extra hour to discuss "generic" babies, chimpanzee mating rituals, or the not insignificant chance that the fellow handing out the "It's a Boy!" cigars isn't actually the daddy of the baby who supposedly looks just like him.

As anyone with a television or a subscription to *People* magazine knows, *Homo sapiens* is not a truly monogamous species. We are also the species with the most labor-intensive, dependent babies on the planet. It's the conflict between the urge to philander and a mother's need to have help taking care of the result that has determined over the eons who our babies really look like—or don't.

Human evolution is driven by the urge to reproduce. You are here because your forebears, every single one of them, successfully passed their genetic material on to a next generation, who in turn passed it on to another and another until at last here you are, warts and all. A single interruption in that chain—a many-great-grandfather trampled by a mastodon before becoming a parent, say—would have resulted in a very different you. Or, more accurately, no you at all.

Once a child is born, a parent is committed, biologically, hormonally, and culturally, to protect and provide for his or her offspring—or gene packet, if you will—until it reaches an age where it can fend for itself. The strength of that commitment, bluntly put, is evolutionarily rooted in how sure a parent is that this child belongs to him or her. (Biological parents aren't always so committed, of course—check the docket of any family court—and adopting parents provide a notable exception to the "biology rules" rule.) A mother's commitment is absolute—she is quite sure this is her baby. The father, on the other hand, sometimes has his doubts.

The direct relationship between paternal certainty and fatherly investment of time and resources in a child's upbringing is borne out in a survey of primate species. At one end of the spectrum is the cotton-top tamarin, a tiny South American monkey named for the tuft of white hair on top of its head, which takes paternal certainty to the ultimate extreme. Once a couple mates, the male doesn't leave her side until she gives birth. They eat together, sleep together in a furry little love-ball, and can often be seen sitting side by side with tails entwined, perfect candidates for a Valentine's Day card.

Since the female never leaves his sight, the cotton-top male is absolutely certain of his paternity. Not coincidentally, he's also the most involved of primate dads. He grooms and plays with his babies (cotton-tops usually have twins), carries them with him wherever he goes, and brings them to their mother for nursing. When she's done he scoops them back up again. This goes on until the babies grow up and set off on their own.

Chimpanzee males, on the other hand, don't sweat the paternity thing. A chimp female often mates with multiple males during her well-advertised fertile period, or estrus—her rump swells and turns an unsubtle pink—so no male knows for sure if a given baby is his. Not that it matters. Guy chimpanzees like to spend their days in multimale packs, hunting, patrolling their territory, and picking fights with rival gangs, so being left out of the childcare loop suits them just fine.

Humans are somewhere in the middle of the primate continuum. As early human childbirth grew more dangerous and babies more dependent, males stayed closer at hand than their chimp cousins. A win/win/sort-of-win situation evolved: mom and baby got protection and material support, thus improving their chances of survival, while dad, since he was around his mate so much, got reasonable assurance that the baby he was spending all that time and energy on was actually his.

"Reasonable" is the key word here, because he couldn't be around her all the time, and since human females don't have a visible estrus, he could never be quite sure when his mate's fertile period was. Human nature conspires against absolute, cotton-top-style paternal certainty. Though we are nominally till-death-do-us-part monogamous, at least in Western societies, people just love to stray from their chosen mates. Yes, we have vows and rings and foil-wrapped pieces of wedding cake smashed in the back of the freezer, but we've also got a promiscuous inner chimp hardwired into our genes, just waiting to cut loose.

And cut loose it often does. "Extra-pair coupling," as the phenomenon is called by euphemism-loving anthropologists, occurs to varying degrees in all cultures. "Mis-assigned paternity"—another anthropological nicety—predictably follows, and more often than one might think. In human populations as diverse as British farmers and the Amazon's Yanomamo Indians, scientists have found that on average, 9 percent of babies studied are not actually the child of the man in the family. That 9 percent isn't a random number; it's a well-honed evolutionary compromise among mother, father, and baby.

How did it come to be? Why would a certain amount of fooling around become so ingrained in human culture? Let's reexamine the situation from the standpoint of the three parties involved. A prehistoric woman needed protection and support; her mate instinctively wanted assurance that he was helping to raise his own biological children; and the baby just wanted to survive, hopefully long enough to get in some "extra-pair coupling" of his or her own. The solution that best served everybody's interests? Generic-looking newborns.

Generic babies make sense. If a newborn *did* look just like his daddy, then about 9 percent of the time a father would see its resemblance to another male—the fellow in the next cave, for example—and most likely reject it, thus decreasing the chances of survival for both the baby and its mother. It might sound like eliminating babies that weren't really his own would enhance the "father's" chance of advancing his genetic line. But it could actually work against him. He might already have other children by the same female, after all, and abandoning his straying mate in a jealous huff would jeopardize his other biological children as well. Plus, our cuckolded male may well have an "adulterine child"—still more euphemisms!—tucked in some other fellow's family, and it would damage his own overall chances of Darwinian success if that child were easily discovered and rejected as well.

The math is complicated, but it turns out that a misassigned paternity rate of about 9 percent actually gives males, as a whole, the best chance of passing on their genes to the next generation. There are babies who really *do* look like their fathers, of course, and in those cases one hopes that it's the right guy. But in general, males owe their reproductive success to generic-looking babies.

Finally, just to seal the deal, humans developed a cultural tweak along the way that helps wrong-dad babies hide even more efficiently. What better way to convince a man he's the father than to tell him so, over and over again, until he believes it, too?

Relatives and friends spontaneously comment on a newborn's resemblance to his father—it's practically universal behavior—and they do so in ways that are telling. A new mother usually points out more paternal than maternal resemblances, and her relatives are more likely to do so than either the father or his family. Mothers also tend to make more looks-just-like-his-daddy comments with first babies, presumably when a man's paternity doubts might be greatest, than with subsequent children, by which time he is hopefully more confident.

So it's true: a baby *does* look like his daddy. And fortunately for him, he looks like a lot of other people, too.

A few years after my first lesson in examining the healthy newborn, I found myself in Tom's role, teaching new medical students about normal baby bodies. One of the students, a scrawny kid with a bushy, swept-back head of '80s hair and a bow tie that was always slightly askew, stood impatiently through my opening lecture, drumming his fingers on a notebook.

When I asked the students to tell me a bit about themselves, he announced that he was headed for a career in neurology; his classmates had long since nicknamed him "B.D.," short for "Brain Doctor," and he seemed to like the name. He considered a pediatrics rotation a waste of his time—he had no desire to become a mere "baby doctor." In fact, he sniffed, once his week in the nursery was done he had no plans ever to touch another baby. Faced with an uninterested, semihostile student, I did what any red-blooded resident would do: I called on him a lot.

I demonstrated the baby origami thing for the students that morning, then I had B.D. do it, too. He was bright, and though he quickly understood the fine points of a baby's womb-to-world transition, he was clearly uncomfortable. He handled the baby awkwardly, and when it began to whimper he jumped back from the bassinet like a man under attack. Once the other students had each had a chance to do an exam, I changed the baby's dirty diaper and asked B.D. to toss it in the trash can by the door. He brought the can to me instead, and I dropped the diaper in.

All done for the morning, I asked if there were any questions.

The students asked about the kinds of things earnest medical students want to know: What's a baby's normal heart rate and blood pressure? How does newborn kidney function compare to an adult's? When do they start walking and talking?

Just as we broke up, B.D. raised his hand. He pointed to the newborn we had just examined. "That doesn't look right," he said, flicking his finger back and forth between the baby's head and chest. "Shouldn't a baby have a neck?" I looked at the baby, with its softball-sized head sitting directly on its shoulders, and I had to admit he had a point. There was nary a neck to be seen.

Contrary to appearances, though, a newborn does indeed have a neck—it's just well hidden. Gently probe under a baby's chin and there among those pudgy skin rolls you'll find a tiny windpipe, only an inch long from jaw to chest. Not much of a neck, as necks go, but it's all the neck a baby needs.

I have learned over the years that comparing anyone's baby to a horse is a losing proposition, but the comparison in this case is useful: a newborn baby at its mother's breast eats just the way a horse drinks. Watch a horse at a water trough—slurp, swallow, slurp, swallow. There's no pausing, because a horse (and most mammals, for that matter) can swallow and breathe at the same time, the better to get away from a water hole quickly, before predators close in. Newborn humans have that same ability, but by four months of age or so we lose it. From then on humans are condemned to a life of either breathing or swallowing, but not both simultaneously. Blame it on an accident of evolution—and on our love of hearing ourselves talk.

Long ago, when we were just spineless worms wallowing in the ancient ooze, nobody ever choked to death. Our slithery ancestors fed by sieving ocean muck through a primitive mouth, and they "breathed" by absorbing oxygen directly through the skin. As bodies got bigger, skin absorption of oxygen became inefficient and impractical. Since oxygen-rich water was already passing through the mouth and gut as the worm fed, it didn't take much evolutionary tinkering to create gills and lunglike structures from outpouchings of the gut.

Unfortunately, as evolution honed and refined this crucial region of the mammalian body, the windpipe wound up in front of the esophagus; the paths for air and food intake thus crisscross one another at the back of the throat. Charles Darwin himself pondered this puzzling arrangement, commenting in 1859 how difficult it was to understand "the strange fact that every particle of food and drink which we swallow has to pass over the orifice of the trachea, with some risk of falling into the lungs, notwithstanding the beautiful contrivance by which the glottis [the opening between the vocal cords in the upper windpipe] is closed."

Darwin's "strange fact," though, is a peculiarly human problem. Other mammals long ago learned to coexist with this peculiar crisscross architecture. The horse seals off its windpipe from its esophagus when drinking. The glottis rises up in the back of a horse's throat and inserts into the rear of its nasal cavity, thus making a sealed tube for air to travel from nose to lungs, even as food and water pass from mouth to stomach.

Human beings are another matter. Darwin's "beautiful contrivance" notwithstanding, the system in humans fails far too often. Food literally tries to "go down the wrong pipe," and we are left at the mercy of a hair trigger system of gags and coughs—and the always handy Heimlich-trained companion—to save us from death by asphyxiation.

Here's where humans went wrong: we talk, therefore we choke. As vocalizations and then actual language grew in importance for our ancestors, we evolved longer necks that allowed us to produce a fabulous array of sounds and tones. The voice box dropped down lower in the neck—better resonance for those bass notes—and the glottis went with it. That changing anatomy forever broke the connection between the windpipe and the back of the nose. (And here's your trivia fact of the day: the original job of the uvula, that hangy-down thing in the back of your throat that doesn't seem to have any function, was to grab on to the windpipe as it rose and seal it tight. Now, sadly, with the trachea sunk down out of its reach, the uvula just hangs there between the tonsils with nothing to do.)

Humans were left with an open, common chamber in the back of the throat, a complicated crossroads for food and water and air. The opera may not be over until the lady in the horned helmet sings, but Brünnhilde will have to hold her breath to swallow before she belts out that final note.

So why does a newborn baby still have that windpipe-to-back-of-the-nose connection? First of all, because it makes for much more efficient eating. Look into the mouth of a crying baby and you'll often see the epiglottis, the flap of cartilage that slaps shut over the windpipe during swallowing, sticking up in the back of the throat like a pink potato chip. When a baby nurses, the epiglottis and the upper part of the windpipe rise up in the back of the throat, thus allowing the baby to feed like a tiny, two-legged Seabiscuit: milk flows around the windpipe and down the esophagus, minimizing the risk of choking. A newborn spends a good part of his day at the breast, and if he had to hold his breath every time he swallowed, his poor mother would never get up out of the rocker.

The other reason is that a newborn has no need of complicated language. A well-timed cry gets his point across quite well: *Hey! Something's wrong! Fix it!* A newborn's squatty neck allows for a horsey feeding technique, something that's a lot more valuable, at least for a few months, than talking.

That tiny little windpipe, along with the newborn throat and nose, is responsible, too, for an often unexpected new-parent scare: weird nocturnal baby noises. One of the working titles for this chapter was "Things That Go Honk in the Night." I chose that title in honor of my daughter Claire and the soft, gooselike noises that came floating from her bassinet the night we brought her home. I bolted from bed the first time I heard her, certain that something awful was happening, and found her sleeping peacefully, her chest rising and falling comfortably. But she was definitely honking. *Ah, I thought to myself. So this is what all those parents worry about!*

Newborn babies are a bit like mockingbirds—they can make an amazing array of clucking, squeaking, and rattling noises, all of them normal, and all guaranteed to scare the dickens out of new parents. There's a reason for the racket: a newborn baby's respiratory tract, from the nose to the throat and on down the windpipe, is quite skinny and very soft.

Start with the nose. Look in your own in the bathroom mirror and you'll no doubt see big, cavernous, adult-sized nostrils with plenty of room for air to pass through. Now look at a newborn's nostrils. The openings are just tiny slits.

It doesn't get much better in the newborn's throat and windpipe. The glottis—the opening between the vocal cords—is only about one-third of an inch wide, and the trachea below the vocal cords is even slightly narrower. The way a newborn's trachea is built complicates things even further. Feel your own windpipe, right at the Adam's apple—it's all cartilage, and hopefully yours is firm and undentable. While still holding on, take a deep breath. Nothing much happens: your trachea is as big and wide as ever.

The cartilage that forms a newborn's trachea is much softer than an adult's, so much so that when a baby takes a quick breath between cries it can partially collapse. This is even truer for the softer tissues of the nose and back of the throat. The combination of sudden air intake and the resulting narrower opening makes for all that nocturnal noise, and depending on which part of this anatomical orchestra is doing the collapsing, the sounds can range from low rumbles to high-pitched squeaks.

Sometimes the cartilage is even softer than usual and collapses during normal breathing, or with crying or feeding, a condition known as *tracheomalacia* (from "trachea" and the Greek word *malakia*, or "softening") or, if the voice box itself is involved, *laryngomalacia*. This can be a serious problem; there may be other abnormalities of the respiratory tract as well. A newborn baby who has *stridor*—a harsh, grunting noise, usually on exhaling—will be thoroughly evaluated before leaving the hospital. Babies with other, more typical breathing noises are free to go home and ruin their parents' sleep. The noisy breathing resolves on its own, usually within a few weeks, when everything in there finally firms up.

The softness of the tissues of the respiratory tract is another consequence of our evolutionary need to birth our big-headed babies in an earlier developmental stage than other primates—to get the boat out of the garage, if you will, while we still can. Given another couple of months in the womb, the trachea would be nice and firm and babies would sleep quietly at night, leaving their parents one less thing to worry about. But no: we think, therefore we honk—at least for a while.

I didn't have all those facts at hand when I did my best to answer B.D.'s question that morning. I couched my reply in terms of neck strength, how a newborn has such poor muscle tone and neurological control that a longer neck would be more prone to injury once that big head started lolling around. It was a pretty good off-the-cuff explanation—he certainly liked the neurological part—but in the end B.D. just nodded and headed off to lunch, his stethoscope draped over his long, skinny, grownup neck.

The windpipe ends in the chest, of course, splitting into a series of bronchial tubes before dead-ending in the alveoli of the lungs, just as in an adult. But a baby's chest is built differently than a grownup's, and in more ways than one.

Start with the prominent breasts, a feature that can be quite unsettling, particularly for the parents of a baby boy—"Are those . . . *boobs?*" being a frequently asked question. My answer—*Yes, they are, and he might even end up making a little breast milk before it's all over*—isn't very comforting. But breast tissue is breast tissue, no matter which sex it belongs to, and given the right combination of hormones, anyone—boys and men included—can produce at least small amounts of milk, a condition known as *galactorrhea.*

In the newborn, milk secreted from the nipple is sometimes called "witch's milk," a nickname whose origin is lost in the mists of time but likely referred to hexes, spells, and other Halloweeny frights in days of yore. As the name implies, the appearance of witch's milk was a very worrisome omen. In Swiss folklore, a newborn producing breast milk was said to "have an imp" inside him, producing milk for its own impish, evil nourishment. Treatment included sucking the milk out—it's not clear whose job this was—thus starving the imp, and then laying a knife in the cradle, sharp edge up, to drive it away for good.

Imps are on the outs nowadays. Breast enlargement is normal in newborns of both sexes. This is due to in utero exposure to the same hormones—estrogen and prolactin in particular—that are responsible for preparing a new mother's breasts for milk production. In about one in twenty babies, the nipples leak a few drops of milk, but since the hormones disappear from a baby's bloodstream shortly after the cord is cut, the breast swelling and milk formation slow down and stop over a few days to weeks, with or without the sharp-knife-in-the-cradle treatment—which, to be clear, I do not recommend.

Once you get past the breasts, you'll notice another difference between babies and adults: babies are barrel-chested; they're built like little dockworkers. Encircle a newborn's chest and your hands will form an almost perfect O. The typical adult chest in cross-section is wider and shallower—more sideways zero than O. The newborn owes his chest shape to the same evolutionary constraints that shaped his head—a round chest is a better fit inside the uterus than a broader, adult-style chest, and it causes less wear and tear coming down the birth canal.

The bones of the newborn chest—the ribs and sternum—are made mostly of cartilage and very little hard bone, an ideal arrangement for a rib-fracture-free birth. But that softness means they're not terribly helpful immediately after birth, when breathing suddenly becomes a big deal. Add in the fact that the intercostal muscles, the muscles between the ribs that do a lot of the work of breathing in adults, are weak from not having been used all that much in utero, and you've got what should be a fairly inefficient breathing mechanism. Fortunately, the newborn diaphragm, the broad sheet of muscle that separates the lungs from the abdominal cavity, picks up the respiratory slack.

The fetal diaphragm gets a decent workout during pregnancy, both from "practice" breathing movements and frequent spasms of the diaphragm muscle itself—all that fetal hiccuping that a pregnant woman feels. Unlike a healthy adult, who uses the muscles of the rib cage to inflate his lungs, the newborn baby practices diaphragmatic breathing, an odd-looking seesaw type of respiration. When the baby inhales, her diaphragm muscle pushes her abdominal contents down, causing the belly to pooch out while the springy chest wall sucks in a bit. The reverse is true when she exhales—the belly flattens while the chest wall springs back.

An adult with a barrel chest and diaphragmatic breathing would be in big trouble—probably suffering from emphysema or some other obstructive lung disease. For a baby, though, it works just fine. Over time the ribs and intercostal muscles grow stronger, the shoulders and chest broaden, and a child grows up to huff and puff just like the rest of us.

A few inches south of the rib cage, smack in the middle of the baby's belly, lies what's left of the umbilical cord—that once crucial placenta-to-fetus lifeline now rendered obsolete by the switchover to air breathing at birth. It isn't a cute, cuddly thing. For most parents the umbilical cord is hands down the most queasy-making part of their baby's body.

The stump of cord left attached to the baby is securely closed with a plastic clamp at birth, a skinny, multitoothed plastic gizmo that snaps together like an alligator's jaws, crushing the cord and its three blood vessels. That clamp plays an important role in the first few hours outside the womb. On the rare occasion that it slips off, blood can leak from the cord. It's usually no more than a drop or two—just enough to make a mess of a baby's fancy new clothes—but if the leak is larger, the bleeding can lead to severe anemia. Thankfully, that's an extremely rare event.

Applied properly, the clamp quickly and permanently seals the end of the cord. Within a few hours the arteries and vein within the cord shrivel and clot, and the risk of bleeding passes. The clamp is removed before the baby is discharged home, usually before I come around to do my discharge exam, typically leaving parents with three questions: *How do I take care of that thing? When will it fall off?* And most critical of all: *Is that an innie or an outie?*

The first two questions are related, since cord care directly affects how long it takes the umbilical stump to fall off. With its oxygen supply gone, the stump dries out, stiffens, and turns black, a process unappealingly known as "dry gangrene." The baby's immune system sends an army of white blood cells to the junction between the dying cord and the abdominal skin; over the course of several days, they slowly toss the cord remnant overboard.

Central to the notion of cord care is one biological fact: as soon as the cord is cut it becomes a piece of decomposing tissue, and bacteria just love to invade tissue that can no longer fight back. Given half a chance, those bacteria will follow the course of the shriveling blood vessels down into the baby's body, leading to a potentially severe infection known as *omphalitis*.

Preventive cord care treatments arose in the 1950s and '60s, when omphalitis was still relatively common in the Western world. The goal of the treatments was to kill the germs that colonized the decomposing cord, thus preventing infection until the cord finally fell off. A pharmacy's worth of chemicals were unleashed on the cord, including soaps, antibiotic ointments, rubbing alcohol, and the once ubiquitous triple dye—a combination of three antiseptic dyes that routinely turned the cord, and often large swaths of a baby's belly, an unearthly midnight blue.

No matter the treatments chosen, they all seemed to work: umbilical cord infections soon became very rare. The remedies themselves, though, were problematic—one of them, hexachlorophene, turned out to be toxic to the newborn nervous system. As researchers sought safer treatments, some began to wonder whether simply keeping the cord clean and dry until it falls off might not work just as well as blasting it with chemicals.

Sure enough, that's what they found. Keep the cord clean and dry, and infections are just as rare as with the chemical warfare approach. Most Western hospitals today either recommend dry cord care or the sparing application of rubbing alcohol to the cord. The dry cord movement is winning more converts every year—it actually takes a day or two longer for the cord to fall off when alcohol is used.

Tragically, umbilical cord infections are still a major threat to mothers and babies in developing countries. As many as 180,000 babies die every year from tetanus, due both to a lack of routine vaccinations for mothers and some very unsanitary cord care practices that promote growth of the toxin-producing germ *Clostridium tetani*. In parts of Africa, charcoal, grease, cow dung, and dried bananas are commonly used as umbilical cord dressings. Not surprisingly, maternal and neonatal deaths are highest in these areas. The World Health Organization today emphasizes maternal tetanus vaccination and sanitary cord care, two low-tech efforts that could save thousands, perhaps millions, of lives.

Back to question number two: When *is* that thing going to fall off? The usual range quoted is anywhere from five to fifteen days, though several factors, including prematurity, cesarean birth, and the way the cord is cared for can keep it attached even longer. Postpartum staff, who don't usually see babies once they've left the hospital, tend to give parents a lowball answer, predicting a fall-off date of about a week. I once overheard a student nurse discussing cord care with a new mother. "One morning you'll go to change her diaper and it'll just be *gone!*" she said, as if the Cord Fairy would come in the middle of the night and snatch it away, perhaps leaving a quarter under her pillow to boot.

The timing of the cord's departure looks different from the clinic end of things. I see a lot of anxious parents in my office at the two week well-baby visit, peeling back their baby's diaper to show me *that thing* is still there, stubbornly hanging on. Not only is it refusing to give up the fight, it's often bloody and sometimes a bit smelly, too. They figure they've failed as parents; the Cord Fairy passed them by.

The first thing I do is reassure them that what they're seeing is normal, that the umbilical cord is, after all, a piece of dying tissue—it's bound to smell a little. The bleeding is normal too. There's an inch or so of blood left in each of the three umbilical cord blood vessels at birth, trapped between where we clamp the cord on the outside and where the baby's body naturally clamps it on the inside. Some of that blood can ooze to the surface as the cord separates.

I go over care of the cord again, reminding them they can pick it up and clean around the base without hurting the baby—there are no pain-sensing nerves in the cord, and the baby won't pop and fly around the room if they dare to move it. Sooner or later, I tell them, all cords fall off. What I usually don't tell them is that my personal cord-hanging-on record in an otherwise healthy baby is eighty-eight parent-torturing days.

The third question, the innie-versus-outie one, is impossible to answer at birth. Ninety percent of adults have innies; no one knows why. The belly button is formed when the skin that surrounded the umbilical cord closes once the cord separates. Sometimes it folds in, sometimes it pooches out—it's a random thing. There's no inheritance pattern, and nothing anyone does seems to affect the outcome.

Not that people don't try. Soranus, the second-century Greek physician, recommended folding the cord remnant on itself at birth, wrapping it in wool, and placing a weight on top of it so that "this part will soon be moulded into a better-shaped cavity." And though I don't see them much anymore, "belly bands" of one kind or another were once employed by nearly every culture on earth. Tied around a newborn's abdomen, the band held an object in place over the navel during the first few weeks of life to ensure a shapely belly button. In my experience these objects have typically fallen into three categories: Coins of Many Countries (quarter-sized or bigger), Vegetables (potato, cucumber, and zucchini slices being the most popular) and Other Stuff (buttons, knotted leather, cotton batting, small stones). Everyone swears by their particular favorite, because they all seem to work. After all, nine out of ten babies will end up with an innie no matter what you do, even if you strap them to a cantaloupe.

So far, so good, in this tour of the newborn body. We've just passed the belly button, its umbilical cord remnant doomed to shrivel and fall off in few days, and not a single controversy has broken out. Sure, a baby's paternity is a big deal, but since that's pretty well disguised it's usually a nonissue in the first day of life. So on to the genitals—girl parts first, since this is probably the only time in life that they're more medically straightforward than boy parts.

Examining a newborn girl's genitalia takes almost no time. There's a pair of prominent, sometimes darkly pigmented *labia majora*, the "large lips" of the vagina, with the smaller *labia minora* peeking from beneath. I spread the labia, take a quick external look at the vagina to make certain there are no rare congenital deformities, and that's it. Though they'll be routinely screened for cancer and infection later in life, and a baby may someday emerge from them, for now there's not much to do but keep them clean. I tell parents to expect a mucous vaginal discharge for a few days, and not to worry if they see a bit of vaginal bleeding, both of which are the result of maternal hormones crossing the placenta. A quick hygiene discussion follows and then we're on to other things.

If only boys were so simple . . .

Looking at it, you wouldn't think a baby boy's penis would be a major source of anxiety for new parents. It's a cute little thing, really, just lying there innocently, a decade and a half or more from getting into any real mischief. But where there's a penis there's a foreskin, and there's the rub: What's a parent to do about circumcision? How are a new mother and father supposed to make an informed decision about taking or leaving it?

It isn't easy. Half the country seems to think a baby is better off without a foreskin, while the other half considers its removal a form of genital mutilation, even a crime against humanity. Stir in opinions from everyone from friends and relatives to the doctor standing at the mother's bedside, circumcision consent form in hand, and it's no surprise that deciding the fate of the foreskin can drive new parents batty.

It can drive whole groups of adults crazy, too, even set them at each other's throats. The World Health Organization is strongly pro-circumcision, for example, while organizations like Doctors Opposing Circumcision are passionately "anti." Dr. Edgar Schoen, in his role as chair of the Task Force on Circumcision of the American Academy of Pediatrics, declared that "the lifetime benefits of circumcision . . . far exceed the risks of the procedure," and scoffed at allegations of diminished sexual pleasure: "Being without a foreskin won't dent [a man's] sex life," he wrote. On the other side of the very deep divide, Dr. Paul Fleiss, an influential Los Angeles pediatrician, invoked the Nuremberg war crimes trials in describing "mass involuntary circumcision" as a "totalitarian concept" that has "no place in modern medicine or the civilized world."

The battle has spanned my pediatrics career. In the mid-1980s, even as several of my pediatric colleagues were revising the circumcision information handout our group gave to expectant parents, others were developing a companion pamphlet they titled "The Rape of the Foreskin." And then there's the man in the white sandwich board I once saw outside a pediatric conference, his message hand-painted in dripping red letters. "Circumcision = Child Abuse!" it said on the front. On the back: "Doctors = Go To Jail!"

The battle isn't limited to doctors. Anticircumcision groups like the National Organization to Halt the Abuse and Routine Mutilation of Males (NOHARMM) and Mothers Against Circumcision (MAC) promote "genital integrity" and distribute flyers with titles like "The Foreskin Advantage." Pro-circumcision organizations like the Internet-based CIRCLIST, founded by a group of American and European men who weren't circumcised at birth and wish they had been, are easy to find, too.

What in the world is going on here? How did such a tiny piece of tissue, the only really controversial part of the newborn body, become such a battleground?

Let's start at the beginning, or as close to the beginning as we can get. Ritual male circumcision has been around a very long time: there are circumcised mummies and six-thousand-year-old Egyptian tomb carvings depicting young men (willing and otherwise) undergoing the procedure. Jews have circumcised their male newborns for thousands of years, in order to fulfill God's covenant with Abraham. Muslims traditionally circumcise their boys, too, though usually not in the newborn period. And circumcision is an ancient rite of adolescent passage throughout the Pacific islands and much of Africa.

The United States, settled largely by Europeans who had no religious or cultural tradition of ritual circumcision, had very low circumcision rates for the first hundred years of its existence. That all changed in the 1890s, when Dr. Peter Charles Remondino, the foreskin-fixated president of the San Diego Board of Health, announced that circumcision was a cure for that peculiarly Victorian obsession, masturbation. In a series of impassioned articles Remondino called the foreskin an "evil genie" and an "outlaw" that irritated and stimulated the underlying *glans,* or "head" of the penis, inducing a young man "to seize the organ" and, well, masturbate.

Remondino declared that the foreskin had outlived its usefulness. He saw it as a primitive throwback, a protector of the penis "necessary of a long past age" when naked humans shinnied up trees for their food, now rendered obsolete by virtue of man's invention of pants. With nothing else to do, the modern, idle foreskin turned on its owner, causing a wide variety of ailments from crossed eyes and crooked spines to asthma and insanity. "Parents cannot make a better paying investment for their little boys [than circumcision]," Remondino wrote, because it "insures them better health, greater capacity for labor, longer life, less nervousness, sickness, loss of time, and less doctor-bills," and even a gentler, more peaceful death.

Remarkably, Remondino's theories were widely praised and quickly adopted by physicians; circumcision as a health measure soon entered the American medical mainstream. By the early twentieth century there was near universal agreement among doctors that routine newborn circumcision was important to good health.

Remondino rode the wave of his popularity for all it was worth. In 1902 he issued a blistering condemnation of his opponents, including Saint Paul, whom Remondino wished were still alive so that he could kill him: "I have been brought up and educated to look upon Saint Paul the founder of Christianity, with awe and admiration," he fumed, "but, by God, Sir, if I had Saint Paul here now, Sir, I would shoot him, yes, Sir, I would shoot him. He had no biblical warrant nor no business to summarily abolish circumcision as he did. . . . I may be wrong about shooting him. He probably did not know the harm he was entailing on gentile humanity by abolishing circumcision. Still, when I think of the agonies I have been made to suffer through his carelessness, I feel he ought to be shot, Sir."

Though the practice began to decline elsewhere as the 1950s dawned—especially in Great Britain, where the new National Health Service questioned its health benefits and cost effectiveness—circumcision remained well entrenched here at home, reaching a peak of more than 90 percent of all boys around mid-century.

The United States is still a particularly circumcision-happy nation. In 1999 nearly 65 percent of all newborn American boys were circumcised, the vast majority for reasons that had nothing to do with religion or culture or anything else other than the trend set in motion by the remarkably insistent Peter Charles Remondino. Compare our rates with those of other countries and regions in that same year: Canada, 35 percent; Australia, 10 percent; England, 6 percent; Scandinavia 2 percent; and less than 1 percent in Germany, Russia, China, and Japan. Worldwide an estimated 10 to 20 percent of boys are circumcised. Once again, as with epidurals and cesareans, we're out ahead of the curve.

Americans are also a circumcision-*un*happy bunch, too, if the growing numbers of organizations devoted to "restoring" the foreskins of men circumcised at birth is any indicator. Citing a number of reasons to re-cover the glans, from issues of sexual pleasure (mainly) to anger and resentment toward one's pro-circumcision parents, groups like RECAP (RE-Cover A Penis) and NORM (the National Organization of Restoring Men) recommend a number of restoration methods. Using weights, cones, or specially designed elastic pulling devices, the skin of the penile shaft is stretched down over the glans, creating a sort of prosthetic foreskin.

In order to understand the controversy, it's necessary to understand what a circumcision really is. In simplest terms, circumcision is the removal of the foreskin, or prepuce, the free fold of skin that covers the glans. That's it. There are a variety of devices for foreskin removal, each with its own boosters, but the end result is the same: when all is said and done, the foreskin is gone, leaving the glans exposed.

If the foreskin were just an ordinary piece of skin, the controversy would no doubt be a bit more muted. But there's more to a foreskin than meets the eye (or scalpel). Despite the name, it's not just a hunk of epidermis. Rich in sensory nerves and blood vessels, the foreskin has been described as a "specific erogenous zone" by the anticircumcision pediatrician Paul Fleiss. It's much more sensitive to touch, motion, and temperature than the glans and the rest of the penis.

The foreskin is two-sided, too, with each side serving a different function, much like the eyelid. The outer surface is an extension of the thin layer of skin that covers the rest of the penis. The inner layer, though, performs several specialized tasks. Sebaceous glands produce smegma, a mixture of natural oils and skin cells that protects and lubricates the glans. Apocrine glands secrete a number of infection-fighting chemicals such as chymotrypsin, which breaks down proteins, and enzymes, too: lysozyme, for one example, destroys bacterial cell walls.

Even so, the foreskin's defenses aren't foolproof, and its failures are the basis of the strongest arguments in favor of circumcision. Uncircumcised boys and men have long been known to be at greater risk of urinary tract infections than those who have been circumcised. And, obviously, only uncircumcised males are at risk to suffer painful foreskin infections.

Uncircumcised men are also more likely to contract certain ulcerating sexually transmitted infections (STIs), such as syphilis, and infection with human papillomavirus, an STI associated with both penile and cervical cancer. New Zealand researchers, for example, followed a group of men from birth to age twenty-five and found that the uncircumcised men in the study were three times more likely to contract an STI than those who had been circumcised.

Circumcision has been shown to reduce HIV risks, too. In March 2007, the World Health Organization (WHO) announced that studies in Kenya, Uganda, and South Africa had shown a marked decrease in HIV transmission among recently circumcised heterosexual men—up to a 60 percent reduction in some areas. WHO is so convinced of circumcision's benefits that its HIV/AIDS website now carries this bold-lettered recommendation: "Male circumcision should be part of a comprehensive HIV prevention package."

Put all the research findings together and it looks as if Peter Charles Remondino was right—maybe not about curing insanity or scoliosis (and probably not masturbation, either), but the reduced risks of infection and cancer seem to make a compelling argument in favor of circumcision.

Still, parents leaning toward not circumcising their sons might look at the same research and wonder about the conclusions. After all, only one in a hundred uncircumcised boys will ever get a bladder infection. Penile cancer is extremely rare, too, on the order of one in a hundred thousand men, and is related to other risk factors, like smoking and poor hygiene. And in the New Zealand study, though circumcision did seem to provide protection from STIs, over 90 percent of the men *didn't* get an STI, whether they were circumcised or not.

And then there's HIV and Africa. I'm not so sure that the apparent HIV protection African men receive from circumcision is applicable to children born in the United States. In Africa, a sizable proportion of HIV infections are spread through heterosexual intercourse; transmission is made easier by the presence of other, untreated sexually transmitted diseases and the reluctance of many men to regularly use condoms. There's no evidence that circumcision would reduce the risks for either gay men or IV drug users— the two groups most at risk of contracting HIV disease in the United States. It's good to keep in mind that the United States had a very high circumcision rate in the 1980s and '90s, a time when the AIDS epidemic exploded.

Full disclosure: I do circumcisions for parents who request them, though at the risk of incurring the wrath of many in my profession, I don't encourage parents to have them done. The fight between the "pro" and "anti" camps makes the issue sound like an all-or-none fight, and it just isn't that clear cut.

I've done hundreds of "circs" over the course of my career, and (though I should probably knock on wood before saying this) I've never had a serious complication with one—no infections or excessive bleeding, no injuries to the glans or the rest of the penis. And though the pain of circumcision is routinely played up in anticircumcision literature, I don't see much of it. I use a combination of oral acetaminophen, a dorsal penile nerve block (a small amount of local anesthetic injected at the base of the penis with a very fine needle), and a sugar-water-filled pacifier, which helps reduce pain by releasing a baby's natural endorphins, much like what occurs during a feeding. Together, those three measures work quite well. The large majority of babies I circumcise show few if any signs of discomfort. Many of them sleep through the whole thing.

I do circumcisions because I don't see this as a black-and-white

Infant Origami · 307

issue. From a public health standpoint, I agree that circumcision is an increasingly important tool in the fight against HIV and other STIs, at least in developing countries, but not so much so that I can personally recommend it for all babies. I can also understand the concerns of parents about pain, complications, or the potential for altering a child's future sexual pleasure. The first two of those concerns are controllable by carefully following standard procedures. The last one is a bit tougher to answer.

Sexual pleasure is an infinitely subjective thing, and whether it's "better" with or without a foreskin is impossible to know—not that that has ever stopped anyone from arguing the point. A quick Internet search pulls up dozens of testimonials from men who were circumcised at birth, circumcised later, or remain "intact." Men in all three groups tend to think their sexual experiences are better (or worse) for having been circumcised (or not). Many long to bring back the foreskin they lost at birth, or to be rid of the one they still have. In a particularly telling study, men who were circumcised as adults spoke unfavorably of a loss of penile sensitivity postcircumcision, but were overall highly satisfied with having had the operation, probably because their partners liked the new "look."

I'm not convinced that circumcision is as sexually disabling as its opponents claim. It's unlikely that circumcision decreases a man's sex drive, since the testicles make testosterone, not the foreskin. The sensations a circumcised man feels may be different, even less than those of his intact brethren, but on a planet with six billion people, most of them sexually active and many of them circumcised, it doesn't seem to be slowing anybody down.

Adding up the risks and benefits here in the early twenty-first-century, I can't recommend circumcision as standard treatment for all boys. Parents have to do the pro-and-con weighing for themselves and decide what's more important to them: HIV risks? a functional foreskin? the very tiny chance of something going wrong with a circumcision?

That process is the same one they will go through with any number of health care decisions they'll be called on to make on their child's behalf—whether to vaccinate or give antibiotics, to name a couple of common examples, or how to deal with cancer or diabetes, to name a couple of rarer ones. If the decision to circumcise or not is the toughest one parents ever have to make for their son, they're getting off very easy in life.

In reality, most brand-new parents don't decide about circumcision based on HIV research or highly subjective pleasure debates; it isn't easy to look down the road to a time when their bouncing baby boy will be big, hairy, and chasing down a mate. Religion plays a deciding role for many families, of course, but the most common reason I hear for circumcising (or not) is family tradition: "We want him to look like his father." I try to point out that today's newborn boy is never *really* going to look like his father—by the time he's old enough to notice things like foreskins, Dad is going to look more like a grandfather than a teenager anyway.

Just south of the genitals lie the much less controversial legs and feet. Still, they're the subject of a lot of questions, because parents holding their newborn for the first time are often startled to find that, when straightened out, their baby's lower extremities form a perfect set of parentheses. Run a finger along the bones of a newborn's leg and you'll trace a graceful arc running from the hip to the toes. That bow-leggedness concerns many parents, but not all. "He looks like a cowboy," a dad once told me as he held his new son. He meant that as a good thing; he raised horses for a living.

A general rule of thumb: the older the relatives present at the first exam, the more questions about the baby's legs. When I started my career in the 1970s, an entire generation of grandparents still had direct experience with rickets, or at least were very aware of it as a disease. The grandparents of today's babies are often the children of my original cadre of grandparents, and so that fear of bowed legs lives on, though in attenuated form.

Rickets is a disease that prevents ossification—the normal hardening, or mineralization, of bone. Rather than firming up in the first months and years of life, the affected bones remain soft and bendy. Once a child with rickets begins to walk, the leg bones curve outward, resulting in stunted, bowed legs by adolescence. (Other bones are affected as well; a pelvis deformed by rickets—child-sized and too misshapen to allow the fetus to pass through the birth canal—was one of the most common indications for a cesarean delivery in the early twentieth century.)

I haven't seen a child with rickets in many years. That's because, except in uncommon inherited cases, rickets is a nutritional disease. The softened bones in nutritional rickets are caused by a lack of vitamin D, a key factor in bone mineralization. Most people in the Western world get their vitamin D from fortified milk (cod-liver oil, another fine source, having long ago passed out of fashion) and sun exposure.

Sunlight was largely unavailable to children born in the slums of nineteenth-century America and soon sent to workhouses; until the 1930s, when milk became fortified with vitamin D, poor urban children with legs stunted by rickets were a common sight. And it was the memory of those children that worried the grandparents I met in the 1970s, when they saw their grandchildren born with bowed legs.

The real reason for a newborn's bowed legs, of course, is the space constraint of the late term uterus. A fetus's bones are soft and flexible; when things get crowded toward the end of pregnancy, they bend and mold to the shape of the womb. Head down, legs folded, a third trimester fetus assumes a space-saving, upside-down, Buddha-like lotus position. It will take a year or two of walking for the leg bones to straighten out; in the meantime, the best thing I can do for parents is counsel patience and talk them out of leg braces and expensive "orthopedic" shoes.

While bowed thigh and shin bones are rarely a problem, curved feet sometimes are. The feet need to move around in the womb to develop properly, and if there's not enough space, the soft bones of the foot can bend too much. *Metatarsus adductus* is a fairly common condition in which the bones in the middle of the foot bend, leaving the foot in an almost C shape when looked at from below. *Metatarsus adductus* can be treated with simple stretching, or, occasionally, with casting to push the bones back into normal shape.

Clubfoot, or *talipes equinovarus,* is more serious. It occurs when in utero space is severely limited, such as when a woman has too little amniotic fluid, a condition known as *oligohydramnios.* The feet don't have room to develop normally; they grow stiff and twisted. Clubfoot can be treated with casts that slowly push the feet back into a more normal shape, or, in more severe cases, with surgery.

Unlike in decades long past, clubfoot today is only rarely a life-altering deformity. Athletes including Olympic gold medal skater Kristi Yamaguchi, professional football hall of famer Troy Aikman, and soccer star Mia Hamm were all born with the condition. But then so, allegedly, was Josef Goebbels, Hitler's propaganda minister. Whatever goals a parent may have for his or her child—hopefully it's the Olympics and not world domination—clubfoot shouldn't get in the way.

By the end of his one-week nursery rotation, B.D.'s people skills and lack of enthusiasm for babies remained unchanged. Early on he alienated a neonatologist when he described a tiny premature baby as looking like a fish. Another resident nearly clobbered him when he refused to attend a delivery on the grounds that he'd already been to one, and one was more than enough. And the nurses, noting the unblanketed babies he imperiously left in his wake, were nearly murderous. ("That's not doctors' work," he sniffed, when a student nurse complained about having to clean up after him.)

But one aspect of the newborn exam did fascinate him. On the final morning of his nursery rotation I found B.D. sitting next to a bassinet, gently stroking a baby's cheek. Every time he touched her, the baby's head turned and she tried to take his finger into her mouth. He did this again and again until he noticed me watching him. I knew better than to mistake all that stroking for a newfound sense of tenderness. "I love primitive reflexes," B.D. said, his eyes shining. He rattled off the names of several: the Moro, stepping, and palmar grasp reflexes. "They're so . . . *neurological!*"

By this time the other students had gathered around us, ready to begin newborn rounds. On overhearing B.D., one of them, a tall, serious young woman who planned to become an obstetrician, raised her hand. "Why are they called primitive reflexes?" she asked. "I mean, what are they actually for?" Before I could answer, B.D. cut in.

"They're not *for* anything," he said with a condescending roll of his eyes. "That's why they're called *primitive.*"

Not so fast, I told B.D. The reflex he'd been toying with clearly had a purpose: the *rooting reflex*—the turning of the head when the cheek is stroked—was obviously designed to help a baby find her mother's nipple, a function as important in modern times as it has been throughout human evolution. But what about the others? Why *does* a baby throw out his arms when he's startled, I asked him, or point his toes when the sole of his foot is stroked? For the first time that week B.D. was stumped, so I gave him an assignment. He already knew the names of all the primitive reflexes, and the movements involved in each of them, but by the following morning I wanted an answer to his colleague's question: *Why do babies have primitive reflexes?* B.D. frowned, then nodded. "You're on," he said.

Primitive reflexes are defined as "reflex actions originating in the brain stem that are exhibited by infants but not adults in response to particular stimuli." In other words, just like an adult's knee-jerk response to a doctor's tapping hammer, they're movements that are preprogrammed and uncontrollable. Stroke the cheek and the newborn turns to what she hopes is a milk-laden breast. Do it again and she'll respond the same way. She can't help herself.

The rooting reflex is present well before birth—a baby born two months prematurely is often already able to turn in the direction of a stroke on the cheek, though at that age she probably won't be able to actually nurse. A full term baby's response, though, is vigorous and searching—her head moves back and forth in smaller and smaller arcs until she locates the nipple. With practice, the searching movements lessen. By three weeks of age a breast-fed baby will zero in on the nipple quickly and accurately.

The two-part *sucking reflex* is linked to the rooting reflex. Once the mother's nipple is placed between the lips and touches the roof of the mouth, the baby's tongue automatically presses it against the hard palate, a movement known as "expression." She then "milks" the nipple, moving her tongue from the areola—the pigmented area that surrounds the nipple—to the tip of the nipple itself. The rooting and sucking reflexes are obviously critical to a newborn's health, and so hardwired that their absence is often the sign of a serious problem: infection, respiratory distress, or perhaps a damaged brain.

The other primitive reflexes are equally hardwired in full term newborns, but not nearly so important to survival as the root and suck—at least not for modern human babies. Several are easily recognizable; others are more subtle and obscure. Chief among the obvious ones is the *Moro reflex*—named for the Austrian pediatrician Ernst Moro, who also discovered the bacteria-killing benefits of breast milk before the Nazis forced him from his position as head of the University of Heidelberg children's clinic for the crime of having a Jewish wife.

The Moro reflex, sometimes called the *startle reflex,* is familiar to just about anyone who has ever held a baby. It appears well before birth—even earlier than the rooting reflex—though it's not fully formed until about thirty-seven weeks. Triggered by sudden movement or loud noise, the Moro is a coordinated series of movements: first the baby's legs straighten and her neck extends; then her arms shoot up and out with fingers spread wide; finally, over a few seconds, she pulls her arms together, clenches her fists, and cries out. The Moro reflex startles parents, too—their natural response is to pick up and comfort the baby.

It's important for a pediatrician to check the Moro reflex at birth, not so much for any function it performs, but because the lack of a Moro can be a symptom of neurological damage. An asymmetric Moro reflex, with only one arm moving as it should, can indicate an injury to the brachial plexus, the trunk of nerves that runs from the spinal cord to the shoulder and controls movement and sensation in the arm. (Kaiser Wilhelm, Queen Victoria's birth-injured grandson whose severe brachial plexus injury permanently paralyzed his left arm, would have had no Moro response on that side at all.) Lack of a Moro reflex on both sides usually points to serious central nervous system damage.

Another familiar reflex is the *palmar grasp:* place your thumbs in a newborn's palms and she'll grip tightly, so tightly that it's sometimes possible to lift a brand-new baby clear off the exam table this way. It's not a trick I'd recommend parents demonstrate to relatives and friends, though, since a baby suspended in the air by her palmar grasp reflex may suddenly let go, triggering a screaming Moro reflex and a first rush of parental guilt. Better to observe this one in the safety of someone's lap.

But then there are a few peculiar, not so obvious reflexes. Take the *plantar reflex:* rub the ball of a baby's foot and her toes curl up while her foot points downward. Then there's the *placing reflex:* touch the top of the foot against the underside of a table and the baby will pull back and place the sole of her foot on the top of the table. And perhaps most odd of all is the *stepping reflex.* Hold a newborn under her arms so that the soles of both her feet touch a flat surface and she'll take a few "steps": one foot placed in front of the other, too weak to actually march, but doing a pretty good imitation.

Looked at in isolation, the primitive reflexes could easily be mistaken for nothing more than interesting little tricks to dazzle new parents: *Look! She's "walking"!* But my challenge to B.D. was to try to connect the primitive reflex dots, to find the common link among them. I wanted him to look past the trees to the forest, or rather, to look up into the trees we came down from millions of years ago.

Long story short: B.D. made a great oral report the next morning, but he missed my point entirely. He laid out the anatomy and physiology of each reflex in great detail, but when he was done the original question remained unanswered: *What are they for?*

What they're for, of course, is to aid a newborn in that first "climb" to his mother's waiting breast. Primitive reflexes are the hardwired neurological responses that were once critical to a newborn's survival. The rooting and sucking reflexes are as important to a newborn's nutrition and health today as they ever were. The placing, stepping, and plantar reflexes, on the other hand, aren't.

Weak though they may be, those "climbing" reflexes still work. The stepping and plantar reflexes power the legs, the palmar reflex aids the hands in finding and grasping the breast, and, once having arrived at the nipple, the root and suck reflexes take care of the rest. Put them all together and a newborn baby's a slow-moving, preprogrammed, breast-seeking missile.

And what's the point of the Moro reflex? Remember that the trigger is something that startles the baby—a loud noise or sudden movement. Her legs straighten, her arms fly out with fingers outstretched; then she pulls his arms inward, hands grasping, and cries out. She's reaching for mama, crying for her attention and protection, and grasping for something her mother no longer has: fur. Consider the chimpanzee newborn, which has all the same primitive reflexes as a human baby, though they're much stronger. By a few days of age it clings unassisted to the fur on its mother's underside, and in the jungle, with the need to flee from predators, the ability to jump up and grab on to mama's fur as she runs from danger is a distinct necessity.

The only part of the Moro reflex a modern human baby still needs, then, is the cry. Even in areas of the world where predators are still an issue, infants are snugly carried in slings or clothing, which have taken the place of our once luxuriant fur.

B.D. was gone before I finished my primitive reflex lecture. He'd been counting down the minutes until noon that Saturday, when his rotation officially ended, and at about a half second past twelve he was gone. He's still out there, I'm sure, happily whacking grownups with his reflex hammer and studiously avoiding babies.

There's much more I go over with new parents—if there's time, that is. The skin alone could take up the whole visit—why it always peels, for example (yours would, too, if you'd just been hot-tubbing for nine months), and those common, usually transient birthmarks with names that hark back to more colorful medical times: the red *angels' kisses* on the forehead and eyelids, or the equally scarlet *stork bite* on the back of the neck. Not to mention the white-dot *milia* sprinkled over the nose and cheeks, the *sucking callus* in the middle of the upper lip, and *erythema toxicum,* the scary-sounding but harmless scattering of red dots that appears all over a newborn's body shortly after birth. Its nickname, "flea bite rash," requires careful explanation lest a family flee the hospital with visions of a vermin-infested maternity ward.

Then there's the question of body hair, summed up nicely by one young father when he asked, *What's with all the fur?* The man was smooth-skinned and baby-faced himself, the stubble of his prematurely receding hairline poking up from his shaved, gleaming scalp. His baby was another story altogether: long, dark, spiky hair shot straight out from her scalp as if she'd gotten a cartoon electric shock in the process of being born. Her eyebrows, thick and lush, met in the middle of her forehead. Tufts of hair sprouted from her ears. Her shoulders and back, with whorls of hair scattered over them, looked like a satellite view of the Atlantic Ocean in a particularly busy hurricane season. She was a pretty little thing, long-lashed and dimpled, but her father was right: she did look, well, *furry.*

There was a time, though, when the man's baby would have been considered freakishly bare-bodied. We were once hairy primates, of course, and furry babies (and adults) were the norm for much of early human history. Then things changed, so much so that humans are now one of only a handful of the world's five thousand species of mammals not covered in fur—and most of the other relatively hairless species spend most of their time in water, like whales and walruses, or in dark burrows, like the naked mole rat. Put another way, human beings are the mammals most at risk for a really nasty sunburn.

We started leaving our hair behind when we left the African forest for the grassy savannah a million or so years ago. A water-repellent full-body rug may have made sense in the shady rain forest, but out on the sun-baked grasslands it made cooling down difficult. Less hair became a big advantage for early hominids—it's estimated that a "naked" ape could travel twice as far on a quart of water as his furry cousin. As an added bonus, the energy once devoted to growing and maintaining that lush crop of body hair could be diverted to other uses, such as nourishing a bigger brain.

We've kept some hair, of course, but compared to yesteryear, our modern bodies look like "after" maps of California's decimated redwood forests, with dense hair growth limited to the equivalent of a few state parks: the top of the head, the male face, the armpits, and the groin. And I'm not sure what it says about us as a species, but what with shaving, waxing, and laser hair removal, we seem awfully determined to finish off what little we still have. Naked mole rat envy, perhaps.

I reassured the furry baby's balding father that this, too, would pass, that the extra body hair is normal, merely an echo of our primate past. No need for shaving or depilatories—it falls out all by itself in the first weeks of life. He was relieved.

I could go on and on with parents, but the limited time I have to spend with a family in the hospital eventually runs out. Plus, there's only so much information brand-new mothers and fathers can absorb. It's well known that immediate postpartum women, and probably their partners, too, don't retain a lot of what they're told in the hospital. It's not surprising, given the intensity of the experience they've just been through. That's why a steady stream of reliable advice and information is so important, from early in pregnancy until well after hospital discharge.

The last thing I do for parents who'll be coming to see me in the outpatient world, then, is to give them my office phone number and my e-mail address. I encourage them to contact me with the questions about their babies that will no doubt pop up in the days and weeks to come. And they do. The "looking at babies" talk that starts in the hospital often becomes an ongoing dialogue as parents and babies slowly settle into a comfortable, if exhausting, home routine.

The hospital stay ends just as it began, with an elevator ride. The scene is repeated several times a day: the doors slide open and a new mother in a wheelchair, her baby bundled in her lap, is rolled inside by a nurse. What follows sometimes looks like one of those twenty-clowns-in-a-taxi circus acts, but in reverse. A gaggle of relatives and friends squeeze in around the wheelchair with suitcases, bouquets, and bunches of "It's a Boy!" balloons in tow. Sometimes the crowd's too big for a single trip. Watching everyone figure out who gets to go with mother and baby and who waits for the next elevator can be an interesting study in budding family dynamics. A foreshadowing, I'm sure, of things to come.

The elevator ride takes all of half a minute—ours is not a very big hospital—but it's a symbolic journey. Just as a fetus has become a baby, and a woman a mother, the move from hospital to home is another kind of birth. The future is uncertain—fate will no doubt dish out a few lumps and bumps in the next couple of decades—but this much is clear: life will never be the same for anyone involved. And that, far more often than not, is a good thing.

Afterword

I first came across the German word *umwelt* in *Arctic Dreams,* a marvelous book by the nature writer Barry Lopez. *Umwelt* translates literally as "environment," the natural world in which people, animals, and plants live. To a biologist, though, the word has a different meaning. *Umwelt* refers to an animal's-eye view of its world—how a polar bear sees the frozen expanse in which it lives, for example, what sense it makes of the midnight sun, the snow-storms, or the seals it pursues on its daily bearish ramblings. The bear's view of its physical world is no doubt very different from that of its wary prey, which in turn is very different from that of the freezing human biologist who observes them both. Every creature's *umwelt* is unique; it's impossible for someone or something else to completely understand it. It's the difference between being a re-searcher and a subject, a spectator and a participant, a doctor and a patient.

Everyone who comes to a birth brings his or her own personal *umwelt* with them. A woman having her first baby carries the sum total of her unique life experiences: her hopes and fears; her life's traumas, both physical and emotional; the love and nurtu-rance she got, or didn't get, from her parents and family; the sup-port, or lack of it, from her partner and friends. Her thoughts and feelings on entering the labor room, and her interpretation of what goes on there, are hers and hers alone. Just as with those proverbial snowflakes, no two labor experiences are ever exactly alike.

Her partner's *umwelt* is by default very different from her own.

He (or she) is not at risk of intense physical pain; there is no doubt that he will physically survive the ordeal. But his hormones have changed over the course of his mate's pregnancy, his feelings about becoming a parent have been more or less intensely thrashed out, and he has some degree of anxiety about what's to come, whether he chooses to express it aloud or let it fester in some couvade-inspired belly pain or toothache.

Then, of course, there's the baby. Who knows what goes on in that tiny cone-shaped head as a newborn takes a first blurry look around the room at the people who will feed her, nurture her, and hopefully protect her from life's rougher edges?

A person's *umwelt* changes over time. A woman returning for her second or third labor is a very different person from the woman she was the first time around. She knows what to expect, more or less, and her earlier experiences, both good and bad, will shape her view of this birth. The people she chooses to have with her at that moment are different, too, irrevocably changed by the ripple effect of a previous child who perhaps bumped them up a generation, turning them into grandparents or aunties, or simply into caring, protective friends. And heaven knows that the worldview of a two-year-old soon-to-be big sister is radically altered from what it was when she was the star of the original show.

My own *umwelt* has changed greatly in the decades since the first time I saw a baby being born. I was barely six years removed from my high school prom when Mitch sat me down at the foot of Tonya's bed. I came to that first childbirth a terrified, woefully unprepared newcomer, a fish so far out of water I might as well have been on the moon. Not so much different, I suppose, from how Tonya's baby Robert must have felt when he blinked up at me from my lap and wondered if this sweaty, wild-eyed creature was the one whose nipple he was supposed to sniff out.

Nearly three thousand births later I am only occasionally terrified, but I'm still in awe of childbirth. I've witnessed just about every permutation of human birth, from "routine" vaginal deliveries—the kind most people expect—to those gone suddenly, terribly wrong.

Yet the most striking thing to me after all these years is how often such an incredibly complicated process goes right. And how often, despite all the pain and fear that can come with having a baby, women come back and do it again.

I never saw Tonya again. I doubt she'd remember me—certainly not with the brain-seared intensity that I remember her. I was just one of many earnest young people in scrubs she no doubt encountered before finally heading home with her son. I can only imagine how I figured into her *umwelt,* her worldview of birthing a baby in a large hospital filled with fledgling doctors.

Tonya's probably a grandmother now, given her three children and the fact that Robert, the baby who nearly scared me to death, would have turned thirty last year. I sometimes wonder how it all turned out for her. Did she have more children? Did they grow up healthy and strong? Did she end up being her daughter's labor coach, drawing on her own experiences to guide her through the pains of having a baby? Or did she tell her daughter the hell with all that, just skip the whole knifing thing and sign up for an epidural?

I think about my early experiences more often these days, as the hospital part of my pediatrics career winds down. Like most pediatricians, I will sooner or later be called on to make a choice: practice in the hospital or in the outpatient clinic, but not both. I can't really disagree with the "hospitalist" trend. Medicine has become too complicated for anyone to be a jack-of-all-illnesses, and doctors who specialize in either hospital or clinic work tend to become better at what they do than those who are spread too thin. Still, I'm proud of being a "dinosaur," grateful that I came of age medically in a time when a pediatrician could do both.

When the time comes, I will choose the outpatient clinic. Though I still enjoy attending births, I can't imagine giving up the relationships I've formed with so many families over the years. I couldn't say good-bye to being a "pediatric grandfather," for one thing, leaving behind the growing numbers of my former patients who now bring their own children to me. And I have to be honest with myself, too. In middle age, dashing through hospital corridors at three in the morning has lost a bit of its allure.

If my most recent call night turns out to be my last, I'll have gone out more or less the way I came in: a witness to a normal birth. The irregular fetal heart rate that prompted the obstetrician to page me had righted itself by the time I got to the labor room, but I decided to wait a few minutes to make sure this particular fetus was serious about entering the world as a healthy baby.

Then came that familiar sequence, the one I'd first seen when Mitch pushed me aside to get to Tonya's baby, the one I've seen so many times since. Out came the head, then the shoulders one by one, then the rest of a healthy baby, cradled in the obstetrician's sure hands. A few seconds and a snip of the cord later, she was cradled in her mother's arms, her bewildered *What just happened here?* eyes slowly coming to focus on her mother's face. And at that moment, with a little girl's life outside the womb safely launched, I left.

Acknowledgments

Many people to thank . . .

First and foremost among them is my wife, Elisabeth Chicoine, for her unerring sense of the right thing to do, for the firm hand with which she guided me back to the writing desk when my confidence flagged, and for marrying me in the first place. I love you, Lis.

While engrossed in my book proposal two years ago, Sarah Jane Freymann nearly missed her Manhattan subway stop. She called me soon after and declared that she would become my agent. She was right. I am grateful to Sarah Jane for her sage advice, her friendship, and, of course, her business savvy. I am also indebted to Jessica Sinsheimer, who first brought my proposal to Sarah Jane's attention.

Sarah Jane in turn introduced me to Susanna Porter, editor extraordinaire at Ballantine Books. I thank Susanna both for her fine editing of my manuscript and for her graceful handling of my sometimes fragile first-time-author ego. Working with her has been a great pleasure. Thanks, too, to Jillian Quint at Ballantine for keeping me on task and on time, and to Emily DeHuff for her superb copyediting.

I was fortunate to meet Robert Asahina, deputy managing editor of *The New York Sun*, and his wife, the novelist Linda Phillips Ashour, at a dinner party in 2005. Bob and Linda kindly offered to have a look at my then nonexistent book proposal and a year later were quite generous in their constructive critique of the real thing.

Their encouragement kept me going in the early, finding-my-way days.

Closer to home . . .

Adair Lara of San Francisco, from whom I learned much about the art of the nonfiction essay, has been my friend and writing mentor for a dozen years. Her support from the very beginning of my writing career has meant a great deal to me.

A heartfelt thank you to Susan Bono, publisher and editor of *Tiny Lights: A Journal of Personal Narrative* in Petaluma, California. Susan helped me polish the rough drafts of several chapters, and as the world's greatest writing group ringmaster, she played a major role in the birth of *Birth Day*.

Speaking of writing groups, I am blessed to belong to the finest I can imagine. Thanks to Christine Falcone, Chuck Kensler, Elizabeth Kern, Margit Liesche (author of *Lipstick and Lies*—a ripping good yarn), Pat Tyler, and, again, Susan Bono. I could not have done this without all of you.

I am grateful, too, to a host of friends who read and offered suggestions on parts of the manuscript: Karen Betaque, Dennis Buchanan, M.D., Colleen Craig, Ann Dubay, Joyce Dutton, Terry Law, Bill LeBlond, Cristie Marcus, Jane Merryman, Susan Milstein, Elliot Morrison, M.D., Sandra Rubin, M.D., Judith Stevenson, and Hazel Whiteoak. In a category all her own is my great friend, personal photographer and number-one fan Jean Porter, who has packed more living into her eighty-five years than most people do in a hundred and seventy.

Several individuals, all experts in their fields, have been very generous with their time and unfailingly patient with my questions:

Judith Rooks, who wears many hats—midwife, epidemiologist, teacher, and tireless advocate for maternal and child health around the globe—was my go-to source for information about nitrous oxide, cesarean statistics, and the state of American childbirth.

When nitrous at long last returns to America's labor rooms—and it will—women will have Judith to thank.

Mark Rosen, M.D., is another multi-hat-wearer. The director of Obstetric Anesthesia, residency director, and vice chair of the Department of Anesthesia and Perioperative Care at the University of California, San Francisco, Mark was kind enough to take me on a tour of the labor and delivery unit at UCSF and to discuss the use of nitrous oxide there in depth. He also was instrumental in helping me understand the intricacies of epidural analgesia.

Donald Caton, M.D., dean of obstetric anesthesia historians and author of *What a Blessing She Had Chloroform: The Medical and Social Response to the Pain of Childbirth from 1800 to the Present,* was an invaluable source of historical information on nineteenth-century obstetrics and anesthesiology.

More people to thank: Dr. James Allen, Wilbour Professor of Egyptology at Brown University, for his personal translation of the Westcar Papyrus; Dr. Ann Hanson of Harvard University, for her description of midwifery practices in ancient Greece; Dr. Christine Moon, who directed me to the story of D. K. Spelt and his fetal learning experiments; Dr. Charles Wysocki, with whom I had fascinating electronic discussion on the chemistry of underarm attraction; Leeni Balogh, for teaching me the art of the efficient literature search; and the librarians of the Wellcome Trust in London, who tried valiantly, if unsuccessfully, to track down Dr. James Barry's operative report from the day of her historic cesarean.

I consider myself incredibly lucky to have worked with a tremendous group of doctors and nurses over the course of my career, at the University of Illinois in Chicago; C. S. Mott Children's Hospital at the University of Michigan in Ann Arbor; and, for the past twenty-six years, Kaiser Permanente in Roseville, Sacramento, and Santa Rosa, California. Thank you all.

Finally, I want to thank my mother, Peg Sloan, for the love of writing she passed on to me in the womb; my father, Barney Sloan, for teaching me what it means to be a real dad; and three people who died long ago but nonetheless greatly influenced the creation of this book: James J. Dalton, my maternal grandfather and a master Irish storyteller; Sister Mary Carola Sellmeyer, S.S.M., the best friend a wide-eyed young boy could ever have had; and Herb Caen, the late, lamented columnist of the *San Francisco Chronicle*—the first person who was neither friend nor relative who told me I could write.

Santa Rosa, California
August 23, 2008

Notes

Chapter 1: Twenty Babies

8 *The female gorilla is a study in childbirthing efficiency* For a detailed analysis of labor and birth in nonhuman primates, and the evolution of modern human childbirth, see the articles by Rosenberg (1992, 1996) and Trevathan (1990, 1999).

9 *Obstetricians divide childbirth into three stages* The mechanics of normal human childbirth are described by Kilpatrick in chapter 12 of Gabbe's *Obstetrics: Normal and Problem Pregnancies*. A discussion of the hormones involved in having a baby can be found in this chapter, as well as in Goldsmith.

9 *The modern human birth canal, though, puts a twist on this ancient design* The history of the dubious pursuit of the "ideal" labor position is worthy of a book of its own. Much of the source material for this part of the chapter is drawn from George Engelmann's *Labor Among Primitive Peoples* (1883). See Bancroft-Livingston (1956) for the story of Louis XIV, his mistress, and the "birth" of flat-on-the-back laboring; for a more modern review see Boyle (2000) and Gupta (2000).

31 *I failed the test* I was apparently the last person in the room to know that Danuta's baby was coming butt-first. Not until much later did I realize Mitch had engaged in an age-old resident pastime: student hazing.

Chapter 2: The First Five Minutes

32 *If we could look inside Amy's body as she hovers between worlds* The incredible cardiovascular changes that occur during and shortly after

a normal birth are described by Alvaro, Fanaroff (chapters 42 and 44), Mercer, and Thompson.

35 *"like the fronds of a sea anemone wafting in the seawater of a rock pool"* Burton's detailed description of the placenta is much more prosaic than this snippet would suggest.

47 *given that I was sure that Sean had Persistent Pulmonary Hypertension of the Newborn* See Ostrea for a detailed explanation of PPHN (the failure of normal womb-to-world transition).

Chapter 3: An Alternate Route

58 *Zeus invented the cesarean section* For more on cesarean birth's legends and myths see Cianfrani, Drife, Pelosi, Sewell, and van Buitenen.

61 *Obstetrical forceps, invented by the medical Chamberlen clan in Britain around 1600* See Sewell and Drife.

62 *the parents decided, in consultation with the doctor and perhaps a clergyman* The Catholic Church played a major role in the promotion of cesarean birth in America. See Ryan and Leavitt (1987, 237–41).

62 *not a single woman survived a cesarean delivery in Paris between 1787 and 1876* A sobering statistic—see Crosby and Sewell.

63 *James Barry stood out like a cub among bears* The remarkable story of James Miranda Stuart Barry is ably told by Hurwitz and Kubba. See also the anonymously bylined *Manchester Guardian* story of August 21, 1865.

66 *A modern cesarean usually begins with a Pfannenstiel skin incision* Cesarean technique is described by Landon (492–97).

70 *In every surgery she performed, Barry faced three monumental obstacles* See Crosby and Sewell for discussion of the dilemma of cesarean-related hemorrhage in the days before blood transfusions.

72 *the struggle to conquer puerperal fever* Puerperal fever's rise from an infrequent childbirth tragedy to an epidemic scourge, and the role of lying-in hospitals in that process, is well documented by Berman, De Costa, and Loudon.

74 *Prominent among them was Louis Pasteur* See De Costa.

74 *Dr. Oliver Wendell Holmes made that connection* To read Holmes's paper in its entirety, see Halsall. See also Viets for an in-depth discussion of Holmes's medical career and the medical climate at the time of his 1843 essay.

75 *"Doctors are gentlemen . . . and gentlemen's hands are clean"* One of my all-time favorite wrongheaded quotes. See De Costa.

75 *Dr. Ignaz Semmelweis*   Semmelweiss's tragic tale is recounted by De Costa and Raju.

76 *introduced by Dr. Joseph Lister of Glasgow*   For more on the concept of antisepsis, see De Costa, and Lister himself; for the full story of Lister and Listerine, see Morgenstern.

77 *more than nine hundred thousand American babies born by cesarean delivery in 1991*   Birth statistics for this section, including cesarean rates, VBAC rates, and the increase in older mothers, were drawn from the websites of the Centers for Disease Control (2002, 2008) (United States statistics) and the World Health Organization (1) (international). See also Landon, Lieberman (2004), Menacker, Menard, and Taffel.

79 *Cesarean's first "golden age"*   See Landon (488–89) for a discussion of the factors that led to the rapid increase in cesarean births in the 1970s and beyond. Freeman writes on fetal monitoring's contribution to that "golden age."

81 *the rise and sudden fall of the VBAC*   See the American College of Obstetricians and Gynecologists (2004), Centers for Disease Control (2002), Cohen, Gregory, and Landon (490–92).

82 *Dr. Edwin Cragin came down firmly on the side of repeat cesareans in 1916*   See Cragin.

83 *elective primary cesarean*   A very controversial topic, and far from settled. For a discussion of the pros and cons from the maternal side of things, see the American College of Obstetricians and Gynecologists (2007), Buhimschi, the International Federation of Gynecology and Obstetrics, Gamble, Klein (2006), Leeman, Minkoff, Morrison, Nygaard, Sharma, Visco, and Young (2003).

84 *"spin doctoring" the research*   See Goer.

85 *the pros of EPC for the baby . . . and its cons*   The short-term outcomes for the fetus and baby are described in the references immediately above. Long-term studies of babies born by EPC are nonexistent. See Salaam regarding the increased incidence of asthma in children born via cesarean to mothers not in labor.

87 *Time to put the lawsuit issue . . . squarely on the table*   See Deutsch, Kershaw, and Chervenak for details of the litigation woes contemporary obstetricians face and changes in clinical practice that have resulted.

88 *Part of that cycle is related to how new obstetricians are trained*   Landon (488–89 and 500–501) outlines recommended changes in training that could help reduce cesarean rates.

Chapter 4: B.E. (Before Epidurals)

94 *In second-century Greece, the famed physician Soranus*   See Temkin's translation of Soranus' *Gynecology* (70–72), Bostock's translation of Pliny's *Natural History,* and Grieve for more historical background on labor pain treatments. Charles Dickens provides a lively, if fictional, account of the subject in chapter 19 of *Martin Chuzzlewit.*

96 *I didn't give much thought to Queen Victoria*   The sources for the fascinating story of Queen Victoria, James Young Simpson, and the rise of chloroform anesthesia include Connor, Dunn (2002), McGowan, the UCLA Department of Epidemiology, and in particular Caton (1999 [2], chapters 3–6) and Leavitt (1986, 116–28). See Ward for background on Victoria's evolving (and souring) view of pregnancy and motherhood, and Farr for a discussion of the moral and religious objections to obstetric anesthesia. Finally, see De Haven Pitcock for a discussion of the rise of consumer demand as it related to obstetric anesthesia in the nineteenth and early twentieth centuries.

105 *chloroform was neither as safe nor as easy to use as Simpson had led the public to believe*   Leavitt (1986, 116–28).

107 *Marguerite Tracy and her companion Constance Leupp journeyed from New York City to Freiburg*   The best accounts of Twilight Sleep and the "Freiburg Miracle" can be found in Tracy's own writing: see Tracy and Leupp (1914), Boyd and Tracy (1914), and Tracy and Boyd's book, *Painless Childbirth* (1915).

112 *Tracy's timing was impeccable*   The rise of feminism provided much of the push for painless childbirth. For contemporary reports, see W. T. George's call for a "sex war," Mrs. John Martin's anti-feminist manifesto, and the anonymously bylined *New York Times* article on a French woman's right to be guillotined.

113 *The National Twilight Sleep Association was formed*   For a contemporary description of the NTSA, see the anonymously bylined *Washington Post* article ("Society women spread Twilight Sleep gospel," 1915).

114 *Dr. Bertha Van Hoosen*   Van Hoosen was America's foremost medical supporter of Twilight Sleep. See Leavitt (1986, 128–36) and Van Hoosen herself.

116 *Van Hoosen's early embrace of Twilight Sleep wasn't typical of American doctors*   For a sampling of American doctors' responses to the public demand for Twilight Sleep, see the anonymously bylined *New York Times* article, "Authority changes its tone" (1914) followed within days by Dr. Claude Wheeler's response.

118 *The Twilight Sleep movement crashed abruptly in the summer of 1915*
The fall of the Twilight Sleep movement, as epitomized by the tragedy
of Mrs. Francis X. Carmody, is well documented in Caton (1999 [2],
129–51) and Leavitt (1986, 139–41).

119 *Twilight Sleep helped doctors accomplish . . . control of the birthing
suite* See Leavitt (1986, 135).

Chapter 5: Nowadays

121 *Opioids, a large group of chemical compounds* For a discussion of the
effectiveness (or lack thereof) of narcotics for labor pain relief, see
Bricker.

122 *Local anesthetic injections can be given in three places as birth nears*
See Rosen (2002 [2]) and Hawkins (2007)

122 *women don't rate these medications very highly* Maternity Center Association (63).

122 *Epidural blockade . . . is infinitely more refined than chloroform ever was*
See Birnbach, Eltzschig, and Hawkins (2007, 414–16) for a description of the technique and mode of action of epidural analgesia.

124 *forceps-assisted deliveries began a steep decline in the mid-twentieth
century* Landon (488–89, 500–501).

125 *Attitudes about labor pain were changing, too* The social connota-
tions of labor pain in the nineteenth century are described in Caton
(1999 [2], chapters 6 and 7); see Hodnett (2002) and Lowe for a
modern review of the topic.

127 *In 1981, Dr. Ronald Melzack and his research team* See Melzack
(1981, 1984).

128 *Labor pain is actually a combination of two distinct kinds of pain* For
a concise review of the physiological and anatomical basis of labor
pain, as well as the contributions of anxiety and a woman's previous
pain experience, see Eltzschig and Lowe.

131 *Women consistently report a high degree of satisfaction with the pain
control an epidural provides during labor* See Maternity Center Association (63).

132 *The chance of paralysis or other severe permanent nerve damage from an
epidural* See Birnbach, D'Angelo (2007 [1] and [2]), and Hawkins
(2003).

132 *First, there's the IV* The common side effects of an epidural are described in Hemminki, Leighton, and Lieberman (2002).

134 *But epidural medications may cause subtler neonatal problems* Murray (1981) was among the first to raise the question of subtle neona-

tal effects from epidural medications. For a sampling of the research on epidurals and breast-feeding, see Baumgarder, Halpern, and Riordan.

135 *Epidural medications can definitely have indirect effects on the newborn* See Leighton and Lieberman (2002).

135 *The combined spinal-epidural block (CSE)* See Birnbach and Hughes for a discussion of the "walking" epidural.

137 *Hospitals outside the United States offer a broader range of . . . treatments* See Bishop, Marmor, Rosen (2002 [1]), and Simkin.

138 *pain relief consistently ranks fourth in postpartum satisfaction surveys* See Hodnett and the Maternity Center Association.

139 *Nitrous oxide is an invisible gas* The remarkable story of the fall of nitrous oxide, and its contemporary usefulness as a labor analgesic, is well told by Bishop, Eger, James, Pearce, Rooks (2007 [1] and [2]), and Rosen (2002 [1]). And, of course, P. L. Travers, in chapter 3 ("Laughing Gas") of *Mary Poppins* (1934).

145 *Though recent animal research has suggested* See McGowan (2008) for an overview of the concerns about general anesthetic agents and fetal brain development.

146 *and the American Society of Anesthesiologists agree* See McGregor.

148 *Drug-free pain relief methods and techniques come in a bewildering variety* For more on complementary and alternative labor pain treatment see Allaire, Lee, Marmor, and Simkin.

Chapter 6: Daddies

161 *My father, Barney Sloan, confirms this* For more about a father's role in 1950s childbirth, talk to my dad. See also Leavitt (2003).

166 *"an unnecessary source of infection, to an essential source of affection"* See Cronenwett and Kunst-Wilson (1981).

166 *There weren't many books written for expectant fathers in the 1970s and '80s* One such book from that era is Gresh's *Becoming a Father*.

169 *Men know all about women and hormones* For a detailed description of male and female reproductive hormones, see Bhasin, Bulun, and Kinsley.

172 *Biologists Sandra Berg and Katherine Wynne-Edwards* and other researchers have done some truly amazing research on the effects of pregnancy on male hormones. See Berg, Delahunty, Fleming, Gray, Storey, Wynne-Edwards, and Ziegler (2000, 2004, 2006).

177 *Dr. Charles Wysocki and his research team* For more on intrepid underarm researchers, see Jacob, Wyart, and Wysocki.

178 *The French have a name for all this . . . couvade* Warren Royal Daw-

son's 1929 book, *The Custom of Couvade,* paired with Nor Hall's "A Psychological Essay on Men in Childbirth," an introductory essay to a 1989 reissue of *The Custom of Couvade,* is well worth a read for anyone interested in cultural couvade. For more on couvade syndrome—a man's physical symptoms during a mate's pregnancy—see Elwood, Klein (1991), Lipkin, and Mason.

Chapter 7: The Gang's All Here

188 *Childbirth hasn't always been like that*   For a refresher on the evolution of human childbirth and the concept of "obligate midwifery," revisit Rosenberg (1992, 1996) and Trevathan (1990, 1999).

191 *"Midwife" is a Middle English term*   To read more on the early history of midwives and other female birth attendants from antiquity through the eighteenth century, see Bostock, Campan, Dunn (2001, 2004), French, Kern, O'Dowd, Rooks (1999), and Temkin. I am also indebted to Dr. James P. Allen of Brown University for his translation of the Westcar Papyrus (personal communication).

198 *That network had been quite extensive and . . . was well documented*   Leavitt's *Brought to Bed* has been a truly indispensable resource in the writing of this book. See also Berman.

201 *an eccentric, yoga-practicing obstetrician by the name of Grantly Dick Read*   See Bender, Caton (1996, 1999 [1]), Cortesi, Goodrich, Moscucci, and, of course, Dick-Read himself, for more on the origins of the natural childbirth movement and the remarkable life of Grantly Dick-Read.

204 *The Read-versus-mainstream-obstetrics battle . . . Fernand Lamaze*   Lamaze didn't live to see his movement come to full fruition. See Bender, Caton (1999, 190–91), De Haven Pitcock, Lamaze International, and Lamaze himself for details of Lamaze's philosophy and the Dick-Read–Lamaze rivalry. Caron-Leulliez describes the politics of painless childbirth in post–World War II France.

211 *The importance of paternal birth attendance . . . moved center stage during the 1960s and '70s*   Ready or not, fathers made their first en masse appearance in labor rooms across the nation. See the 1974 paper by Greenberg that set much of it in motion, and the studies by Draper, Gbininigie, Greenhalgh, Johnson, Shapiro, and Szeverenyi. The work of Palkovitz (1985, 1986, 1987) was especially important in shaping more reasonable expectations of fathers in the delivery room, and raised the question of whether the father is really the best support person for a laboring woman.

214 *The vanishing delivery room nurse*   See Freeman for a discussion of the unfulfilled promise of electronic fetal monitoring.

218 *But if dads weren't the best coaches, then who?*   The return of the experienced female birth companion, whether friend, relative, or professionally trained doula, is a welcome trend. The work of Klaus and Kennell was and is critical to convincing the medical world of the benefits of continuous labor support. For more, see Campbell, Hodnett, Jannsen, Kayne, Kitzinger, Rooks (1999), Scott (1999 [1] and [2]), and Young (1998).

Chapter 8: Inside Looking Out

227 *a Power Ranger (the red one)*   A complete history of the Red Power Ranger can be found at: http://en.wikipedia.org/wiki/Red_Ranger.

230 *The ability of light to reach the fetal eye*   Fetal visual development is described by Birch, Edward, Lecanuet (1996), Ruben (1992), and Wright.

231 *a team of obstetrics researchers at the University of New Mexico*   See Caridi.

232 *The human fetus went deaf in 1885*   Early fetal hearing research was ingenious back then and entertaining to read today. See Kisilevsky (1998), Moon, and Preyer. In particular, see Lecanuet (1996) for an excellent review of the research that led to current understanding of the fetus's sensory capabilities.

232 *the fetal Jesus "leaped in my womb for joy"*   Luke 1:39–44.

233 *fetal hearing research entered a remarkably productive "golden age"*   For detailed discussions of fetal hearing, voice recognition, and other aural learning abilities, see Gerhardt (1996, 2000), Kisilevsky (1998, 2003, 2004), Lecanuet (1993, 1996), Moon, Philbin, and Ruben (1992).

235 *The first studies of the uterine noise floor*   The transmission of sound from the extrauterine world and the "noise floor" of the uterus are discussed in Abrams, Gerhardt (2000), Lecanuet (1996), Richards, and Sohmer.

237 *In 1948, D. K. Spelt of Pennsylvania's Muhlenberg College*   For a fascinating account of conditioning the human fetus by means of buzzing doorbell parts and thwacking wood boxes, see Spelt himself.

240 *respond to sounds as diverse as* Peter and the Wolf *and jet noise from a nearby airport*   Ruben (1992).

240 *"teach the fetus" materials*   See Moon for a discussion of some of the

dubious programs that tout prenatal learning via "belly phones," patterned heartbeats, and such.

241 *Adding even more noise to that environment, even if it's "good" noise* Too much noise in the uterus can lead to permanent hearing damage. See Etzel, Gerhardt (2000), Pierson, and Ruben (1997).

242 *Let's start with smell* The details of the structure and functioning of the fetal and neonatal olfactory system are discussed in Lecanuet (1996), Meredith, and Schaal.

243 *when the amniotic fluid was withdrawn from the womb for testing, it smelled strongly of garlic* Mennella (1995).

244 *their babies showed a preference for carrots* Mennella (2001).

244 *The fetus tastes the same things it smells* Fomon describes the taste abilities of the fetus and newborn.

246 *when placed on his mother's abdomen . . . a freshly born baby will make a remarkable journey* That journey is beautifully captured in chapter 2 of Marshall and Phyllis Klaus's *Your Amazing Newborn* (1998).

247 *He knows what he's looking for* See de Haan, Easterbrook, Slater, and Turati for more on the newborn's ability to recognize facelike features.

249 *the newborn's sense of smell is actually the key to finding his mother's nipple* See Klaus (1998, chapter 2) and Porter.

251 *The physical benefits of touch have been proven in research* See Beachy's study of infant massage and hospitalized premature babies.

Chapter 9: "The Newborn Worth Rearing"

255 *Apgar scores are assigned today at one minute and five minutes of age* For details of the Apgar scoring system see Kattwinkel.

257 *Dr. Virginia Apgar was born in 1909* The complete story of this remarkable woman can be found in Baskett (2000) and James (1975).

259 *The evaluation of the newborn in the first minutes of life is a process as old as human history* See Baskett (2001); Kattwinkel; O'Donnell; and Rodkinson's translation of the Talmud for more on newborn resuscitation in ancient times.

260 *At birth the baby was subjected to a quick check for congenital deformities* See Galanakis for the similarities of Soranus' and Apgar's evaluations of the newborn.

261 *Next up on Soranus' neonatal checklist: baby salting* Temkin (79–80).

261 *I learned about mouth-to-mouth resuscitation when I was ten or eleven*

years old O'Donnell provides a concise and entertaining history of the rise and fall (and rise) of mouth-to-mouth breathing.

266 *The Schulze Method wasn't as crazy as it sounds* The Schulze Method, with diagrams of Schulze himself and a baby in full swing, can be found in Baskett (2001). See also O'Donnell.

268 *A look at the medical texts of the time is instructive* See Crosse, Holt, Sheldon, and Stone.

270 *Virginia Apgar turned her attention to that gray zone of neonatal assessment* To read Apgar's landmark study, See Apgar (1953).

271 *The algorithm goes by the official, humdrum name* See Kattwinkel for a discussion of the NRP guidelines. Higgins explains the rationale for using lower oxygen concentrations in modern resuscitation.

Chapter 10: Infant Origami

281 *It was Konrad Lorenz* For more on Lorenz and his geese and Eckhard Hess and his pupil measuring experiments, see Lorenz, Maestripieri, and Waite.

282 *researchers at the University of Wisconsin have found* See Nitschke.

283 *Science used to be so much simpler* Duffy provides, in mind-boggling detail, an explanation of the increasingly complicated understanding of the genetics of eye color. See Laeng for his theory about the desirability of a blue-eyed mate to a blue-eyed man.

285 He looks just like his daddy, doesn't he? I found the subject of a newborn's resemblance to his or her (putative) father fascinating, and a completely unexpected aspect of writing this book. Bredart and Bressan convincingly argue for anonymous-looking newborns and the benefits of "misassigned paternity" in human societies. Alexander and Yogman discuss the concept of paternity certainty in nonhuman primates and how human babies evolved to look like nobody in particular—for their own good. Daly's study shows that the looks-just-like-his-daddy comments made by friends and relatives help convince a father of his paternity.

290 *Our slithery ancestors fed* Nesse provides a concise and very readable history of the evolution of the odd relationship of the human respiratory and gastrointestinal tracts.

291 *Charles Darwin himself pondered this puzzling arrangement* Read of Darwin's puzzlement in *The Origin of Species* (page 191 of the first edition).

291 *we talk, therefore we choke* The changes in the position of the

human larynx, resulting in our rich vocal talents but also the loss of our ability to drink like a horse, is described by Morris and Nesse.

292 *"Things That Go Honk in the Night"* The newborn windpipe is a scarily soft and skinny thing, prone to all kinds of noisemaking. See Bluestone, Briscoe, and Hollinger.

295 *In the newborn, milk secreted from the nipple is sometimes called "witch's milk"* The folklore surrounding birth and newborns is incredibly rich. Forbes relates some of the legends surrounding newborn galactorrhea. Leung provides a modern review of the subject.

295 *babies are barrel-chested* The newborn body is very different from that of the older child and adult; ignoring the dissimilarities can lead to any number of medical misadventures. Kovarik and Kliegman describe those differences from the perspectives of an anesthesiologist and a pediatrician.

296 *A few inches south of the rib cage* Pomeranz (who, by the way, was my senior resident when I was an intern at the University of Michigan) provides an excellent review of the underappreciated umbilicus and its care. Holve's 1955 paper is a sobering account of omphalitis in the mid-twentieth century. Roper details the global effort to eliminate maternal and neonatal tetanus. See Zupan for a summary of current research on umbilical cord care.

300 *If only boys were so simple* Ah, circumcision—easily the most polarizing newborn-body topic. See Aggleton and Alanis for an excellent history of the procedure. Fleiss and Taylor describe the structure and function of the foreskin. For strong "anti" arguments, see Denniston, Fleiss, Milos, and Ray; on the adamantly "pro" side, see Schoen and the World Health Organization (2007). For a valiant attempt to reach a middle ground, see Benatar. Fink's study of sexual satisfaction following adult circumcision, in which men were found to have less sensitive penises, more problems with erections—and overall *increased* satisfaction—highlights the complexity and contradictions of the issue.

The debate over circumcision's merits as an HIV/STD prevention tool is well covered by the American Academy of Pediatrics (1999 and 2005), Fergusson (the New Zealand study), Flynn, Russell, and WHO. Edouard provides an African perspective.

Finally, I highly recommend Peter Charles Remondino (1891, 1902) to anyone interested in understanding nineteenth-century circumcision mania. Remondino's attack on his opponents—and his willingness to shoot a saint in the bargain—is a medical classic of a kind we'll not likely see again.

308 *Rickets is a disease that prevents ossification*   See Williams for a vivid
    picture of the scourge of rickets in eighteenth-century England, and
    Chesney for a concise history of the disease.

311 Why do babies have primitive reflexes?   For an illustrated descrip-
    tion of primitive reflexes in the newborn, see the National Library of
    Medicine (2007). Weirich tells the story of Ernst Moro and the Nazis.

Bibliography

Abrams, R., and K. Gerhardt (2000). The acoustic environment and physiological responses of the fetus. *Journal of Perinatology* 20(8, Pt. 2): S31–6.

Aggleton, P. (2007). "Just a Snip"?: A social history of male circumcision. *Reproductive Health Matters* 15(29): 15–21.

Alanis, M., and R. Lucidi (2004). Neonatal circumcision: A review of the world's oldest and most controversial operation. *Obstetrical and Gynecological Survey* 59(5): 379–95.

Alexander, R. D. (1990). How did humans evolve? *University of Michigan Special Publications* 1:1–38.

Allaire, A. (2001). Complementary and alternative medicine in the labor and delivery suite. *Clinical Obstetrics & Gynecology* 44(4): 681–91.

Allen, J. (2007). Papyrus Westcar (personal communication).

Alvaro, R., and H. Rigatto (2005). Part III: Transition and Stabilization. *Avery's Neonatology: Pathophysiology and Management of the Newborn.* Philadelphia: Lippincott Williams & Wilkins.

American Academy of Pediatrics, Task Force on Circumcision (1999). Circumcision policy statement of reaffirmation—2005. *Pediatrics* 103(3): 686–93.

American College of Obstetricians and Gynecologists (2004). Vaginal birth after previous cesarean delivery. ACOG Bulletin No. 54, 1–10.

——— (2007). ACOG Committee Opinion: Cesarean delivery on maternal request. *Obstetrics & Gynecology* 110(6): 1501.

Anonymous (August 21, 1865). A strange story. *Manchester Guardian.*

——— (March 16, 1913). Women demanding guillotine "rights": French feminists say it is unjust to deprive sex of "privilege" of execution. *New York Times.*

——— (August 27, 1914). Authority changes its tone. *New York Times.*

——— (January 3, 1915). Society women spread Twilight Sleep gospel to prevent future suffering by the mothers of the United States. *Washington Post.*

Apgar, Virginia (1953). A proposal for a new method of evaluation of the newborn infant. *Current Researches in Anesthesia and Analgesia,* July–August, 260–67.

Bancroft-Livingston, G. (1956). Louise de Valliere and the birth of the man-midwife. *Journal of Obstetrics and Gynocology of the British Commonwealth* 63:261–67.

Baskett, Thomas (2000). Virginia Apgar and the newborn Apgar Score. *Resuscitation* 47:215–17.

Baskett, T. F., and F. Nagele (2001). Bernhard Schultze and the swinging neonate. *Resuscitation* 51(1): 3–6.

Baumgarder, D., and P. Muehl (2003). Effect of labor epidural anesthesia on breastfeeding of healthy full-term newborns delivered vaginally. *Journal of the American Board of Family Practitioners* 16(1): 7–13.

Beachy, J. (2003). Premature infant massage in the NICU. *Neonatal Network* 22(3): 39–45.

Benatar, F., and D. Benatar (2003). Between prophylaxis and child abuse: The ethics of neonatal male circumcision. *American Journal of Bioethics* 32(2): 35–48.

Bender, M. (May 16, 1967). History of natural childbirth: From mysticism to practicality. *New York Times.*

Berg, Sandra J., and Katherine E. Wynne-Edwards (2001). Changes in testosterone, cortisol, and estradiol levels in men becoming fathers. *Mayo Clinic Proceedings* 76(6): 582–92.

Berman, P. (1995). The practice of obstetrics in rural America, 1800–1860. *Journal of the History of Medicine* 50:175–93.

Bhasin, S. (2008). Physiologic regulation of testicular function: Sex-steroid production and action. *Williams Textbook of Endocrinology,* 645–52. Philadelphia: Saunders Elsevier.

Birch, E. E., and A. R. O'Connor (2001). Preterm birth and visual development. *Seminars in Neonatology* 6:487–97.

Birnbach, D., and I. Browne (2005). Chapter 58: Anesthesia for Obstetrics. *Miller's Anesthesia.* Philadelphia: Churchill Livingstone, Elsevier.

Bishop, J. (2007). Administration of nitrous oxide in labor: Expanding the options for women. *Journal of Midwifery & Women's Health* 52(3): 308–9.

Bluestone, C. (2005). Humans are born too soon: Impact on pediatric otolaryngology. *International Journal of Pediatric Otorhinolaryngology* 69:1–8.

Bostock, J. (trans.) (2007–2008). Pliny the Elder, *Natural History* (1855). http://www.perseus.tufts.edu/cgi-bin/ptext?lookup=Plin.+Nat.+toc.

Boyd, Mary, and Marguerite Tracy (1914). More about painless childbirth. *McClure's Magazine* 43(6): 56–70.

Boyle, Mary (2000). Childbirth in bed: The historical perspective. *The Practising Midwife* 3(11): 21–24.

Bredart, S., and R. French (1999). Do babies resemble their fathers more than their mothers? A failure to replicate Christenfeld & Hill (1995). *Evolution and Human Behavior* 20(3): 129–35.

Bressan, P. (2002). Why babies look like their daddies: Paternity uncertainty and the evolution of self-deception in evaluating family resemblance. *Acta Ethology* 4:113–18.

Bricker, L. (2002). Parenteral opioids for labor pain relief: A systematic review. *American Journal of Obstetrics and Gynecology* 186(5): S81–93.

Briscoe, M., S. Ulualp, and F. Quinn (2007). Pediatric congenital subglottic stenosis. Paper presented at the Grand Rounds Presentation, University of Texas Medical Branch, Dept. of Otolaryngology, Galveston.

Buhimschi, C., and I. Buhimschi (2006). Advantages of vaginal delivery. *Clinical Obstetrics* 49(1): 167–83.

Bulun, S., and E. Adashi (2008). The physiology and pathology of the female reproductive axis. *Williams Textbook of Endocrinology,* 541–66. Philadelphia: Saunders Elsevier.

Burton, G., C. Sibley, and E. Jauniaux (2007). Section I: Physiology. Chapter 1: Placental Anatomy and Physiology. Gabbe, *Obstetrics: Normal and Problem Pregnancies* 3–25. Philadelphia: Churchill Livingstone.

Campan, Madame (2006). *The Private Life of Marie Antoinette.* Warick, NY: 1500 Books.

Campbell, D., K. Scott, M. Klaus, and M. Falk (2007). Female relatives or friends trained as labor doulas: Outcomes at 6 to 8 weeks postpartum. *Birth* 34(3): 220–27.

Caridi, B., J. Bolnick, B. Fletcher, and W. Rayburn (2004). Effect of halogen light stimulation on nonstress testing. *American Journal of Obstetrics and Gynecology* 190(5): 1470–72.

Caron-Leulliez, M. (2006). Childbirth without pain: Politics in France during the cold war. *Canadian Bulletin of Medical History* 23(1): 69–88.

Caton, Donald (1999). *What a Blessing She Had Chloroform: The Medical and Social Response to the Pain of Childbirth from 1800 to the Present.* New Haven and London: Yale University Press.

———(1996). Who said childbirth is natural? The medical mission of Grantly Dick Read. *Anesthesiology.* 84(4): 955–64.

Centers for Disease Control (2002). Vaginal birth after cesarean: California, 1996–2000. *Morbidity and Mortality Weekly Report* 51(44): 996–98.

—— (2008). Vital Statistics: Births. http://209.217.72.34/vitalstats/ReportFolders/ReportFolders.aspx.

Chervenak, J. (2007). Overview of professional liability. *Clinics in Perinatology* 34:227–32.

Chesney, R. (2002). Rickets: The third wave. *Clinical Pediatrics* 41, no. 3 (April 2002): 137–39.

Cianfrani, T. (1960). *A Short History of Obstetrics and Gynecology.* New York: Thomas.

Cohen, B. (2001). Brief history of vaginal birth after cesarean section. *Clinical Obstetrics & Gynecology* 44(3): 604–8.

Connor, H., and T. Connor (1996). Did the use of chloroform by Queen Victoria influence its acceptance in obstetric practice? *Anaesthesia* 51(10): 955–57.

Cortesi, A. (January 8, 1957). Pope sanctions painless childbirth. *New York Times.*

Cragin, E. B. (1916). Conservatism in obstetrics. *New York Medical Journal* 104:1–3.

Cronenwett, L., and William Kunst-Wilson (1981). Stress, social support and the transition to fatherhood. *Nursing Research* 30(4): 196–201.

Crosby, W. (1989). Cesarean section's rise to respectability. *Contemporary OB/GYN,* May, 32–49.

Crosse, V. M. (1946). *The Premature Baby.* London: J. & A. Churchill Ltd.

Daly, M., and M. Wilson (1982). Whom are newborn babies said to resemble? *Ethology and Sociobiology* 3:69–78.

D'Angelo, R. (2007). Anesthesia-related maternal mortality: A pat on the back or a call to arms? *Anesthesiology* 106(6): 1096–1104.

—— (2007). Death and injury resulting from epidural analgesia, personal correspondence.

Darwin, Charles (1859). *The Origin of Species.* London: John Murray. First edition.

Dawson, Warren R. (1929). *The Custom of Couvade.* Manchester: Manchester University Press.

De Costa, C. (2002). "The contagiousness of childbed fever": A short history of puerperal sepsis and its treatment. *Medical Journal of Australia* 177(11/12): 668–71.

de Haan, M., K. Humphreys, and M. Johnson (2002). Developing a brain specialized for face perception: A converging methods approach. *Developmental Psychobiology* 40:200–212.

De Haven Pitcock, C. (1992). From Fanny to Fernand: The development of consumerism in pain control during the birth process. *American Journal of Obstetrics and Gynecology* 167(3): 581–87.

Delahunty, K., D. McKay, and D. Noseworthy (2007). Prolactin responses to infant cues in men and women: Effects of parental experience and recent infant contact. *Hormones and Behavior* 51(2): 213–20.

Denniston, G. (2007). Doctors Opposing Circumcision (D.O.C.). http://www.doctorsopposingcircumcision.org/.

Deutsch, A., J. McCarthy, K. Murray, and R. Sayer (2007). Why are fewer Florida medical students choosing obstetrics and gynecology? *Southern Medical Journal* 100(11): 1095–98.

Dickens, Charles (1843). *Martin Chuzzlewit*. New York: Penguin Classics, 2000.

Dick-Read, Grantly (2004). *Childbirth Without Fear*. London: Piner & Martin Ltd.

Draper, J. (1997). Whose welfare in the labour room? A discussion of the increasing trend of fathers' birth attendance. *Midwifery* 13(3): 132–38.

Drife, J. (2002). The start of life: A history of obstetrics. *Postgraduate Medical Journal* 78:311–15.

Duffy, D., G. Montgomery, W. Chen, Z. Zhao, M. Le, L. James, et al. (2007). A three-SNP haplotype in the intron 1 of OCA2 explains most human eye color variation. *American Journal of Human Genetics* 80:241–52.

Dunn, P. M. (2001). Jacob Rueff (1500–1558) of Zurich and the expert midwife. *Archives of Disease in Childhood Fetus & Neonatal Edition* 85:222–24.

——— (2002). Sir James Young Simpson (1811–1870) and obstetric anaesthesia. *Archives of Disease in Childhood Fetal & Neonatal Edition* 86:F207–9.

——— (2004). Louise Bourgeois (1563–1636): Royal midwife of France. *Archives of Disease in Childhood Fetal & Neonatal Edition* 89:185–87.

Easterbrook, M., B. Kisilevsky, D. Muir, and D. Laplante (1999). Newborns discriminate faces from scrambled faces. *Canadian Journal of Experimental Psychology* 53(3): 231–41.

Edouard, L., and F. Okonofua (2006). Male circumcision for HIV prevention: Evidence and expectations. *African Journal of Reproductive Health* 10(3): 7–9.

Edward D. & Kaufman L. (2003). Anatomy, development and physiology of the visual system. *Pediatric Clinics of North America* 50:1–23.

Eger, I. E. (1985). *Nitrous oxide*. New York: Edward Arnold, Ltd.

Eltzschig, H., E. Lieberman, and W. Camann (2003). Regional anesthesia and analgesia for labor and delivery. *New England Journal of Medicine* 348:319–32.

Elwood, R., and C. Mason (1994). The couvade and the onset of paternal care: A biological perspective. *Ethnology and Sociobiology* 15:145–56.

Engelmann, George (1883). *Labor Among Primitive Peoples.* St. Louis: J. H. Chambers & Co.

Etzel, R., and S. Balk (1997). Noise: A hazard for the fetus and newborn. *Pediatrics* 100(4): 724–27.

Fanaroff, A., and R. Martin (2005). Chapter 42: The respiratory system. *Neonatal-Perinatal Medicine.* St. Louis: Mosby.

———— (2005). Chapter 44: The Blood and Hematopoietic System. *Neonatal-Perinatal Medicine.* St. Louis: Mosby.

Farr, A. D. (1980). Early Opposition to Obstetric Anaesthesia. *Anaesthesia* 35:896–907.

Fergusson, D., J. Boden, and L. Horwood (2006). Circumcision status and risk of sexually transmitted infection in young adult males: An analysis of a longitudinal birth cohort. *Pediatrics* 118(5): 1971–77.

Fink, K., C. Carson, and R. DeVellis (2002). Adult circumcision outcomes study: Effect on erectile function, penile sensitivity, sexual activity and satisfaction. *Journal of Urology* 167(5): 2113–16.

Fleiss, Paul, F. Hodges, and R. Van Howe (1998). Immunological functions of the human prepuce. *Sexually Transmitted Infections* 74(5): 364–67.

Fleming, A. S., C. Corter, J. Stallings, and M. Steiner (2002). Testosterone and prolactin are associated with emotional responses to infant cries in new fathers. *Hormones and Behavior* 42(4): 399–413.

Flynn, P., P. Havens, and M. Brady (2007). Male circumcision for prevention of HIV and other sexually transmitted diseases. *Pediatrics* 119:821–22.

Forbes, T. (1950). Witch's milk and witches' marks. *Yale Journal of Biology and Medicine* 22:219–25.

Fomon, S. (2000). Taste acquisition and appetite control. *Pediatrics* 106(5, Supp.): 1278.

Freeman, R. (1990). Intrapartum fetal monitoring: A disappointing story. *New England Journal of Medicine* 322:624–26.

French, V. (1986). Midwives and maternity care in the Greco-Roman world. *Helios* 13:69–84.

Galanakis, E. (1998). Apgar score and Soranus of Ephesus. *Lancet* 352:2012–13.

Gamble, J. A., and D. K. Creedy (2000). Women's request for a cesarean section: A critique of the literature. *Birth* 27(4): 256–63.

Gbinigie, N. I., M. L. Alderson, and P. M. Barclay (2001). Informed consent, and fainting fathers. *Anaesthesia* 56(6): 603–4.

George, W. L. (December 14, 1913). What the feminists are really fighting for. *New York Times.*

Gerhardt, K. (1996). Fetal hearing: Characterization of the stimulus and response. *Seminars in Perinatology* 20(1): 11–20.

Gerhardt, K., and R. Abrams (2000). Fetal exposures to sound and vibroacoustic stimulation. *Journal of Perinatology* 20:S21–30.

Goer, H. (2003). "Spin doctoring" the research. *Birth* 30(2): 124–29.

Goldsmith, L., G. Weiss, and B. Steiner (1995). Relaxin and its role in pregnancy. *Endocrinology & Metabolism Clinics of North America* 24(1): 171–86.

Goodrich, F. W. (1953). The theory and practice of natural childbirth. *Yale Journal of Biology and Medicine* 23:529–34.

Gray, P., C.-F. Yang, and H. Pope (2006). Fathers have lower salivary testosterone levels than unmarried men and married non-fathers in Beijing, China. *Proceedings of the Royal Society of London, Series B: Biological Sciences* 273(1584): 333–39.

Greenberg, M., and N. Morris (1974). Engrossment: The newborn's impact on the father. *American Journal of Orthopsychiatry* 44(4): 520–31.

Greenhalgh, R., P. Slade, and H. Spiby (2000). Fathers' coping style, antenatal preparation, and experiences of labor and the postpartum. *Birth* 27(3): 177–84.

Gregory, K., L. Korst, and P. Cane (1999). Vaginal birth after cesarean and uterine rupture rates in California. *Obstetrics & Gynecology* 94:985–89.

Gresh, S. (1980). *Becoming a Father.* New York: Butterick Publishing.

Grieve, M. (1971). *A Modern Herbal.* New York: Dover Publications, Inc.

Gupta, J. K., and C. Nikodem (2000). Maternal posture in labor. *European Journal of Obstetrics, Gynecology, & Reproductive Biology* 92:273–77.

Hall, N. (1989). *A Psychological Essay on Men in Childbirth.* Dallas: Spring Publications, Inc.

Halsall, P. (1998). Modern History Sourcebook: Oliver Wendell Holmes (1809–1894): Contagiousness of Puerperal Fever, 1843. http://www.fordham.edu/halsall/mod/1843holmes-fever.html.

Hanson, A. (2007). Greek translation of "iatrine" (personal communication).

Hawkins, J. L. (2003). Anesthesia-related maternal mortality. *Obstetric Anesthesia* 46(3): 679–87.

Hawkins, J. L., L. Goetzl, and D. Chestnut (2007). Obstetric anesthesia. Gabbe, *Obstetrics: Normal and Problem Pregnancies,* 5th ed., 396–425. Philadelphia: Churchill Livingstone.

Hemminki, E. (2006). Why do women go along with this stuff? *Birth* 33(2): 154–58.

Higgins, R., E. Bancalari, M. Willinger, and T. N. Raju (2007). Executive summary of the workshop on oxygen in neonatal therapies: Controversies and opportunities for research. *Pediatrics* 119(4): 790–96.

Hodnett, E. (2002). Pain and women's satisfaction with the experience of childbirth: A systematic review. *American Journal of Obstetrics and Gynecology* 186(5): S160–72.

Hodnett, E., S. Gates, G. Hofmeyr, and C. Sakala (2005). Continuous support for women during childbirth: Selected Cochrane Systematic Reviews. *Birth* 32(1): 72.

Hollinger, L. (1998). Evaluation of stridor and wheezing. *The Child's Doctor: Journal of Children's Memorial Hospital, Chicago,* Spring 1998, electronic edition.

Holt, L. Emmett, and R. McIntosh (1940). *Holt's Diseases of Infancy and Childhood.* New York and London: D. Appleton–Century Co.

Holve, L., and F. Smith (1955). Omphalitis and peritonitis in the neonatal period. *U.S. Armed Forces Medical Journal* 6(4): 491–99.

Hughes, D., S. W. Simmons, J. Brown, and A. M. Cyna (2004). Combined spinal-epidural versus epidural analgesia in labour. *Birth* 31(1): 71.

Hurwitz, B., and R. Richardson (1989). Inspector General James Barry MD: Putting the woman in her place. *British Medical Journal* 298(6669): 299–305.

International Federation of Gynecology and Obstetrics (2007). FIGO statement on cesarean section. http://www.figo.org/Caesarean.asp.

Jacob, S., M. McClintock, B. Zelano, and C. Ober (2002). Paternally inherited HLA alleles are associated with women's choice of male odor. *Nature Genetics* 30:175–79.

James, L. (1975). Fond Memories of Virginia Apgar. *Pediatrics* 55(1): 1–4.

James, William (1882). Subjective effects of nitrous oxide. *Mind* 7.

Jannsen, P. A., E. Ryan, D. Etches, M. Klein, and B. Reime (2007). Outcomes of planned hospital birth attended by midwives compared with physicians in British Columbia. *Birth* 34(2): 140–47.

Johnson, M. P. (2002). The implications of unfulfilled expectations and perceived pressure to attend the birth on men's stress levels following birth attendance: A longitudinal study. *Journal of Psychosomatic Obstetrics and Gynecology* 23(3): 173–82.

Kattwinkel, J. (2008). *Neonatal Resuscitation Textbook.* Elk Grove, IL: American Academy of Pediatrics.

Kayne, M., M. Greulich, and L. Albers (2001). Doulas: An alternative yet complementary addition to care during childbirth. *Clinical Obstetrics & Gynecology* 44(4): 692–703.

Kennell, John, and S. McGrath (2001). Commentary: What babies teach us: The essential link between baby's behavior and mother's biology. *Birth* 28(1): 20–21.

Kern, E. A. (1996). *The Minister, the Mother, the Midwife, and the Physician:*

Childbearing in Colonial and Revolutionary New England. Stanford University, Palo Alto, CA.

Kershaw, S. (May 29, 2003). In insurance cost, woes for doctors and women. *New York Times.*

Kilpatrick, S., and E. Garrison (2007). Chapter 12: Normal Labor and Delivery. Gabbe, *Obstetrics: Normal and Problem Pregnancies,* 5th ed.: 303–17. Philadelphia: Churchill Livingstone, Elsevier.

Kinsley, C., and K. Lambert (2006). The maternal brain. *Scientific American* 294(1).

Kisilevsky, B. S., S.M.J. Hains, A.-Y. Jacquet, C. Granier-Deferre, and J. P. Lecanuet (2004). Maturation of fetal responses to music. *Developmental Science* 7(5): 550–59.

Kisilevsky, B. S., S.M.J. Hains, K. Lee, X. Xie, and H. Huang (2003). Effects of experience on fetal voice recognition. *Psychological Science* 14(3): 220–24.

Kisilevsky, B., and J. Low (1998). Human fetal behavior: 100 years of study. *Developmental Review* 18:1–29.

Kitzinger, S. (2001). Letter from Europe: Awake, aware—and action! *Birth* 28(3): 210–12.

Klaus, Marshall (1997). The doula: An essential ingredient of childbirth rediscovered. *Acta Paediatrica* 86(10): 1034–36.

——— (1998). Mother and infant: Early emotional ties. *Pediatrics* 102(5, Supp.): 1244–46.

Klaus, M., and J. Kennell (2001). Commentary: Routines in maternity units: Are they still appropriate for 2002? *Birth* 28(4): 274–75.

Klaus, M., and P. Klaus (1998). *Your Amazing Newborn.* New York: Perseus Books.

Klaus, M., P. Klaus, and G. Berkowitz (1992). Maternal assistance and support in labor: father, nurse, midwife, or doula? *Clinical Consultations in Obstetrics and Gynecology* 4(4): 211–17.

Klein, H. (1991). Couvade syndrome: Male counterpart to pregnancy. *International Journal of Psychiatry in Medicine* 21(1): 57–69.

Klein, M. C. (2006). Epidural analgesia: Does it or doesn't it? *Birth* 33(1): 74–6.

Kliegman, R. (2007). Part XI. Chapter 94.2: Physical Examination of the Newborn Infant, 675–79; and Chapter 101: Respiratory Tract Disorders, 728–52. *Nelson Textbook of Pediatrics,* 18th ed. St. Louis: Saunders.

Kovarik, W. (2005). Chapter 76: Pediatric and Neonatal Intensive Care: Mechanics of Breathing. *Miller's Anesthesia.* Philadelphia: Churchill Livingstone, Elsevier.

Kubba, A., and M. Young (2001). The life, work and gender of Dr. James Barry MD (1795–1865). *Proceedings of the Royal College of Physicians, Edinburgh* 31:352–56.

Laeng, B., R. Mathisen, and J.-A. Johnsen (2007). Why do blue-eyed men prefer women with the same eye color? *Behavioral Ecology and Sociobiology* 61:371–84.

Lamaze, Fernand (1972). *Painless Childbirth: The Lamaze Method.* New York: Pocket Books.

Lamaze International (2007). History of Lamaze. http://www.lamaze.org/AboutLamaze/History/tabid/104/Default.aspx.

Landon, M. B. (2007). Cesarean Delivery. Gabbe, *Obstetrics: Normal and Problem Pregnancies,* 5th ed., 486–520. Philadelphia: Churchill Livingstone.

Leavitt, Judith W. (1986). *Brought to Bed: Childbearing in America, 1750–1950.* New York: Oxford University Press.

——— (1987). The growth of medical authority: Technology and morals in turn-of-the-century obstetrics. *Medical Anthropology Quarterly* 1(3): 230–55.

——— (2003). What do men have to do with it? Fathers and mid-twentieth century childbirth. *Bulletin of the History of Medicine* 77:235–62.

Lecanuet, J.-P., I. Capponi, and L. Ledru (1993). Prenatal discrimination of a male and a female voice uttering the same sentence. *Early Development and Parenting* 2(4): 217–28.

Lecanuet, J.-P., and B. Schaal (1996). Fetal Sensory Competencies. *European Journal of Obstetrics, Gynecology, & Reproductive Biology* 68:1–23.

Lee, H. (2004). Acupuncture for labor pain management: A systemic review. *American Journal of Obstetrics and Gynecology* 191:1573–79.

Leeman, L. (2005). Patient-choice cesarean delivery. *American Family Physician* 72(4).

Leighton, B., and S. Halpern (2002). The effects of epidural analgesia on labor, maternal, and neonatal outcomes: A systematic review. *American Journal of Obstetrics and Gynecology* 186(5): S69–77.

Leung, A., and D. Pacaud (2004). Diagnosis and management of galactorrhea. *American Family Physician* 70(3).

Lieberman, E. (2002). Unintended effects of epidural analgesia during labor: A systematic review. *American Journal of Obstetrics and Gynecology* 186(5): S31–68.

Lieberman, E., E. K. Ernst, and J. P. Rooks (2004). Results of the national study of vaginal birth after cesarean section. *Obstetrics & Gynecology* 104:933–42.

Lipkin, Mark, and Gerri Lamb (1982). The couvade syndrome: An epidemiologic study. *Annals of Internal Medicine* 96:509–11.

Lister, Joseph (1870). The antiseptic system of treatment in surgery. *Lancet* 2:287.

Lorenz, Konrad (1971). Part and parcel in animal and human societies. *Studies in animal and human behaviour,* vol. II, 115–95. Cambridge, MA: Harvard University Press.

Loudon, I. (1986). Deaths in childbed from the eighteenth century to 1935. *Medical History* 30:1–41.

Lowe, Nancy (2002). The nature of labor pain. *American Journal of Obstetrics and Gynecology* 186(5): S16–24.

Maestripieri, D. (2004). Developmental and evolutionary aspects of female attraction to babies. *Psychological Science Agenda* 18(1).

Marmor, T., and D. Krol (2002). Labor pain management in the United States: Understanding patterns and the issue of choice. *American Journal of Obstetrics and Gynecology* 186(5): S173–80.

Martin, Mrs. John (August 29, 1915). The woman movement and the baby crop. *New York Times.*

Martin, R. D. (1990). *Primate Origins and Evolution: A Phylogenetic Reconstruction.* Princeton: Princeton University Press.

Mason, C., and R. Elwood (1995). Is there a physiological basis for the couvade and onset of paternal care? *International Journal of Nursing Studies* 32(2): 137–48.

Maternity Center Association (2004). Recommendations from *Listening to Mothers: The First National U.S. Survey of Women's Childbearing Experiences. Birth* 31(1): 61–65.

McGowan, F., and P. Davis (2008). Anesthetic-related neurotoxicity in the developing infant: of mice, rats, monkeys, and, possibly, humans. *Anesthesia & Analgesia* 106(6): 1599–1602.

McGowan, S. W. (1997). Sir James Young Simpson Bart: 150 years on. *Scottish Medical Journal* 42:185–87.

McGregor, D. (1999). Waste anesthetic gases: An update on information for management in anesthetizing areas and the postanesthesia care unit. *American Society of Anesthesiologists Newsletter* 63(7).

Melzack, Ronald (1981). Labour is still painful after prepared childbirth training. *Canadian Medical Association Journal* 125:357–63.

Melzack, R., R. Kinch, P. Dobkin L. Lebrun, and P. Taenzer (1984). Severity of labour pain: influence of physical as well as psychologic variables. *Canadian Medical Association Journal* 130, no. 5 (March 1, 1984): 579–84.

Menacker, F., E. Declercq, and M. Macdorma (2006). Cesarean delivery:

Background, trends and epidemiology. *Seminars in Perinatology* 30(5): 235–41.

Menard, M. K. (1999). Cesarean delivery in the United States. *Obstetrics and Gynecology Clinics of North America* 26(2): 275–85.

Mennella, J. (1995). Garlic ingestion by pregnant women alters the odor of amniotic fluid. *Chemical Senses* 20(2): 207–9.

Mennella, J., C. Jagnow, and G. Beauchamp (2001). Prenatal and postnatal flavor learning by human infants. *Pediatrics* 107(6): e88.

Mercer, J. S., and R. L. Skovgaard (2002). Neonatal transitional physiology: A new paradigm. *The Journal of Perinatal and Neonatal Nursing* 15(4): 56–75.

Meredith, M. (2001). Human vomeronasal organ function: A critical review of best and worst cases. *Chemical Senses* 26(4): 433–45.

Milos, M., and D. Macris (1992). Circumcision: A medical or a human rights issue? *Journal of Nurse-Midwifery* 37(2, Supp.): 87–96.

Minkoff, H., and F. Chervenak (2003). Elective primary cesarean delivery. *New England Journal of Medicine* 348:946–50.

Moon, C., and W. Fifer (2000). Evidence of Transnatal Auditory Learning. *Journal of Perinatology* 20:S37–44.

Morgenstern, L. (2007). Gargling with Lister. *Journal of the American College of Surgeons* 204(3): 495–97.

Morris, S. (1982). *The Normal Acquisition of Oral Feeding Skills: Implications for Assessment and Treatment.* New York: Therapeutic Media, Inc.

Morrison, J., and I. Z. MacKenzie (2003). Cesarean section on demand. *Seminars in Perinatology* 27(1): 20–33.

Moscucci, O. (2003). Holistic obstetrics: The origins of "natural childbirth" in Britain. *Postgraduate Medical Journal* 79:168–73.

Murray, A., R. Dolby, R. Nation, and D. Thomas (1981). Effects of epidural anesthesia on newborns and their mothers. *Child Development* 52(1): 71–82.

National Library of Medicine (2007). Infantile reflexes. http://www.nlm.nih.gov/medlineplus/ency/article/003292.htm.

Nesse, R., and G. Williams (1994). Legacies of Evolutionary History. *Why We Get Sick,* 123–27. New York: Times Books.

Nitschke, J., J. Nelson, and B. Rusch (2001). Motherly love: An fMRI study of mothers viewing pictures of their infants. *NeuroImage* 13(6): 450.

Nygaard, Ingrid, and D. Cruikshank (2003). Should all women be offered elective cesarean delivery? *Obstetrics & Gynecology* 102(2): 217–19.

O'Donnell, C., A. Gibson, and P. Davis (2006). Pinching, electrocution, ravens' beaks, and positive pressure ventilation: A brief history of neonatal resuscitation. *Archives of Disease in Childhood Fetal & Neonatal Edition* 91(5): F369–73.

O'Dowd, M., and P. Elliott (2000). *The History of Obstetrics and Gynecology.* New York: Parthenon Publishing Group.

Ostrea, E., and E. Villanueva-Uy (2006). Persistent pulmonary hypertension of the newborn. *Pediatric Drugs* 8(3): 179–85.

Palkovitz, Rob (1985). Fathers' birth attendance, early contact, and extended contact with their newborns: a critical review. *Child Development* 56(2): 392–406.

———— (1986). Laypersons' beliefs about the "critical" nature of father-infant bonding: Implications for childbirth educators. *Maternal-Child Nursing Journal* 15(1): 39–46.

———— (1987). Father's motives for birth attendance. *Maternal-Child Nursing Journal* 16(2): 123–29.

Pearce, D. (2008). Humphry Davy. *BLTC Research.* http://www.general anaesthesia.com/people/humphry-davy.html.

Pelosi, Marco A., and Marco A. Pelosi (1997). Historical perspective: Cesarean section. *ACOG Clinical Review,* January/February, 13–16.

Philbin, M., and P. Klaas (2000). Hearing and behavioral responses to sound in full-term newborn. *Journal of Perinatology* 20:S67–75.

Pierson, L. (1996). Hazards of noise exposure on fetal hearing. *Seminars in Perinatology* 20(1): 21–29.

Pomeranz, A. (2004). Anomalies, abnormalities, and care of the umbilicus. *Pediatric Clinics of North America* 51:819–27.

Porter, R., and J. Winberg (1999). Unique salience of maternal breast odors for newborn infants. *Neuroscience & Behavioral Reviews* 23(3): 439–49.

Preyer, Erklärung von W. (1937). Embryonic motility and sensitivity (trans. G. E. Coghill & W. K. Legner). *Monographs of the Society for Research in Child Development* 2(6, serial no. 13).

Raju, T. N. (1999). Ignác Semmelweis and the etiology of fetal and neonatal sepsis. *Journal Perinatology* 19(4): 307–10.

Ray, M. (2007). Mothers Against Circumcision. http://www.mothers againstcirc.org.

Remondino, Peter C. (1891). *History of Circumcision from the Earliest Times to the Present: Moral and Physical Reasons for Its Performance.* London: F. A. Davis.

———— (1902). Circumcision and its opponents. *American Journal of Dermatology and Genito-Urinary Diseases* 6:73.

Richards, D., B. Frentzen, K. Gerhardt, M. McCann, and R. Abrams (1992). Sound levels in the human uterus. *Obstetrics & Gynecology* 80(2): 186–90.

Riordan, J., and A. Gross (2000). The effect of labor pain medication on neonatal suckling and breastfeeding duration. *Journal of Human Lactation* 16(1): 7–12.

Rodkinson, M. (trans.) (1903). Chapter XVIII: Regulations Regarding the Clearing Off of Required Space, the Assistance to Be Given Cattle When Giving Birth to Their Young and to Women About to Be Confined. *The Babylonian Talmud, Tract Sabbath*, bk. I, vol. II. New York: New Talmud Publishing Company: 282.

Rooks, Judith P. (1997). *Midwifery and Childbirth in America*. Philadelphia: Temple University Press.

———— (2007). Nitrous oxide for pain in labor: Why not in the United States? *Birth* 34(1): 1–5.

———— (2007). Use of nitrous oxide in midwifery practice: Synergistic, and needed in the United States. *Journal of Midwifery and Women's Health* 52(3): 186–89.

Roper, M., J. Vandelaer, and F. Gasse (2007). Maternal and neonatal tetanus. *Lancet* 370:1947–59.

Rosen, Mark (2002). Nitrous oxide for relief of labor pain: A systematic review. *American Journal of Obstetrics and Gynecology* 186(5): S110–26.

———— (2002). Paracervical block for labor analgesia: A brief historic review. *American Journal of Obstetrics and Gynecology* 186(5): S127–130.

Rosenberg, K. (1992). The evolution of modern human childbirth. *Yearbook of Physical Anthropology* 35:89–124.

Rosenberg, K., and Wenda Trevathan (1996). Bipedalism and human birth: The obstetrical dilemma revisited. *Evolutionary Anthropology* 4:161–68.

Ruben, R. J. (1992). The ontogeny of human hearing. *Acta Otolaryngologica* 112:192–96.

———— (1997). A time frame of critical/sensitive periods of language development. *Acta Otolaryngologica* 117(2): 202–5.

Russell, S. (2007). Circumcision pushed in AIDS fight: Millions of lives could be saved in Africa, U.N. says. *San Francisco Chronicle*, March 27, 2007.

Ryan, J. (2002). The chapel and the operating room: The struggle of Roman Catholic clergy, physicians, and believers with the dilemma of obstetric surgery, 1800–1900. *Bulletin of the History of Medicine* 76:461–94.

Salaam, M., H. Margolis, and R. McConnell (2006). Mode of delivery is associated with asthma and allergy occurrences in children. *Annals of Epidemiology* 16:341–46.

Schaal, B. (2004). Olfaction in the fetal and premature infant: Functional status and clinical implications. *Clinics in Perinatology* 31(2): 261–85.

Schoen, Edgar (1997). Is circumcision healthy? Yes. *American Council on Science and Health* 9(4).

Scott, K., G. Berkowitz, and M. Klaus (1999). A comparison of intermittent and continuous support during labor: A meta-analysis. *American Journal of Obstetrics and Gynecology* 180:1054–59.

Scott, K., P. Klaus, and M. Klaus (1999). The obstetrical and postpartum benefits of continuous support during childbirth. *Journal of Women's Health & Gender-Based Medicine* 8(10): 1257–64.

Sealey, R. (2003). The Digesta (personal communication).

Sewell, J. E. (1993). *Cesarean section: A brief history*. Paper presented at the History of Cesarean Section exhibition at the National Library of Medicine: April 30, 1993.

Shapiro, J. (1987). The Expectant Father. *Psychology Today* 21(1): 36–42.

Sharma, G., and H. Minkoff (2004). Ethical dimensions of elective primary cesarean delivery. *Clinical Obstetrics & Gynecology* 103(2): 387–92.

Sheldon, Wilfred (1936). Chapter II: Some Affections of the Newborn. *Diseases of Infancy and Childhood*. London: J. & A. Churchill Ltd.

Simkin, Penny, and Mary Ann O'Hara (2002). Nonpharmacologic relief of pain during labor: Systematic reviews of five methods. *American Journal of Obstetrics and Gynecology* 186(5): S131–59.

Slater, A., and R. Kirby (1998). Innate and learned perceptual abilities in the newborn infant. *Experimental Brain Research* 123:90–94.

Sohmer, H., R. Perez, J. Sichel, and R. Priner (2001). The pathway enabling external sounds to reach and excite the fetal inner ear. *Audiology and Neuro-Otology* 6(3): 109–16.

Speert, H. (1956). Thomas Wharton and the jelly of the umbilical cord. *Obstetrics & Gynecology* 8(3): 380–82.

Spelt, D. K. (1948). The conditioning of the human fetus in utero. *Journal of Experimental Psychology* 38:338–46.

Stone, Emerson L. (1945). *The New-Born Infant: A Manual of Obstetrical Pediatrics*. London: Henry Kimpton.

Storey, A. E., C. J. Walsh, R. L. Quinton, and K. E. Wynne-Edwards (2000). Hormonal correlates of paternal responsiveness in new and expectant fathers. *Evolution and Human Behavior* 21:79–95.

Szeverenyi, P., R. Poka, M. Hetey, and Z. Torok, (1998). Contents of childbirth-related fear among couples wishing the partner's presence at delivery. *Journal of Psychosomatic Obstetrics and Gynecology* 19:38–43.

Taffel, S. M., P. Placek, M. Moien, and C. Kosary (1991). 1989 U.S. cesarean rate steadies—VBAC rises to nearly one in five. *Birth* 18(73): 77–81.

Taylor, J. R., A. Lockwood, and A. Taylor (1996). The prepuce: Specialized mucosa of the penis and its loss to circumcision. *British Journal of Urology* 77(2): 291–95.

Temkin, O. (1956). *Soranus' Gynecology.* Baltimore: Johns Hopkins Press.

Thompson, M., and C. Hunt (2005). Part V: The Newborn Infant: Control of Breathing. *Avery's Neonatology: Pathophysiology and Management of the Newborn.* Philadelphia: Lippincott Williams & Wilkins.

Tracy, Marguerite, and Mary Boyd (1915). *Painless Childbirth.* New York: Frederic A. Stokes Co.

Tracy, Marguerite, and Constance Leupp (1914). Painless childbirth. *McClure's Magazine* 43(2): 37–52.

Travers, P. L. (1934). Chapter 3: Laughing Gas. *Mary Poppins.* New York: Harcourt, Brace.

Trevathan, Wenda (1990). The evolution of helplessness in the human infant and its significance for pre- and peri-natal psychology. *Pre- and Peri-Natal Psychology* 4(4): 267–80.

———— (1999). Evolutionary Obstetrics. *Evolutionary Medicine* Chapter 8: 183–207. New York: Oxford University Press.

Turati, C. (2004). Why faces are not special to newborns: An alternative account of the face preference. *Current Directions in Psychological Science* 13(1): 5–8.

UCLA Department of Epidemiology, School of Public Health (2001). Anesthesia and Queen Victoria. http://www.ph.ucla.edu/epi/snow/victoria.html.

van Buitenen, J.A.B. (trans.) (1973). *Mahabharata,* vol. 1. Chicago: University of Chicago Press.

Van Hoosen, Bertha (1915). The new movement in obstetrics. *Women's Medical Journal* 25(6): 121–23.

Viets, H. R. (1943). A mind prepared: O. W. Holmes and "The Contagiousness of Puerperal Fever," 1843. *Bulletin of the Medical Library Association* 31(4): 319–25.

Visco, A., M. Vishwanathan, and K. Lohr (2006). Cesarean delivery on maternal request: maternal and neonatal outcomes. *Obstetrics & Gynecology* 108(6): 1517–29.

Waite, J. (1999). Eckhard Hess. http://www.muskingum.edu/~psych/psycweb/history/hess.htm#Biography.

Ward, Y. M. (1999). The womanly garb of Queen Victoria's early motherhood, 1840–42. *Women's History Review* 8(2): 277–93.

Weirich, A., and G. Hoffman (2005). Ernst Moro (1874–1951): A great pediatric career started at the rise of university-based pediatric research but was curtailed in the shadows of Nazi laws. *European Journal of Pediatrics* 164(10): 599–606.

Wheeler, C. (August 30, 1914). "Twilight Sleep": Editor of medical journal states his position on new treatment. *New York Times.*

Williams, G. (1986). *The Age of Agony: The Art of Healing, 1700–1800.* Chicago: Academy Chicago Publishers.

World Health Organization (2007). The World Health Report 2005: Make Every Mother and Child Count. http://www.who.int/whr/2005/annexes -en.pdf.

——— (2007). Male Circumcision in HIV Prevention. http://www.who.int/ hiv/topics/malecircumcision/en/.

Wright, K., and P. Spiegel (2002). *Pediatric Ophthalmology and Strabismus,* 2nd ed., Springer Publishing, New York.

Wyart, C., W. Webster, and J. Chen (2007). Smelling a single component of male sweat alters levels of cortisol in women. *Journal of Neuroscience* 27(6): 1261–65.

Wynne-Edwards, Katherine E. (2001). Hormonal changes in mammalian fathers. *Hormones and Behavior* 40(2): 139–45.

Wysocki, Charles, and G. Preti (2004). Facts, fallacies, fears, and frustrations with human pheromones. *The Anatomical Record Part A: Discoveries in Molecular, Cellular, and Evolutionary Biology* 281A (1): 1201–11.

Yogman, M. (1990). *Male Parental Behavior in Humans and Nonhuman Primates.* Oxford: Oxford University Press.

Young, D. (1998). Doulas: Into the mainstream of maternity care. *Birth* 25(4): 213–14.

——— (2003). The push against vaginal birth. *Birth* 30(3): 149–52.

Ziegler, T. E., S. L. Prudom, and N. J. Schultz-Darken (2006). Pregnancy weight gain: Marmoset and tamarin dads show it too. *Biology Letters* 2(2): 181–83.

Ziegler, T. E., and C. T. Snowdon. (2000). Preparental hormone levels and parenting experience in male cotton-top tamarins, *Saguinus oedipus*. *Hormones and Behavior* 38(3): 159–67.

Ziegler, T. E., K. Washabaugh, and C. T. Snowdon. (2004). Responsiveness of expectant male cotton-top tamarins, *Saguinus oedipus*, to mate's pregnancy. *Hormones and Behavior* 45:84–92.

Zupan J., P. Garner, and A. Omari (2004). Topical umbilical cord care at birth. *Cochrane Database of Systematic Reviews*, Issue 3. Art No.: CD001057. DOI: 10.1002/14651858.CD001057.pub2.

Index

ABOUT THE AUTHOR

Mark Sloan, M.D., has been a pediatrician and a fellow of the American Academy of Pediatrics for more than twenty-five years. He is an assistant clinical professor in the Department of Family and Community Medicine at the University of California, San Francisco. He is one of the highest-rated pediatricians (by patients and peers) in Kaiser Permanente's Northern California region. His writing has appeared in the *Chicago Tribune* and *San Francisco Chronicle,* among other publications. He lives in Santa Rosa, California, with his wife and two teenage children, who continue to provide him with a wealth of practical pediatric experience.